AF540814

PHARMACOKINETICS

ENCYCLOPAEDIA OF PHARMACEUTICAL TECHNOLOGY

Vol. 4
PHARMACOKINETICS

By
Dr. G.P. Garg
&
Dr. M. Prakash

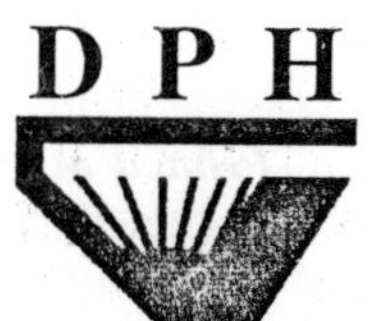

DISCOVERY PUBLISHING HOUSE PVT. LTD.
NEW DELHI-110 002

First Published-2010

ISBN: 978-81-8356-595-0 (Set)

Published by:

DISCOVERY PUBLISHING HOUSE PVT. LTD.

4831/24, Ansari Road, Prahlad Street

Darya Ganj, New Delhi-110002 (India)

Phone: 23279245, 43764432 • Fax: 91-11-23253475

E-mail: parul.wasan@gmail.com • dphbooks@rediffmail.com

web: www.discoverypublishinggroup.com

Printed at

Mehra Offset Press

Preface

The present title "Encyclopaedia of Pharmaceutical Technology" has been written for those in the pharmaceutical research and those responsible for the education and training in pharmaceutical science and technology of graduate and undergraduate students. Medicine is an ever changing science. As new research and clinical experience broaden our knowledge, changes in treatment and drug therapy are required. This branch of life science has progressed enormously in recent years and the significant advances in therapeutics and an understanding of the need to optimize during delivery in the body have brought about an increased awareness of the valuable role played by the dosage forms. This statement is as true as it was back in ninteenth century and perhaps more so, given the increasing emphasis being placed on discovery, development, and use of large molecular entities as therapeutic and diagnostic agents. Development of these abilities requires an integration of knowledge, skills, attitudes, and values that can be acquired only through structured learning process including independent study, hands on practice and the availability of advanced literature. This tittle has designed to meet such needs of learners in the health professions.

In the last two decades, the pharmaceutical industry has experimented and successfully adopted several integrated and multidisciplinary approaches in the research areas of dring compound screening, toxicological evaluation, and pharmaceutical product development. The book is written in a concise style that facilitates an in-depth level of understanding of the essential concepts. The objectives of the present title are three folds: (i) to serve as a useful tool to help guide scientists in research and development by outlining the theory and successful practice of in vitro - in vivo correlation, (ii) to help formulators apply the tool in designing and developing prototypes that enable selection of clinical formulations, and (iii) to help formulate strategy(ies) for product life-cycle management.

To make the work more comprehensive and informative, the author has consulted many authoritative books, research journals, abstracts, monographs etc., so there can be no claim to originality except in the manner of treatment.

The author expresses his thanks to his friends and colleagues whose continue inspirations have initiated him to bring out this book.

The author expresses his gratitude to Mr. Wasan and staff of M/s Discovery Publishing House Pvt. Ltd. for their whole hearted co-operation in the publication of this book.

Author

Contents

1

INTRODUCTION

Recombinant DNA technology produced many protein drugs in large scale and many important protein drugs like erythropoietin (EPO) for anemia-associated diseases, granulocyte-colony stimulating factor (G-CSF) for leucopoenia, and insulin for diabetes are now clinically available. In addition, peptide hormones like leuprolide [an agonist of luteinizing hormone-releasing hormone (LHRH)] are also clinically used. However, these peptide/protein drugs are unstable because of hydrolytic degradation in the body. Peptide/protein drugs also have a barrier for their administration because of low absorption efficiency. Therefore, their is parenteral preparation, *main dosage form* in which case intravenous (i.v.) or subcutaneous (s.c.) injection is used. After i.v. injection of these drugs, the administered drug molecules are completely available to the systemic circulation (i.e., bioavailability (BA) is 100%). On the other hand, BA becomes lower when these drugs are injected s.c. or i.m. In some protein drugs like interferon gamma, BAs after s.c. and i.m. injection are greater than 100% (i.e., 200% and 300%, respectively. Furthermore, it is recognized that protein drugs whose molecular weight is larger than about 20 kDa are absorbed into the systemic circulation via lymphatic route. As a result, a large T_{max} value is obtained, when peak serum or plasma drug level appears after administration; for example, T_{max} is approximately 8 h for s.c.-injected EPO. After the serum drug level reached its maximum level, C_{max}, serum drug concentration decreases. In the case of organic compound drugs, the elimination process is composed of hepatic metabolism and renal excretion pathways. However, for peptide/protein drugs, we must consider the hydrolytic degradation process because of poor tolerability of these drugs to endogenous hydrolytic enzymes. Therefore, the elimination half-life of peptide/protein drugs is generally shorter than that of organic compound drugs. To increase the stability of peptide/protein drugs, several approaches have been performed and second- generation peptide/protein drugs have been developed and launched on the market, including PEGylated protein drugs (i.e., pegylation) and attachment of polyethylene glycol (PEG) to protein molecules.

In the case of PEG-EPO, the administration frequency has decreased to once per week as compared with three times per week for the conventional EPO preparations; although almost the same serum EPO levels are obtained in the two types of EPO preparations. Most of the current peptide/protein drugs are injectable, and there is great commercial potential for delivery systems that use alternative administration routes like the pulmonary route and the nasal route, as suggested from insulin new dosage forms. In these cases, the pharmacokinetic profile of the peptide/protein drugs shows a completely different pattern as compared with that obtained after i.v. injection. In this section, the pharmacokinetics of clinically important peptide/protein drugs, such as insulin, EPO, G-CSF, interferon, growth hormone, leuprolide, desmopressin, and antibodies, are described in relation to their administration routes and formulations (i.e., dosage forms).

INSULIN

The finding of insulin in 1922 by Ranting and Best is one of the greatest discoveries in the history of medicine, and now it has been already proven that adequate control of blood glucose delays or prevents the progression of diabetic complications. To achieve the suggested targets for glycemic control necessary to reduce the incidence of diabetic complications, it has been established that a more intensive insulin regimen requiring multiple insulin injections is required for patients with type 1 diabetes mellitus. From a patient's point of view, however, noninvasive insulin delivery systems have been required for a long time. Indeed, a major limitation for advancing to intensive insulin therapy is that the only viable way to administer insulin is through injection. Several other methods of insulin delivery are now available or in development, including: continuous subcutaneous insulin infusion by a wearable infusion pump; total or segmented transplantation of a pancreas; transplantation of isolated islet cells; implantation of a programmable insulin pump; oral, nasal, rectal, and transdermal mechanisms of insulin delivery; insulin analogs; implantation of polymeric capsules that give continuous or time-pulsed release of insulin; and implantation of a biohybrid artificial pancreas, which uses encapsulated islets. Many of these methods of insulin delivery are aimed at achieving a more physiological means of delivery of the insulin, at improving glycemic control, and, hopefully, at minimizing the secondary complications of diabetes.

On the other hand, during the nearly 80 years of insulin therapy, insulin preparations have undergone dramatic changes in their purification, production, and formulation. Despite these changes, and despite the development of different injection regimens and delivery systems, normalizing glycemic control still has not been adequately achieved. Recently, specific amino acid substitutions of the β-chain of the insulin molecule by recombinant DNA techniques have resulted in insulin analogs that have different pharmacokinetic properties than currently available insulins. Some of these insulin analogs appear to have less variation in absorption than conventional insulins, and analogs have been developed with both very rapid and delayed absorption. Those analogs with a very rapid absorption may be useful in better mimicking the physiological insulin profiles seen postprandially than currently available native insulins. All of these advances have been accomplished through protein engineering to produce insulin analogs with a decreased tendency for self-association (monomeric insulin), which in turn increases the subcutaneous absorption of these insulins. These monomeric insulin analogs have been found to have a faster onset of action and are better able to reduce postprandial glucose excursions than conventional human insulin preparations, which sub cutaneously become hexamers and slow absorption. These insulin analogs, especially the monomeric types, appear to be less immunogenic and antigenic where the pharmacokinetic aspects of human insulin and an analog insulin of aspart and lispro are described. In addition, other delivery options for insulin besides subcutaneous administration, such as transdermal and nasal approaches, are described.

Pharmacokinetics of Human Insulin after Intravenous Administration

In the 1970s, pork insulin had been widely used for the treatment of diabetics. In the 1980s, biosynthetic and recombinant DNA technology came to be introduced. In 1981, Halban et al. compared the biologic potency of pancreatic human insulin with that of biosynthetic human insulin, which was manufactured by recombinant DNA techniques in bacteria, after intravenous injection in rats. The metabolic clearance rates of A14-mono-^{125}I-insulin (pork) were found to be similar to those observed for semi-synthetic [^{3}H]insulin (pork), being 20.8 ± 0.8 mL/min/kg and 23.6 ± 1.0 mL/min/kg, respectively. On the other hand, the metabolic clearance rates for A14-mono-^{125}I-biosynthetic human insulin was 24.6 ± 2.2 mL/min/kg, which was significantly higher than the value for A14-mono-^{125}I-pork insulin. In addition, the specific activity of the pancreatic human insulin was 32 U/mg, whereas that for biosynthetic human insulin was 27 U/mg. These values were not significantly different but were higher than the value for pancreatic pork insulin (25 U/mg). Biosynthetic human insulin is thus no less active than pork insulin in rats, and possibly somewhat more active. Moreover, in 1987, Brogden and Heel reviewed that human insulin, whether produced by recombinant DNA techniques (biosynthetic, insulin crb) or enzymatic modification of porcine insulin (semi-synthetic, insulin emp) is equivalent in biological activity to porcine insulin after intravenous administration. There were no differences in the pharmacokinetic profiles among them. However, slight differences between human and porcine insulin in hypoglycemic activity after subcutaneous injection appear to be related to differences in absorption and are unlikely to be of major clinical importance.

Turnheim and Waldhausl characterized pharmacokinetic aspects of recombinant human insurin in human. After intravenous injection, the plasma concentration of insulin declines with at least two exponentials. Inslin distributes rapidly from the intravascular space to tissue compartments with a distribution half-life of 2.4 min, whereas insulin disappears slowly with an elimination half-life of 50–130 min, which is reflecting the elimination from the interstitial fluid and the tissues that use insulin. Total body clearance of insulin, which is the result of metabolic degradation, ranges between 700 and 800 mL/min. The sites of degradation are primarily the liver (hepatic insulin clearance: 320–400 mL/min) and the kidneys (renal insulin clearance: 190–270 mL/min); hence, insulin disposal depends on the function of these organs. The apparent volume of distribution for insulin is approximately equal to the extracellular space. Insulin kinetics appears not to be altered in diabetes mellitus, except in cases with insulin antibodies or in insulin-resistant patients, in which insulin removal may be retarded.

Pharmacokinetics of Human Insulin after Subcutaneous Administration

There is a continuing search for improved insulin formulations to imitate the physiological pattern of insulin secretion as closely as possible, and thereby to minimize the complications of diabetes mellitus. The major advances achieved to date are in the area of human insulin analog synthesis resulting from the introduction of recombinant DNA techniques and in improved delivery systems that use noninvasive or minimally invasive modes of administration. Usually, insulin is administered subcutaneously to control blood sugar levels in type 1 and type 2 diabetics. There are plenty of insulin pharmaceutics, and insulin's physico-chemical differences provide different profiles in the insulin pharmacokinetics after subcutaneous injection. Kang et al., investigated absorption mechanisms of insulins with different physico-chemical properties after subcutaneous administration in humans. Based on a single-blind randomized comparison study of seven healthy male volunteers 22–43 years of age, equimolar dosages of ^{125}I-labeled forms of soluble hexameric 2 Zn^{2+} human insulin and human insulin analogs with differing association states at pharmaceutical concentrations (AspB10, dimeric; AspB28, mixture of monomers and dimers; AspB9, GluB27, monomeric) were administred. The initial fractional disappearance rates for the four insulin preparations were 20.7 ± 1.9 (hexameric soluble human insulin), 44.4 ± 2.5 (dimeric analog AspB10), 50.6 ± 3.9 (analog AspB28), and 67.4 ± 7.4%/h (monomeric analog AspB9, GluB27). The absorption of the dimeric analog was significantly faster than that of hexameric human insulin, and the absorption of monomeric insulin analog AspB9, GluB27 was significantly faster than that of dimeric analog AspB10. There was a negative linear correlation between association state and the initial fractional disappearance rates ($r = -0.98$, $p < 0.02$). A log-linear scale analysis for the elimination of insulin showed that only the monomeric analog had a monoexponential elimination. On the other hand, two phases in the rates of absorption were identified for the dimer and three for hexameric human insulin. The fractional disappearance rates calculated by log-linear regression analysis were monomer 73.3 ± 6.8%/h; dimer 44.4 ± 2.5%/h from 0 to 2 h and 68.9 ± 3.5%/h from 2.5 h onward; and hexameric insulin 20.7 ± 1.9%/h from 0 to 2 h, 45.6 ± 5.0%/h from 2.5 to 5 h, and 70.6 ± 6.3%/h from 5 h onward. The author concluded that the lag phase and the subsequent increasing rate of subcutaneous soluble insulin absorption can be explained by the associated state of native insulin in pharmaceutical formulation and its progressive dissociation into smaller units during the absorption process.

Pharmacokinetics of Rapid-acting Insulin Analog after Subcutaneous Administration

By the end of the 1980s, to accommodate postprandial hyperglycemia, monomeric insulin formulations, insulin lispro (the Lys-Pro analog) and insulin aspart (the Asp-Pro analog) had been developed for clinical use.

Formulations including insulin lispro have a rapid rate of absorption after subcutaneous injection and, therefore, have to be administered at meal time. Their residence time is also about two fold shorter than regular human insulin, minimizing the risk of the excessive hypoglycemic effect that characterizes regular human insulin formulations. Becker et al. compared the pharmacokinetics and pharmacodynamics of insulin lispro with regular human insulin after subcutaneous injection in obese subjects in a single-dose, randomized, double-blind, cross-over euglycemic clamp study. Insulin lispro had more rapid-acting profiles than regular human insulin. Fractional glucose infusion rate (GIR)-area under the curve (AUC) of the GIR curve and maximum GIR were greater for insulin lispro compared with regular human insulin. Time to 20% (early glucose disposal) and 80% (bulk of activity) of total GIR-AUC were shorter for insulin lispro than regular human insulin, which was corroborated by more rapid and shorter residing pharmacokinetic profiles of insulin lispro than regular human insulin, evidenced by shorter times to 20% of total AUC of insulin, C_{max} of insulin, and mean residence time. On the other hand, Osterberg et al. compared the pharmacokinetics and pharmacodynamics of insulin aspart with regular human insulin in healthy subjects in a cross-over trial. There were statistically significant differences between most of the human insulin and insulin aspart pharmacokinetic parameters, including the sigmoidicity of the time-course of absorption (1.5 for human insulin vs. 2.1 for insulin aspart), elimination rate constant (0.010 min^{-1} vs. 0.016 min^{-1}, respectively). In addition, the pharmacodynamic model parameters were mostly not different, except for the rate of insulin action (0.012 min^{-1} vs. 0.017 min^{-1}, respectively). Moreover, Homko et al. compared insulin levels and actions in patients with type 1 diabetes after subcutaneous injection of insulin analogs, aspart and lispro. Both insulin

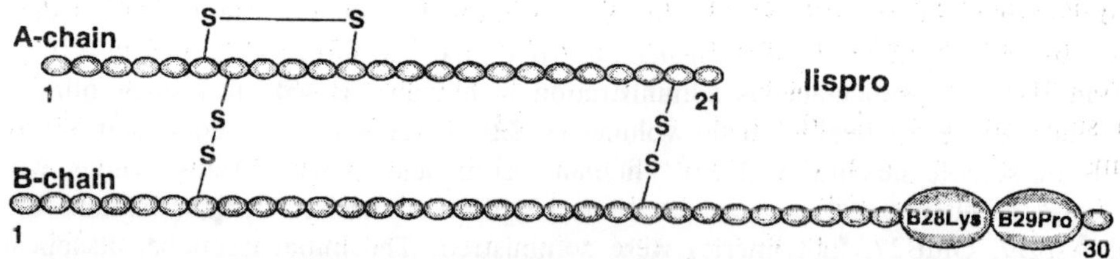

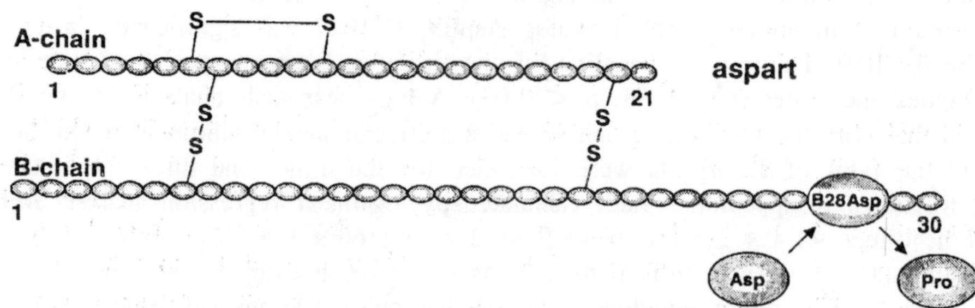

Fig. 1.1. Schematic presentation of primary structure of human insulin lispro and aspart.

analogs produced similar serum insulin levels (250–300 pmol/l) at approximately 30 min and disappeared from serum after approximately 4 h. Insulin aspart and lispro had similar effects on glucose and fat metabolism. Effects on carbohydrate metabolism (glucose uptake, glucose oxidation, and endogenous glucose production) peaked after approximately 2–3 h and disappeared after approximately 5–6 h. Effects on lipid metabolism (plasma free fatty acid, ketone body levels, and free fatty acid oxidation) appeared to peak earlier (at approximately 2 h) and disappeared earlier (after approximately 4 h) than the effects on carbohydrate metabolism. The author concluded that both insulin aspart and lispro are indistinguishable from each other with respect to blood levels and that they are equally effective in correcting abnormalities in carbohydrate and fat metabolism in patients with type 1 diabetes.

Other Formulations of Human Insulin

Inhaled insulin

Subcutaneous insulin has been used to treat diabetes since the 1920s; however, despite a number of different formulations, intensive insulin therapy with multiple daily injections has not gained widespread clinical acceptance. Great efforts have been made in searching for noninvasive administration modes of insulin that will avoid the need for parenteral administration of subcutaneous injection. Attempts to find effective, well-tolerated, nonenteral routes for delivering insulin began in the 1920s, and, over the years, have included ocular, buccal, rectal, vaginal, oral, nasal and uterine delivery systems, where various enhancers or formulations have been tested to increase the bioavailability of insulin from each route. Until recently, it was believed that insulin delivered noninvasively was associated with a bioavailability that was too low to offer a realistic clinical approach. However, progress in the pharmaceutical approach of insulin suggests that inhaled insulin is an effective, well-tolerated, noninvasive alternative to subcutaneous regular insulin.

Oral inhalation of insulin potentially offers noninvasive treatment and better glycemic control in diabetes by virtue of its apparently faster absorption into the systemic circulation compared with subcutaneous injection. However, the pharmacokinetics of inhaled insulin in the human lung has yet to be fully clarified because of the complexity of insulin-glucose physiology and the difficulty in approximating the inhaled dose. In 2004, Sakagami conducted a meta-analysis of insulin pharmacokinetics in the lung after oral inhalation of insulin in humans, where, based on the data from well-controlled clinical studies of inhaled insulin published in the literature, a physiologically realistic insulin-glucose kinetic model was derived. The model defined the first-order absorption ($k_{a,L}$) and parallel non-absorptive loss ($k_{mm,L}$), the latter primarily occurring via metabolism and mucociliary clearance in the lung with two systemic compartments. The significant estimate for $k_{a,L}$ was found to be from 0.020 to 0.032 h^{-1}, effectively unchanged across doses (from 0.3 to 1.8 IU/kg), formulations (powder vs. liquid), and subjects (healthy vs. diabetic), suggesting passive diffusive absorption of insulin from the lung. In contrast, the values for $k_{mm,L}$ were much larger (from 0.5 to 1.6 h^{-1}) and decreased with increasing inhaled dose. From this perspective, the author considered that a dose-dependent saturable lung metabolism regulates the value of $k_{mm,L}$, alongside mucociliary clearance. As a result, the absolute bioavailability of insulin through the oral inhalation ranged from 1.5% to 4.8%.

Henry et al. evaluated the AERx insulin Diabetes Management System (AERx iDMS) to the deep lung for systemic absorption, which was an aerosol of liquid human insulin produced by Aradigm. This study examined the effects on pulmonary function, pharmacokinetics, and pharmacodynamics of inhaled insulin in asthmatic and nonasthmatic subjects without diabetes, where a total of 28 healthy and 17 asthmatic subjects were enrolled in a two-part, open-label trial. The area under the time versus concentration curve (AUC) of insulin after inhalation showed significantly greater value for healthy subjects than for asthmatic subjects, whereas no difference was observed for maximum concentration in the two groups. In addition, a greater reduction of serum glucose level was observed in healthy subjects. Moreover, asthmatic subjects had greater intra-individual variations in insulin AUC, maximum concentration values, and glucose levels than healthy subjects. In this report, the author concluded that, after inhaling insulin using the AERx iDMS, asthmatic subjects absorbed less insulin than healthy subjects, resulting in less reduction of serum glucose.

The rationale behind developing a pulmonary drug delivery system is to ensure that insulin powder is delivered deep into the lungs, where it is easily absorbed into the bloodstream, in a handheld inhalation device. More recently, Nektar Therapeutics has developed a pulmonary drug delivery system for insulin. This device converts the insulin powder particles into an aerosol cloud for the patient to inhale. The inhaler requires no power source, and the clear chamber ensures that the patient knows immediately when all the insulin has been inhaled. In addition, Nektar Therapeutics is using its Advanced PEGylation technology to develop a dry powder-inhaled polyethylene glycol (PEG) formulation for delivering peptides efficiently across the lungs and to promote prolonged serum concentration of the peptide. PEGylation is designed to increase the size of the active molecule and ultimately improve drug performance by optimizing pharmacokinetics, increasing bioavailability, and decreasing immunogenicity and dosing frequency. The investigation has begun with inhaled, long-acting (PEGylated) insulin, and is funded by Pfizer.

Intranasal insulin

Insulin administered nasally has considerable potential for the treatment of both type 1 and type 2 diabetes. Using enhancers or novel delivery systems such as adequate bioadhesive microspheres, it is believed that the low bioavailability of simple formulations of insulin can be greatly improved. Therefore, several efforts on developing the nasal delivery system of insulin with nontoxic and nonirritant properties have been done.

In 1992, Drejer et al. investigated the pharmacokinetics of intranasal insulin containing a medium-chain phospholipid (didecanoyl-L-alpha-phosphatidylcholine) as absorption enhancer in 11 normal volunteers. Intranasal insulin was absorbed in a dose-dependent manner with a mean plasma insulin peak 23 $\pm$ 7 min after administration. Mean plasma glucose nadir was seen after 44 $\pm$ 6 min, 20 min after intravenous injection. Moreover, intranasal administration of insulin resulted in a faster time-course of absorption than subcutaneous injection, and the bioavailability for the nasal formulation was 8.3% relative to an intravenous bolus injection when plasma insulin was corrected for endogenous insulin production estimated by C-peptide.

On the other hand, there are negative opinions on the nasal delivery of insulin. In 1995, Hilsted et al. evaluated metabolic control and safety parameters (hypoglycemia frequency and nasal mucosa physiology) in 31 insulin-dependent diabetic patients treated with intranasal insulin in an open, cross-over randomized trial. Serum insulin concentrations increased more rapidly and decreased more quickly during intranasal as compared with subcutaneous insulin administration. Metabolic control deteriorated, as assessed by hemoglobin A1c concentrations, slightly but significantly after intranasal as compared with subcutaneous insulin therapy. The bioavailability of intranasally applied insulin was low; therefore, intranasal insulin doses were approximately 20 times higher than subcutaneous doses. The frequency of hypoglycemia was similar during intranasal and subcutaneous insulin therapy, and nasal mucosa physiology was unaffected after intranasal insulin. The author concluded that because of low bioavailability and a high rate of therapeutic failure, intranasal insulin treatment was not a realistic alternative to subcutaneous insulin injections.

In the early twenty-first century, nanoparticles based on nanotechnology have altered the direction of investigation in the drug delivery system. Nanoparticles, an evolvement of nanotechnology, are increasingly considered as a potential candidate to carry therapeutic agents safely into a targeted compartment in an organ, particularly a tissue or a cell. In 2002, Dyer et al. investigated effects of chitosan-formulated nanoparticles on the insulin pharmacokinetics and pharmacodynamics as a nasal drug delivery system. The nasal absorption of insulin after administration in chitosan nanoparticle formulations and in chitosan solution and powder formulations was evaluated in rats and in conscious sheep. Insulin-chitosan nanoparticle formulations produced a pharmacological response in the two animal models, although in both cases the response in terms of lowering the blood glucose levels was less than that of the nasal insulin-chitosan solution formulation. The insulin-chitosan solution formulation was found to be significantly more effective than the complex and nanoparticle formulations. The authors concluded that chitosan nanoparticles did not improve the nasal absorption.

Erythropoietin

Erythropoietin (EPO), a glycoprotein hormone with a molecular mass of 30 KDa, is mainly synthesized by the kidney in response to hypoxia. Serum EPO concentrations in humans normally range from 6 to 32 U/L. The plasma half-life of EPO is reported to range from 2 to 13 hours, with a volume of distribution close to plasma volume. As expected for a large sialoglycoprotein, less than 10% of EPO is excreted in the urine. EPO is known to stimulate the proliferation and differentiation of erythrocytic progenitors in the bone marrow, leading to reticulocytosis and increased erythrocyte numbers in the blood.

Recombinant human EPO (rHuEPO) has proven beneficial for treating renal anemia as well as anemia of other chronic disorders, including auto immune diseases, malignancies, and AIDS. Evidence from clinical trials indicates that anemia associated with cancer chemotherapy generally responds well to a standard rHuEPO regimen of 150 IU/kg subcutaneous (s.c.) three times per week. Several dosage recommendations have been made for surgery patients depending on the type of surgery and practicality of an autologous blood donation program. In patients scheduled for major orthopedic surgery, three weekly 600 IU/kg s.c. doses of rHuEPO, with the last one on the day of the surgery, have been suggested. Goldberg et al. present here pharmacokinetic/pharmacodynamic (PK/PD) modeling from four comparable, placebo-controlled, parallel-group studies in healthy subjects who were administered single rHuEPO doses of 300 to 2400 IU/kg as well as multiple doses of 600 IU/kg/wk and 150 IU/kg/tiw for 4 weeks.

Clinical trials of recombinant product began in Seatle and London in 1986, and its efficacy was established at an early stage. The early studies confirmed that intravenously administered EPO was highly effective in correcting the anemia of end-stage renal failure in hemodialysis. The intravenous route was, however, clearly impractical for patients maintained on continuous ambulatory peritoneal dialysis (CAPD) who had no ready vascular access, which necessitated an examination of the intraperitoneal and subcutaneous routes of administration, and several pharmacokinetic studies have compared these in CAPD patients. These three routes of erythropoietin administration are the only ones to have been investigated either from a pharmacokinetic or a therapeutic point of view. Although Storring et al. and Charles et al. compared the two forms of rHuEPO (i.e., EPO-alpha and EPO-beta), they reported that the volume of distribution after intravenous EPO-beta compared with EPO-alpha and that delayed subcutaneous absorption of EPO-beta compared with EPO-alpha. They believed the pharmacokinetic differences were caused by their glycosylation.

Pharmacokinetics of Erythropoietin in Healthy Subjects

Intravenous administration in the dialysis center has been practical and effective for patients undergoing hemodialysis, but impractical for patients without vascular access who are receiving peritoneal dialysis. Studies of subcutaneous administration showed lower but more sustained peak plasma EPO concentrations (C_{max}) than occurred using the intravenous route. The efficacy of subcutaneous administration supports the concept of a sustained minimal effective EPO concentration. High C_{max}

values after intravenous administration appear unnecessary; the dose response relationship seen with intravenous administration most likely correlates with serum EPO concentrations maintained above a minimal effective level.

Flaharty et al. presented data on the pharmacokinetics of EPO in healthy normal subjects. To assess phamacokinetics to human recombinant erythropoietin (EPO-beta), single intravenous doses (10, 50, 150, and 500 IU/kg) were administered at monthly intervals to 16 healthy subjects in a two-panel, placebo-controlled, double-blind ascending-dose trial. A 1000-IU/kg dose was subsequently administered in an open manner. EPO concentrations were detemined in serum by radioimmunoassay. Mean EPO apparent half-lives ranged fiom 4.42 to 11.02 hours. The apparent volume of distribution was between 40 and 90 mL/kg, consistent with plasma water, and the apparent clearance values ranged from 4 to 15 mL/kg/hr, with both parameters having the highest values at the 10-IU/kg dose level. Clearance tended to decrease as a function of dose. The use of EPO in healthy individuals will have clinical relevance if EPO is found to be effective for use in autologous transfusion programs. Although EPO was well tolerated in this study, clinical trials in patients with end-stage renal disease have shown adverse effects, including hypertension, seizures, and thrombocytosis, related to the increase in erythropoiesis. These effects are not expected in normal subjects, but careful monitoring should be performed if EPO is used in repeated doses in healthy subjects.

Salmonson et al. also described the pharmacokinetics of rHuEPO after intravenous and subcutaneous administration of 50 U/kg to six healthy male volunteers. The calculated mean values for volume of distribution at steady state and clearance after an i.v. dose were 76 ± 33 mL/kg and 12.0 ± 3.0 mL/h/kg, respectively. Serum concentrations of rHuEPO peaked at 13.0 ± 6.0 h after the s.c. dose and the bioavailability over 72 h was 36 ± 23%. The mean residence time and half-life of rHuEPO were 6.2 ± 1.0 and 4.5 ± 0.9 h after i.v. and 46 ± 18 and 25 ± 12 h after s.c. administration. They found that the serum concentration time profiles after i.v. adminisitaration followed a mono- or bi-exponential decline, and the elimination after s.c. dose was described by a mono-exponential decline.

McMahon et al. reported a double-blind, placebo-controlled study of the pharmacokinetics and safety of multiple doses of rHuEPO 150 or 300 U/kg, either by i.v. bolus or s.c. in normal male subjects, which demonstrated that rHuEPO had a dose-related effect on the hematocrit independent of the route of administration, and that multiple doses of rHuEPO had no direct pressor effects. When rHuEPO was injected by i.v. route, a mono-exponential decrease in serum EPO level was observed for 18 to 24 hours postdose. Absorption of s.c.-injected rHuEPO occurred more slowly with relatively low serum EPO levels being maintained for 48 hours. As a result of the prolonged elevation in serum EPO concentrations with s.c. injection, with injections every 48 hours, s.c. resulted in higher preinjection serum EPO concentrations than with i.v. injection of the same dose.

Moreover, Ramakrishnan et al. described the pharmacokinetic and pharmacodynamic modeling of rHuEPO after single and multiple doses in healthy volunteers. A one-compartment model with limited distribution and nonlinear elimination characterizes the data from the i.v. dosing. Most of the rHuEPO after s.c. dosing was rapidly absorbed within 2 to 3 days by zero-order rate constant. A dual-absorption model (fast zero-order and slow first-order inputs) with nonlinear disposition characterized the pharmacokinetics of s.c. rHuEPO. A similar pharmacokinetic model describes the time-course of plasma concentrations of rHuEPO on monkeys. On the other hand, Cheung et al. demonstrated the pharmacokinetics of rHuEPO after single s.c. doses of 300, 450, 600, 900, 1200, 1350, 1800, and 2400 IU/kg and in multiple s.c. dose regimens: 150 IU/kg three times a week for four weeks and 600 IU/kg once per week for four weeks in open-label, randomized placebo-controlled studies in healthy volunteers. The absorption rate of rHuEPO after s.c. administration was independent of dose, whereas clearance was dose-dependent, in which it decreased with increasing dose. In an advanced investigation,

Cheung et al. further described the comparison of the pharmacokinetics administered s.c. once weekly (qw), 150 IU/kg, and three times weekly (tiw), 40,000 IU. The C_{max} values for serum rHuEPO qw were six times and AUC values three times that of the tiw regimen. Sub sequent study reported by Krzyzanski et al. showed that a phamacokinetic and pharmacodynamic (PK/PD) model for rHuEPO in healthy subjects was developed to describe the time profiles of changes in serum rHuEPO and the pharmacological responses of percent reticulocytes, total red blood cell counts, and hemoglobin after single and multiple subcutaneous administration of rHuEPO. Data used is the same data as Wing Cheung et al. A dual-absorption model (fast zero-order and slow first-order inputs) with linear disposition kinetics was used to characterize the pharmacokinetics of erythropoietin after subcutaneous administration. Flip-flop kinetics was apparent in the pharmacokinetics as the absorption rate was slower (ka = 0.7 day^{-1}) than the elimination rate (CL/Vd = 1.2 – 9.2 day^{-1}).

Pharmacokinetics of Erythropoietin in Patients

rHuEPO is established as an effective therapeutic agent for anemia in patients undergoing long-term hemodialysis. After an intravenous dose of EPO 24 to 240 U/kg, serum clearance was 0.66 ± 0.42 L/h; terminal elimination half-life was 6 to 9 h and did not change after repeated doses given for more than two months. In hemodialysis patients, the pharmacokinetics of rHuEPO was studied by Brockmöller et al. They investigated in 12 patients under chronic hemodialysis on a thrice weekly intravenous rHuEPO treatment. The pharmacokinetics of rHuEPO was also assessed after a subcutaneous injection during the initial period and during maintenance treatment. After the first i.v. dose, plasma EPO concentrations were best described by a mono-exponential disposition function with a mean (±s.d.) elimination half-life of 5.4 ± 1.7 h. The volume of distribution was 70 ± 5.2 mL/kg, and the clearance was administered intravenously as 10.1 ± 3.5 mL/h/kg. After three months of continuous therapy, the plasma half-life of rHuEPO decreased by 15% (mean half-life during steady state: 4.6 ± 2.8 h), while mean clearance and volume of distribution remained constant. On the other hand, the absorption of rHuEPO after s.c. injection was prolonged and flip-flop kinetics applied. The extent of systemic availability of the s.c. dose ranged from 28% to 100% (mean 44%).

Gladziwa et al. described the pharmacokinetics of rHuEPO after long-term therapy in patients undergoing hemodialysis and hemofiltration. In 17 patients with end-stage renal disease (ESRD), studies were performed in three groups to assess pharmacokinetics during the intertreatment interval and during hemofiltration and dialysis treatment. After an intravenous bolus injection of EPO 150 U/kg, the half-life was 7.7 h, steady-state volume of distribution was 0.066 L/kg, and total plasma clearance was 5.4 mL/min. The mean steady-state serum concentration during multiple-dose administration was 656 U/L. The drug was not eliminated by hemofiltration or dialysis. Therefore, long-term treatment of ESRD patients with EPO does not significantly alter the pharmacokinetic profile of the drug. EPO dosage adjustment or substitution after hemofiltration and dialysis is not necessary. On the other hand, peritoneal dialysis (PD) has gained recognition worldwide as an alternative to hemodialysis in the management of patients with end-stage renal disease. The most common is continuous ambulatory peritoneal dialysis (CAPD) in which most patients perform four to five exchanges daily. As the peritoneal catheter provides direct access to the peritoneum, intraperitoneal drug administration has become widely used for the administration of certain drugs. The instillation and drainage of PD fluids contribute to the total body clearance of drugs, in which peritoneal clearance is low. Taylor III et al. reported the pharmacokinetic studies after rHuEPO administration to patients receiving PD. Intraperitoneal (i.p.) drug administration, via a PD catheter, produces a concentration gradient between the peritoneal and vascular compartments, favoring drug absorption. Absorption is enhanced if the plasma concentration of drug is low relative to the concentration of drug in the peritoneal fluid. Lymphatics draining the diaphragm contribute to the absorption of albumin and dextrans from the peritoneum and may be important in the absorption of protein drugs or other large-molecular-weight compounds like rHuEPO. The pharmacokinetic parameters observed in patients undergoing CAPD following i.v. and s.c. administration are similar to those determined for hemodialysis patients. s.c. adminisitration was found efficacious in several studies of PD patients, and allows reduction of the dose of EPO to 50–60% of the i.v. dose. i.p. administration is convenient and circumvents any pain associated with s.c. administration. In several studies, EPO was administered i.p. 1L to 2L of dialysate and allowed to dwell for varying time periods. Low absorption of EPO from the peritoneal cavity is seen if dialysate is present. Hematological response similar to those observed with either s.c. or i.v. administration were seen following i.p. administration using this technique, but substantially higher doses were required. Other investigators have reported poor efficacy, although this may result partly from the low doses administered. Based on these observations, the i.p. administration of EPO in large volumes of dialysate appears prohibitively costly to achieve the desired results. An improved bioavailability was observed in humans after administration of undiluted EPO 400 U/kg followed by an 8-hour dry dwell. A greater than nine fold increase in bioavailability was observed with dry administration, compared with diluting the dose in 2-L dialysate followed by an 8-hour dwell. The dry-dose administration area under the concentration-time curve (AUC) approached that seen with s.c. dosing. Ateshkadi et al. administered EPO 100 U/kg IP to eight patients undergoing CAPD using a 4-hour dry dwell followed by an infusion of 2-L dialysate that was allowed to dwell for 6 hours. The i.p. EPO serum-concentration time profiles were similar to those observed with s.c. administration, with a mean bioavailability of 11.4% compared with 22.8% for s.c. administration. Ongoing studies are examining the pharmacokinetics and efficacy of administration using an 8-hour dry dwell. Single-dose pharmacokinetics of EPO were studied in pediatric dialysis patients. EPO appears to be better absorbed and more rapidly cleared in children than it is in adults. Differences in the volume of distribution of EPO have also been noted between children and adults. These differences may be result of methodological differences between studies or true physiological differences relating to the plasma volume or tissue distribution of the drug. A recent study of i.p. administration in five children on continuous cycling peritoneal dialysis (CCPD) suggests that this route is safe and efficacious.

Erythropoietin Formulation

Humoral factors and cytokines are glycosylated with variable numbers of carbohydrate chains, each of which has variable carbohydrate structures. Although the biological function is typically determined by the protein component, carbohydrate can play a role in molecular stability, solubility, *in vivo* activity, serum half-life, and immunogenicity. The sialic component of carbohydrate, in particular, can extend the serum half-life of protein therapeutics. One aspect of glycoengineering is to introduce N-linked glycosylation consensus sequences into desirable positions in the peptide backbone to generate proteins with increased sialic acid-containing carbohydrate, thereby increasing *in vivo* activity because of a longer serum half-life.

DarbEPO alfa (DA) is a hyperglycosylated analog of recombinant human erythropoietin (rHuEPO) generated by glycoengineering. This rHuEPO is used to treat the anemia associated with chronic kidney disease and cancer. The discovery that the sialic acid-containing carbohydrate content of rHuEPO was directly proportional to the serum half-life and *in vivo* bioactivity led to the hypothesis that additional carbohydrate on rHuEPO might further enhance *in vivo* activity. DA contains two additional N-linked glycosylation sites and has increased *in vivo* activity and prolonged duration of action because serum half-life is increased three fold above rHuEPO, which allows for less frequent dosing with subsequent increased convenience for the patient and caregiver and improved patient compliance.

Allon et al. investigated the pharmacokinetics of darbEPO alfa and rHuEPO after repeated intravenous dosing in patients with chronic kidney disease receiving hemodialysis. Overall, 47 patients were randomized to receive darbEPO alfa administered once weekly or three times weekly or EPO administered three times weekly for up to 52 weeks. Pharmacokinetic profiles were measured during weeks 1 and 12. The terminal half-life of darbepoietin alfa was 17.8 hours, which was approximately two to three times longer than that of EPO (6.3 hours). The clearance of darbepoietin alfa (2.00 mL/h/kg) was approximately four times slower than those of EPO (8.58 mL/h/kg). They conclude that darbepoietin alfa can be administered- less frequently than EPO in patients with chronic kidney disease receiving hemodaialysis.

Lerner et al. also studied the pharmacokinetics of darbepoietin alfa in pedisatric patients with chronic kidney disease (CKD). Twelve patients 3-16 years of age with CKD were randomized and received a single 0.5 μg/kg dose of darbepoietin alfa administered i.v. or s.c. After a 14- to 16-day washout period, patients received an identical dose of darbepoietin alfa by the alternate route. After i.v. administration, the mean clearance of darbepoietin alfa was 2.3 mL/h/kg with a mean terminal half-life of 22.1 h. After s.c. administration, absorption was rate limiting, with a mean terminal half-life of 42.8 h and a mean bioavailability of 54%. Comparison of these results with those from a previous study of darbepoietin alfa in adult patients indicated that the disposition of darbepoietin alfa administered i.v. or s.c. is similar in adult and pediatric patients, although absorption may be slightly more rapid in pediatric patients after s.c. dosing.

Granulocyte Colony Stimulating Factor (G-CSF)

Colony stimulating factors (CSFs) as well as hematopoietic growth factors are a group of glycoproteins regulating the survival, proliferation, and differentiation of hematopoietic progenitor cells as well as the function and activation of the mature cells. The CSFs are produced by a variety of cells and range in molecular mass from 14 to 90 kDa. Recently, these factors have been purified, cloned, and produced through recombinant DNA techniques. The recombinant factors have been shown to have biologic properties and actions that are similar to the naturally occurring factors. The availability of quantities of the recombinant factors has resulted in their introduction into clinical trials and into the market.

The pharmacokinetics of CSFs has been evaluated widely in animals and in man. Early studies, however, used impure or poorly characterized fractions and the interpretation of these results is difficult. With the availability of recombinant proteins, these limitations were overcome and definitive studies have been completed. In general, the biologic effects of these factors can be quantitated by measuring the effects on the target hematopoietic cell population, which has provided a basis for relating the pharmacokinetic profile of the factor to the pharmacodynamic response. As clinical trials and the therapeutic applications of these factors are expanded, the knowledge and understanding of the pharmacokinetics of the drug will be critical to guide the clinician in the choice of dosing routes and schedule.

The generation of granulocytes from immature hematopoietic progenitor cells depends on the presence of several hormone-like glycoproteins. CSFs are acidic glycoproteins required for the survival, proliferation, and differentiation of hematopoietic progenitor cells. Granulocyte-colony stimulating factor (G-CSF) was identified because it induced differentiation in a murine myelomonocytic leukemic cell line and stimulated granulocyte colony formation by normal progenitor cells. The hematopoietic actions of this regulator are restricted exclusively to cells of neutrophilic granulocyte lineage. Murine and human G-CSFs have been purified from various sources and the genes encoding human and murine G-CSF have been isolated. This factor supports the growth and proliferation of relatively late granulocyte progenitor cells already committed to the neutrophil lineage and enhances the function and activation of mature neutrophils. This factor has also been cloned and expressed in both bacterial cells and mammalian cells. Characterization of the gene encoding G-CSF has led to the production of this protein by recombinant DNA techniques. The recombinant form of human G-CSF, rhG-CSF, is also capable of supporting the formation of granulocytic colonies from committed precursor cells. The availability of large quantities of molecularly homogeneous and biologically active human G-CSF by recombinant DNA technology has made it possible to explore the use of human G-CSF as a therapeutic agent. rhG-CSF shows broad species cross-reactivity with respect to its characteristic biologic response, a rapid and dose-dependent neutrophilia. The potential clinical applications for rhG-CSF include myelorestoration after bone marrow transplantation, mitigating chemotherapy-induced neutropenia, boosting host defense against infections, and augmenting effecter cell purpose.

Pharmacokinetics of G-CSF in Animals

Cohen et al. also reported biexponential clearance of *E. coli*-derived rhG-CSF administrated intravenously to hamsters; the α and β serum half-lives were 0.5 and 3.8 hr, respectively (all data were normalized to the amount recovered at 5 min after injection). Tanaka and Kaneo reported the pharmacokinetics of rhG-CSF (KRN8601) in male Sprague-Dawley rats at a dose of 5 μg/kg as a pre-clinical investigation. The serum concentrations of rhG-CSF were monitored using a specific sandwich enzyme immunoassay. For i.v. administration, the serum concentration-time curve showed a rapid disappearance of rhG-CSF from the systemic blood with a mean residence time (MRT) of 1.34 hr. For s.c., i.m., and i.p. administration, lower peak serum levels were observed; but after 2 to 3 hr, rhG-CSF levels were higher than those for i.v. administration with the MRTs of 3.92, 2.90, and 3.54 hr, respectively. Moreover, Tanaka et al. examined the influence of dose level and route of administration on the pharmacokinetics of *E. coli*-derived G-CSF after i.v. administration to Sprague-Dawley rats at doses of 10 or 100 μg/kg. Biexponential plasma clearance was noted after an i.v. dose of 100 μg/kg; the half-lives at distribution phase (α) and elimination phase (β) were 25 and 102 min, respectively. In addition, the total body clearance of rhG-CSF in the rat after i.v. administration showed an approximate 30% decrease from 80 to 56 mL/h/kg as the dose was increased from 1 to 10 μg/kg; no further decreases in the total body clearance were noted up to 100 μg/kg. However, the volume of distribution calculated was equivalent at each dose. For the serum concentration profiles of rhG-CSF after extravascular administration, an i.m. injection gave slightly faster absorption kinetics of rhG-CSF from the injection site into systemic blood than did s.c. and i.p. injections. After s.c. administration, biological effects were noted at 2 h and were sustained for 36 h, suggesting rapid absorption. Peak serum concentrations were seen at approximately 2–3 h postdose. The calculated bioavailability of the subcutaneous dose was approximately 78%. There were nonproportional increases in the AUC value; a 100-fold increase in the dose resulted in a 164-fold increase in the AUC. Bioavailability after subcutaneous dosing ranged from approximately 50% to 70%. The results of this study suggested that two mechanisms may be involved in the clearance of G-CSF. One pathway is saturated at low concentrations and represents high-affinity, low-capacity receptor-mediated uptake by target cells (neutrophils). The other mechanism represents clearance by nonspecific pathways such as renal excretion.

In multiple-dose studies, rhG-CSF was injected into animals by i.v. and s.c. at 5 μg/kg/day for 7 days. When the serum concentration-time profiles on day 7 after multiple dosing of rhG-CSF were compared with single dosing, the AUC after i.v. multiple dosing decreased by 17.4%. However, the half-lives and the volume of distribution were not significantly different between single and multiple dosing groups. In addition, the AUC after s.c. multiple dosing decreased by 25.6% without significant differences in the bioavailability and observed maximum serum concentration of rhG-CSF. These results showed that the clearance of rhG-CSF increased after multiple dosing, although the mechanism of increased clearance was not apparent.

Moreover, Tanaka et al. reported the effect of sex differences and hepatic or renal failure on the pharmacokinetics of rhG-CSF in the rats. After i.v. and s.c. administration of rhG-CSF to male and female Sprague-Dawley rats at a dose of 5 and 100 μg/kg, area under the concentration versus time curve and elimination half-lives of rhG-CSF in female rats were smaller than those for male rats. The volume of distribution of rhG-CSF in female rats was not significantly different from that in male rats. After s.c. administration, the values of AUC, MRT, and half-lives of elimination phase in female rats were smaller than those for male rats. In the *in vitro* biological activities of rhG-CSF using [^{3}H]thymidine uptake assay in cultures of bone marrow cells obtained from male and female rat femur, female rat bone marrow cells showed a similar dose-response profile to rhG-CSF to that of male rat bone marrow cells. The effect of rhG-CSF administration in rats was a specific activity on the neutrophil lineage with an increase of neutrophils in peripheral blood. On the other hand, the *in vivo* effects of rhG-CSF after i.v. and s.c. adrninistration to male and female rats at 5 and 100 μg/kg doses, namely the neutrophil count in female rats, was similar to that in male rats in the early period; however, the neutrophil count in female rats was lower than that in male rats 24 h after administration. These results indicate the sex differences in pharmacokinetics and the *in vivo* effects of rhG-CSF as well as the close relationship between pharmacokinetics and the *in vivo* effects of rhG-CSF. In rats with experimental renal and hepatic failure, the total body clearance of rhG-CSF after i.v. administration at a dose of 10 μg/kg was 44.48 mL/h/kg in sham-operated rats compared with 9.429 mL/h/kg in bilaterally nephrectomized rats. In sham-operated rats, the elimination half-life of rhG-CSF at β phase was 1.51 h, and it increased to 5.33 h after nephrectomy. In contrast, the volumes of distribution were identical in both rats. In rats with acute renal failure induced by uranyl nitrate, the total body clearance and volume of distribution were identical to those of control rats, but the elimination half-life at β phase was slightly shorter. In 70% hepatectomized rats, the clearance of rhG-CSF decreased from 42.08 mL/h/kg to 31.93 mL/h/kg, and similar half-lives were observed in rats in both the sham-operated and hepatectomized groups. However, the volume of distribution decreased after hepatectomy. In rats with hepatic failure induced by CCl_4, the pharmacokinetic changes were similar to those observed in hepatectomized rats. These results suggest that renal clearance makes a major contribution to total body clearance compared with hepatic clearance.

Pharmacokinetics of G-CSF in Humans

In the early period, the pharmacokinetics of *E. coli*-derived rhG-CSF as part of phase I and II clinical trial was evaluated by Layton et al. The protein was administered by i.v. or s.c. routes at dose levels of 3 to 30 μg/kg. The elimination half-life after i.v. dosing was 1.4 h at a dose of 1 μg/kg, and increased to 4.2 h at a dose of 60 μg/kg. These results indicated saturation mechanisms in the total body clearance at doses greater than 10 μg/kg. When a continuous s.c. infusion was performed for 5 days, steady state was not achieved and there was a rapid reduction in serum G-CSF levels during the last 2 days of administration. Neutrophil levels increased during this period, and these results were interpreted as neutrophil receptor-mediated regulation of G-CSF uptake and degradation. The peak levels of G-CSF after initiation of s.c. dosing were achieved at 6 h, and these levels were maintained for up to 16 h. When high doses of melphalan were coadministered with G-CSF, the neutrophil levels did not increase and serum G-CSF levels remained constant.

For the pharmacokinetics of rhG-CSF in humans, it has been reported that the absorption and clearance of rhG-CSF follow first-order kinetics without any apparent concentration dependence. When rhG-CSF was administered by 24-h constant i.v. infusion at a dose level of 20 μg/kg, the mean serum concentration achieved 48 ng/mL. Constant i.v. infusion for 11 to 20 days produced steady-state serum concentrations over the infusion period. Sub cutaneous administration of rhG-CSF at doses of 3.45 and 11.5 μg/kg resulted in peak serum concentrations of 4 and 49 ng/mL, respectively. The mean value of volume of distribution was 150 mL/kg. The elimination half-life was 3.5 h after either i.v. routes or s.c. routes, with a clearance rate of 0.5–0.7 mL/min/kg. The administration of a daily dose for 14 consecutive days did not affect the half-life.

More recently, Hayashi et al. reported the results of pharmacokinetic and pharmacodynamic (PK/PD) analysis for rhG-CSF (lenograstim) after s.c. administration. A total of 72 adult healthy volunteers were administered 1 μg/kg of rhG-CSF. There was no correlation between the maximal plasma concentration (C_{max}) and an increase in peripheral neutrophil count, whereas a negative correlation between AUC and this increase was observed. It is considered that the mechanism of this phenomenon is probably based on the correlation between the elimination rate constant (ke) and neutrophil increase, because the ke probably has a close relationship with uptake by neutrophil and its progenitor the G-CSF receptor. Indeed, a volunteer with higher ke showed a greater increase in neutrophil count. Therefore, AUC is proportional to the rhG-CSF remainder, that is, the proportion that is not consumed in the course of increasing the neutrophil count. From this perspective, the bioavailability calculated from the AUC is unlikely to indicate the absorbed amount. A two-compartment pharmocokinetic model with zero-order absorption and first-order elimination provided a good curve fit, suggesting that the absorption process is not a first-order process but is a zero-order process.

As the clearance of rhG-CSF is known to decrease with a rise in dose and is known to be saturable, the average clearance after i.v. administration will be lower than that after s.c. administration. Therefore, the apparent absolute bioavailability with subcutaneous administration calculated from the AUC ratio is expected to be a conservative estimate. In a second study by Hayashi et al., the estimation of rhG-CSF absorption kinetics after s.c. administration with a nonlinear elimination pharmacokinetic model using a modified Wagner–Nelson method was studied, and the results of the bioequivalency study between two rhG-CSF formulations with a dose of 2 μg/kg were described. The apparent absolute bioavailability for s.c. administration was 56.9% and 67.5% for each formulation, and the ratio between them was approximately 120%. The true absolute bioavailability was, however, estimated to be 89.8% and 96.9%, respectively, and the ratio was approximately 108%. The absorption pattern was applied to other doses, and the values of predicted clearance for s.c. and i.v. administrations were then similar to the values for several doses reported in the literature. Using this pharmacokinetic model, the underestimation of bioavailability was around 30%, and the amplification of difference was 2.5 times, from 8% to 20%, because of the nonlinear pharmacokinetics. The neutrophil increases for each formulation were identical, despite the different bioavailabilities. Therefore, it is considered that there is an upper limit to the transfer rate of rhG-CSF from subcutaneous tissue to blood, and that the amount eliminated through the saturable process, which indicates the amount consumed by the G-CSF receptor, was identical for each formulation.

Wang et al. also reported the PK/PD relationship of the granulopoietic effects of r-metHuG-CSF (filgrastim) in healthy volunteers through a population pharmacokinetic approach. Healthy male volunteers were enrolled into a four-way crossover clinical trial. Subjects received four single doses of r-metHuG-CSF (375 and 750 μg for i.v. and s.c., respectively) with an intervening washout period of 7 days, and an absolute neutrophil count (ANC) was determined. Data analysis was performed using mixed-effects modeling as implemented in the NONMEM software package. The final PK/PD model incorporates a two-compartment PK model with bisegmental absorption from the s.c. site, first-order and saturable elimination pathways, and an indirect PD model. A sigmoidal E_{max} model for the stimulation of ANC input rate (k_{in}) was superior to the conventional E_{max} model (E_{max} = 12.7 ± 1.7; EC_{50} = 4.72 ± 0.72 ng/mL; Hill = 1.34 ± 0.19). In addition, a time-variant scaling factor for ANC observations was introduced to account for the early transient depression of ANC after r-metHuG-CSF administration. The absolute bioavailability after s.c. administration of r-metHuG-CSF was estimated to be 0.619 ± 0.058 and 0.717 ± 0.028 for 375 μg and 750 μg s.c. doses, respectively. The time profiles of concentration and ANC, as well as the concentration approximate ANC relationship of r-metHuG-CSF in healthy volunteers, were well described by the developed population PK/PD model.

On the other hand, Hernandez-Bernal et al. evaluated the equivalence of the pharmacokinetic, pharmacodynamic, and safety properties of two commercially available recombinant G-CSF formulations in 24 healthy male volunteers using a standard two-way randomized crossover double-blind study, with a 3-week washout period. A single 300-μg G-CSF dose was administered subcutaneously. Absolute neutrophils (ANC), white blood cells (WBC), and $CD3^{4+}$ cell counts were the pharmacodynamic variables measured up to 120 h. Other clinical and laboratory determinations were used as safety criteria. The pharmacokinetic parameters for formulation A and B were very close to each other (i.e., AUC, 235.9 vs. 270.0 ngh/mL; C_{max}, 29.2 vs. 33.4 ng/mL; T_{max}, 4.2 vs. 4.7 h; half-life, 3.2 vs. 2.8 h; CL, 260.9 vs. 277.2 mL/h; Vd, 1.2 vs. 1.1 L; and MRT, 7.58 vs. 7.38 h). The pharmacodynamics showed high similarity because ANC and WBC had the same profiles for both products and no differences were detected for the estimated parameters. The $CD3^{4+}$ cell count increments were evident for both formulations in a similar way as well. According to the overall results, these formulations could be considered as clinically comparable.

G-CSF Formulation

Generally, peptide/protein drugs undergo extensive hydrolysis in the gastrointestinal tract and have short circulating half-lives in the blood. For optimal clinical efficacy, therefore, they must be given by daily injections. Recently, it has been found that attaching a polyethylene glycol (PEG) moiety (PEGylation) improves the pharmacokinetic and pharmacodynamic profiles of peptide/protein drugs. Conjugating peptide/protein drugs with PEG, a process known as pegylation, is now an established method for increasing the circulating half-life of protein and liposomal pharmaceuticals. PEGs are nontoxic water-soluble polymers that, owing to their large hydrodynamic volume, create a shield around the pegylated drug, thus protecting it from renal clearance, enzymatic degradation, and recognition by cells of the immune system.

For the formulation of G-CSF, PEGylated filgrastim (pegfilgrastim) has a longer half-life than unmodified filgrastim and, when administered as a single dose, has been shown to be at least as efficacious as daily filgrastim. As a result of its reduced renal clearance, the elimination of pegfilgrastim is predominantly neutrophil-mediated, so its clearance is self-regulated. In addition, pegfilgrastim can be administered at a fixed dose instead of in weight-based doses. For these reasons, pegfilgrastim can potentially increase patient adherence and acceptance of treatment, thus having a beneficial effect on their quality of life. Furthermore, treatment is likely to cost less because of the reduced need for medical interventions. Similarly, pegylated liposomal doxorubicin has a longer half-life than unmodified doxorubicin and has been shown, because of its reduced reticuloendothelial system clearance, to produce higher concentrations of doxorubicin in tumors and to have greater clinical efficacy than doxorubicin in the treatment of some solid tumors. Pegylated liposomal doxorubicin is also associated with less myelosuppression and febrile neutropenia.

For the pegylated formulation for subcutaneous route, van Der Auwera et al. produced a pegylated G-CSF formulation, Ro25-8315, which is produced by conjugation of rhG-CSF mutant with PEG, where the pharmacodynamics and pharmacokinetics of Ro25-8315 was evaluated in comparison with rhG-CSF (filgrastim). Subjects received single subcutaneous doses of Ro25-8315 ranging from 10 to 150 μg under a double-blind, randomized, placebo-controlled design. Filgrastim was administered as a single dose (5 or 10 μg/kg) and, following a 14-day washout period, daily for 7 days. Ro25-8315 increased absolute neutrophil count (ANC) by six- to eight-fold and $CD3^{4+}$ cell count more than 30-fold at the highest doses tested. Single doses (60–150 μg) of Ro25-8315 and multiple doses of filgrastim had similar effects on ANC and $CD34^{+}$. The phamacokinetic profile of Ro25- 8315 was dose-dependent, with peak concentrations and the AUC increasing 100-fold over the range of doses studied. Time to reach peak concentration (T_{max}) and half-life of Ro25-8315 averaged 20–30 h at all doses, approximately three times longer than with filgrastim. Adverse events were not serious and occurred with similar frequency with both products. Pegylation of rhG-CSF mutant results in more desirable pharmacokinetic properties and a longer duration of action with effective increases in ANC and measures of peripheral blood progenitor cell mobilization for at least 1 week.

More recently, Maeda et al. developed a new sustained-release formulation of rhG-CSF. The formulation is a double-layer minipellet (DL-MP) that is designed to maintain a sustained release of rhG-CSF without an initial burst. The DL-MP is composed of a core of collagen matrix and a coating layer with collagen. This formulation of rhG-CSF was then prepared, and its characteristics were determined, in normal rats. After subcutaneous administration, it was found that blood rhG-CSF concentration was maintained for about 1 week. Moreover, after administration of the DL-MP rhG-CSF formulation with additional condroitin sulfate, a persistent increase in white cell count was found. Therefore, the DL-MP formulation system was useful as a long-acting formulation of rhG-CSF characterized by excellent long-acting properties without an initial burst.

In general, an oral route is most popular form of administration; however, peptide/ protein drugs without some pharmaceutical modifications should not be applicable because of poor absorption based mainly on extensive hydrolysis in the gastrointestinal tract. Taking this background into consideration, Eiamtrakarn et al. designed a new formulation of G-CSF for oral administration, where a new gastrointestinal mucoadhesive patch system (GI-MAPS) has been designed for the oral delivery of G-CSF in beagle dogs. The system consists of four layered films, 3.0×3.0 mm^2, contained in an enteric capsule. The 40-μm backing layer is made of a water-insoluble polymer, ethyl cellulose (EC). The surface layer is made of an enteric pH-sensitive polymer such as hydroxypropylmethylcellulose phthalate (HP-55), Eudragit L100 or S100, and was coated with an adhesive layer. The middle layer, a drug-containing layer, made of cellulose membrane is attached to the EC backing layer by a heating press method. Both drug and pharmaceutical additives including an organic acid, citric acid, and a non-ionic surfactant, polyoxyethylated castor oil derivative (HCO-60), were formulated in the middle layer. The surface layer was attached to the middle layer by an adhesive layer made of carboxyvinyl polymer. The same three kinds of GI-MAPSs containing 125 μg of rhG-CSF were prepared and orally administered to dogs, and the increase in total white blood cell (WBC) counts were measured as the pharmacological index for G-CSF. Comparison with the total increase of WBCs after i.v. injection of the same amount of G-CSF (125 μg) indicated the pharmacological availabilities (PA) of G-CSF were 23%, 5.5%, and 6.0% for Eudragit L100, HP-55, and Eudragit S100 systems. By decreasing the amount of HCO-60 and citric acid, the PA of G-CSF decreased. These results suggest the usefulness of GI-MAPS for the oral administration of protein.

For pulmonary drug delivery, the opportunity for systemic administration of peptides and proteins that are, at present, usually administered parenterally has been available. As a result of the large surface area, good vascularization, immense capacity for solute exchange, and ultra-thinness of the alveolar epithelium are unique features of the lung, which can facilitate systemic delivery via pulmonary administration of peptide/protein drugs. Physical and biochemical barriers, lack of optimal dosage forms, and delivery devices limit the systemic delivery of biotherapeutic agents by inhalation. Current efforts exist to overcome these diffi- culties to deliver metabolic hormones. Systemic delivery of rhG-CSF can readily induce an increase in circulating levels of natural GCSF to approximately three to five times greater than baseline. Niven et al. showed that rhG-CSF induced systemic response after delivery by aerosol in hamsters. The absorption from the lung was rapid, with a concomitant increase in white blood cells to four times baseline. The bioavailability was 45.9% of the administered dose and 62.0% of the dose reached the lung lobes. In a study that compared pulmonary administration of rhG-CSF powder with solution, a normal systemic response was obtained, indicating that rhG-CSF retains its activity in the solid state after formulation. Dissolution and absorption of rhG-CSF from powders were not rate limiting because the plasma concentration versus time profiles peaked at similar times in both powder and solution administration.

More recently, Miyamoto et al. developed the *in vivo* nasal absorption system of the FITC-dextrans with a mean molecular weight ranging from 4.3 to 167 kDa and rhG-CSF, in which the effect of poly-L-arginine (poly-L-Arg) on the *in vivo* nasal absorption in rats were studied. When FITC-dextrans were coadministered intranasally with 1.0 w/v% poly-L-Args of different molecular weight [MW, ca. 45.5 and 92 kDa, poly-L-Arg (50) and poly-L-Arg (100)], the bioavailability increased markedly compared with that after administration of FITC-dextran alone. However, the bioavailability decreased exponentially with the increasing molecular weight of FITC-dextrans. There was no significant difference between the enhanced nasal absorption of FITC-dextrans achieved by the coadministration of poly-L-Arg (50) and poly-L-Arg (100). Moreover, the relationship between the bioavailability and the molecular weight of FITC-dextrans indicated that the molecular weight of protein drugs, which exhibited efficient absorption with poly-L-Arg, was about 20 kDa, whereas the lower limit of bioavailability for developing a potent transnasal delivery system was assumed to be about 10%. Indeed, the nasal absorption of rhG-CSF, which has a molecular weight of 18.8 kDa, was also increased after coadministration of 1.0 w/v% poly-L-Arg (50) and the bioavailability was about 11%. It seems likely that poly-L-Arg can be used to provide adequate nasal absorption of various protein drugs, which have a molecular weight of about 20 kDa, thereby allowing the successful development of a variety of trans- nasal drug delivery systems.

Interferon

Interferons (IFNs) are classified into three major groups that reflect antigenic and structural differentiation. IFN-α (leukocytic interferon) is produced by B lymphocytes, null lymphocytes, and macrophages; its production can be induced by foreign, virus-infected, tumor or bacterial cells. Human IFN-α is a family of more than 15 subtypes, with molecular masses of 17.5–23 kDa. These proteins are composed of 165–166 amino acid residues and show approximately 80% sequence homology. The secondary structure of human IFN-a consists of 55–70% α-helix and less than 16% β-sheet. In general, human IFN-α does not contain N-linked glycosylation sites. There are 13 species of subtype IFN-α, and each IFN-α subtype has a different affinity for IFN receptor or a different antiviral activity. These IFNs tend to be acidic, with isoelectric points of 5.7–7.0. In commercial settings, native IFN-α (Ly-IFN-Ly) and recombinant IFNs (IFN-α2a, IFN-α2b, and IFN-α con) are available. IFN-β (fibroblast interferon) is a product of fibroblasts, epithelial cells, and macrophages that can be induced by viral and other nucleic acids.

Human IFN-β is a single species with the molecular size of the natural glycoprotein 23 kDa with 166 amino acid residues. IFN-β shows 29% structural homology to IFN-α. The secondary structure consists of 36% α-helix and 33%-β sheet. The isoelectric point falls between 6.8 and 7.8. Now, native IFN-β and recombinant IFN-β, IFN-β 1b are available. IFN-γ (immune interferon) is a product of activated T lymphocytes stimulated by foreign antigens and is composed of 143 amino acids. Human IFN-γ is heterogeneous, the molecular size depending on glycosylation and possibly oligomerization. Higher molecular sizes of 50–70 kDa have been reported, suggesting oligomerization. It shows no statistically significant sequence homology to IFN-α or IFN-β. IFN-γ is acid-labile and highly basic, with an isoelectric point of 8.6–8.7.

A lot of works involving IFNs has been done with natural or cloned human IFN preparations. In the 1970s, human testing of IFNs was restricted by their limited availability, purity, and specific activity; however, recombinant DNA technology has provided high-purity (>99%) and high-specific-activity preparations for large-scale human testing. Human leukocyte interferon was the first preparation available.

Early phase I studies, intending to establish the safety, tolerance, pharmacokinetics, and efficacy of interferons, targeted a host of viral and oncologic diseases using animal species. In clinical use, the results were often disappointing. However, the importance of the route and rate of administration as treatment variables had been identified. On the other hand, the pharmacokinetics of conventional drugs commonly demonstrates species specificity. In case of IFNs, however, the catabolism and excretion of IFNs are similar across most species. Therefore, animals may serve as suitable models for the pharmacokinetics of IFNs in humans.

Pharmacokinetics of Interferon in Animals

Absorption of IFN-α from intramuscular, subcutaneous, intraperitoneal, intradermal, duodenal, and rectal sites has been reported. In general, IFN-α absorption from these sites is prolonged, and maximum serum concentrations occur 1–6 h post injection, followed by measurable concentrations through 8–24 h post injection. The concentration-time profile appears to be independent of the purity or source of IFN-α, namely, partially purified, natural, or recombinant. In addition, the disposition profiles were similar across the tested species, including mice, rabbits, dogs, and monkeys. Several of these studies have determined the absolute bioavailability from the intramuscular site to be 42% in dogs and 93% and 56% in monkeys.

The absorption of IFN-β from intramuscular, subcutaneous, and intraperitneal sites is similar to that observed for IFN-α. The concentration-time curves are also similar to those seen with IFN-α, namely, prolonged absorption with concentrations persisting from 9 to 24 h after the injection. Estimates of absolute bioavailability from the intramuscular site can be obtained from published data: 60% in rats, 33% and 60% in rabbits, and 43% in monkeys. Recently, a bioavailability of 2.2% was reported for IFN-β after intranasal administration to rabbits. However, absorption appears to be independent of species and interferon source. Contraly to this appearance, the absorption of IFN-γ has not been studied as extensively as that of IFN-α or -β. According to the results of Weck et al., serum concentrations of IFN-γ were very low or nondetectable after intramuscular injection of nonglycosylated IFN-γ in monkeys.

After bolus injection, the initial decline in serum concentrations following intravenous administration is rapid for IFN-α, -β, and -γ for all species tested with the half-lives of initial distribution on the order of minutes. Serum concentrations initially decrease rapidly, then decline more slowly, with terminal elimination half- lives ranging from minutes (30–40 min for IFN-α in mice) to hours (7–12 h for IFN-β in rabbits) depending on the species selected and the type of interferon.

Both IFN-α and IFN-β have a volume of distribution after intravenous administration that ranges from 20% to 100% of body weight in mice, rats, rabbits, dogs, and monkeys, suggesting distribution into a volume that approximates total body water. Similar data for IFN-γ are not available. The tissue content of the interferons generally parallels that found in serum or plasma. Measurable concentrations or titers of interferons have been demonstrated in the brain, spleen, lung, liver, and kidney. For IFN-β and -γ, the amount of interferon determined in specific organs or tissues reflected the amount found in the serum or plasma, suggesting no uptake of these interferons into the sample organs or tissues. For IFN-α, the uptake results on tissue distribution studies have been mixed. Heremans et al.reported the uptake of IFN-α by liver, lung, and spleen after intraperitoneal administration of homologous mouse IFN-α to mice. In contrast, Bohoslawec et al. showed no appreciable uptake of murine IFN-α into brain, liver, lung, or spleen after intravenous administration to mice. However, the kidney showed an appreciable uptake of murine IFN-α. Two human IFN-α subtypes, A and D, and one human hybrid, A/D, displayed a tissue distribution profile similar to that of biologically active mouse IFN-α.

The catabolism of interferons has been the most widely researched area of pre- clinical IFN pharmacokinetics. Undoubtedly, the gastrointestinal tract is the most effective and efficient system for catabolizing proteins. The liver has also been shown to play a role in the catabolism of dycosylated proteins, and the kidney is the major catabolic organ for circulating low-molecular-mass (<60 kDa) proteins. In addition, other organs and tissues, such as the lungs and muscles, are thought to play minor roles in protein catabolism. For the catabolism of interferons, IFN-α has been the most extensively studied of the three types of interferons. In general, IFN-α is filtered through the glomeruli of the kidney followed by luminal endocytosis and proximal tubular reabsorption. During reabsorption, IFN-α undergoes proteolytic degradation by lysosomal enzymes; therefore, negligible amounts of intact IFN-α are excreted in the urine. In nephrectomized animals (rats and rabbits), therefore, the clearance was significantly decreased. In addition to the above findings, Bocci et al. demonstrated that the liver has been shown to play a small role in the catabolism of IFN-α. On the other hand, both IFN-β and IFN-γ undergo renal catabolism, but to a much smaller extent than IFN-α. Natural IFN-β and -γ are glycoproteins that contain sialic acid groups; they are therefore subject to the liver catabolism characteristic of this class of proteins. For recombinant IFN-a, there is an evidence that it reduces hepatic drug metabolism activity in mice. Moreover, it has been demonstrated that the greater the antiviral activity of a given IFN in murine cells, the greater its ability to depress hepatic microsomal cytochrome P450 content in mice.

Pharmacokinetics of Interferon in Humans

The pharmacokinetics of interferons has been evaluated using a variety of dosing regimens varying from intermittent to continuous administration. Although definitive pharmacokinetics has not been reported in all cases, enough information is available to define their basic disposition characteristics. Serum interferon concentrations after intravenous administration decline rapidly in a biexponential manner for IFN-α and IFN-β. On the other hand, monoexponential decline has been observed for IFN-γ. IFN concentrations fall several orders of magnitude over the measurable serum concentration-time course. Terminal half-lives range from 4 to 16 h for IFN-α, 1 to 2 h for IFN-β, and 25 to 35 min for IFN-γ. At the doses tested, serum concentrations are generally measurable for between 8 and 24 h after dosing of IFN-α and up to 4 h after injection for IFN-β and -γ. The total body clearance of IFN-α has been reported to range from 4.9 to 21 liters/h or 24 liters/h per/m^2. For IFN-β, the total body clearance is much higher, 19–38 liters/h per/m^2, whereas that of IFN-γ falls between the two at 12.66–32.4 liters/h.

Oral absorption of intact proteins has met with limited success because of the natural proteolytic capabilities of the gastrointestinal tract. The systemic absorption of interferons from sites other than the gastrointestinal tract has been remarkably good, considering the size of these molecules. Intramuscularly and subcutaneously administered IFN-α and nonglycosylated IFN-γ are well absorbed, >80% for IFN-α and 30–70% for IFN-γ. These routes exhibit protracted absorption, which results in maximum serum or plasma concentrations occurring after 1 to 8 h. Concentrations are measurable for 4 to 24 h after injection for both IFN-α and IFN-γ. Maximum serum concentrations following these routes of administration are at least an order of magnitude less than the highest concentration observed after intravenous administration of an equal dose. The absorption of IFN-β from muscle or skin has not been sufficient to produce much greater serum concentrations because of the limits of assay detection.

The volume of distribution is similar for both IFN-α and IFN-γ, ranging from 12 to 40 liters. Although this volume is not physiological, it is approximately 20% to 60% of body weight. Information regarding IFN-β has not been established. On the other hand, the penetration of interferons across the human blood-brain barrier has been actively studied. Partially purined, natural, and recombinant interferons do not readily cross the blood-brain barrier intact after intravenous, intramuscular, or subcutaneous administration. These data suggest that direct effect of parent interferon for the nervous system is not responsible for the occurrence of neurotoxicity, a common side effect of interferon therapy.

Interferon Formulation

Other routes of administration have been evaluated, such as inhalation, intralesional, intranasal, intraperitoneal, intraventricular, and intraocular rates, in clinical studies. For the most part, these alternative routes were attempts to improve the delivery of interferon to sites not easily accessible via the systemic circulation. These dosing strategies have provided adequate concentrations of interferon in cerebrospinal fluid, lymph, nasal mucosa, and peritoneal fluid, but have not led to clinical success, undoubtedly reflecting the lack of understanding of the inherent mechanism of interferon action.

The recommended twice-weekly administration of IFN-α does not maintain sustained plasma concentrations of the drug, thereby adversely affecting the potential biological response. During the last few years, "*pegylation technology*" has been used to develop long-acting forms of IFN-α that help to avoid most of these problems. Polyethylene glycols are nontoxic water-soluble polymers that, owing to their large hydrodynamic volume, create a shield around the pegylated drug, thus protecting it from renal clearance, enzymatic degradation, and recognition by cells of the immune system. Two separate compounds, peginterferon α-2a (PEGASYS) and peginterferon α-2b (PEG-Intron), are now both approved for use alone or in combination with ribavirin for the treatment of chronic hepatitis C. Interferon therapy for chronic hepatitis C is not a cure, but it is able to decrease the viral load and may decrease the risk of complications (e.g., cirrhosis, liver failure, and liver cancer). Pegylation of the interferon increases the amount of time the interferon remains in the body by increasing the size of the interferon molecule. Increasing molecule size slows the absorption, prolongs the half-life, and decreases the rate of interferon clearance.

Thus the duration of biological activity is increased with pegylated INF over nonpegylated INF. The pegINF-α products offer an advantage over nonpegylated INF-α products because of less frequent administration. Tolerability of the pegylated INF is comparable with the nonpegylated formulations. Monotherapy with these agents produces a better response in some patients than monotherapy with the nonpegylated formulation. Combination therapy with ribavirin is more effective than monotherapy. In 1995, Nalin et al. demonstrated that conjugation of IFN-α 2a to a linear polyethylene glycol (PEG) (M, 5000) via a urea linkage increased the half-life, and plasma residence time parameters of IFN-α 2a were one and one-half fold and two fold greater than those corresponding to the native IFN-α 2a in rats, with reduced immunogenicity in mice. In humans, a twice-weekly dosing of PEG_{5K}-IFN-α 2a is required to achieve antiviral levels similar to those attained with unconjugated IFN, as shown in a phase II trial involving chronic hepatitis C patients. Ramon et al. reported that the conjugation of INF-α 2b (IFN-α 2b) to a branched-chain (40,000) polyethylene glycol ($PEG_{2,40K}$-IFN-α 2b) markedly improved the resistance to tryptic degradation and the thermal stability of IFN-α 2b. The serum half-life of $PEG_{2,40K}$-IFN-α 2b showed 330-fold longer, whereas plasma residence time was increased 708 times compared with native IFN. Pegylation alters the pharmacokinetic properties of IFN-α and allows for once-weekly administration. Pegylated IFNs contain either linear PEG chains of small molecular weight, as in pegylated IFN-α-2b (12 kD), or larger branched moieties, as in pegylated IFN-α-2a (40 kD). There are pharmacokinetic and pharmacodynamic differences between these two IFNs. The much-increased sustained virological response rates observed with pegylated IFN-α-2a (40 kD) and pegylated IFN-α-2b (12 kD) support the rationale for pegylation of IFN.

The absorption half-life of standard IFN-α is 2.3 h, whereas absorption half- lives for pegylated IFN-α-2a and α-2b are 50 h and 4.6 h, respectively. The volume of distribution for pegylated IFN-α-2a is considerably restricted, whereas the volume of distribution for pegylated IFN-α-2b is only approximately 30% lower than that for conventional IFN. As a result of its large size, the 40-kD pegylated IFN-α-2a has a more than 100-fold reduction in renal clearance compared with conventional IFN-α. Clearance of pegylated IFN-α-2b is about one tenth that of unmodified IFN-α. Although data are limited, both drugs appear to show differences in the initial viral decay pattern in patients with chronic hepatitis C. However, it remains unknown whether these differences in the initial viral decline predict differences in the primary clinical endpoint, sustained virological response.

The development of new IFN-α delivery strategies is a key issue to simplify its administration and improve its therapeutic effects while reducing its dose-related side effects. One of the most attractive approaches toward this purpose is the encapsulation of IFN-α into microspheres by a biodegradable polymer, poly(lacticglycolic acid) (PLGA). Sanchez et al. developed the method of encapsulation of IFN-α into biodegradable microparticles and nanoparticles using PLGA and poloxamer 188, which is a stabilizing agent, and encapsulated IFN-α within PLGA/ poloxamer blend microspheres or nanospheres where their preparation techniques led to the efficient encapsulation of IFN-α and the modulation of their particle size ranging from 280 nm to 40 gm. The antiproliferative activity of the IFN-α varied depending on the formulation. Moreover, PLGA/poloxamer blend microspheres were able to provide significant amounts of active IFN-α for up to 96 days.

In 2004, Peleg-Shulman et al. developed a new type of pegylated INF-α-2 conjugate, peg_{40}-FMS-IFN-α-2, which is capable of regenerating native INF-α-2 at a slow rate under physiological conditions. A 2-sulfo-9-fluorenylmethoxycarbonyl (FMS)-containing bifunctional reagent, MAL-FMS-NHS, has been synthesized, enabling the linkage of a 40-kDa peg-SH to IFN-α-2 through a slowly hydrolyzable bond. The *in vitro* rate of regeneration of native interferon from this preparation was estimated to have a half-life of 65 h. Following subcutaneous administration to rats and monitoring of circulating antiviral activity, active IFN-α-2 levels peaked at 50 h, with substantial levels still being detected 200 h after administration. This value contrasts with a half-life of about 1 h measured for unmodified interferon. The concentration of active IFN-α-2 scaled linearly with the quantity injected. Comparing subcutaneous to intravenous administration of peg40-FMS-IFN-α-2, the long circulatory lifetime of IFN-α-2 was affected both by the slow rate of absorption of the pegylated protein from the subcutaneous volume and by the slow rate of discharge from the peg in circulation.

More recently, Ito et al. demonstrated the usefulness of the oral patch preparations for INF-α. The patch preparations were composed of three layers; a water-insoluble backing layer, a drug-containing layer with an absorption enhancer, and a surface layer containing pH-dependent polymer were prepared. As absorption enhancer, three surfactants, Gelucire44/14 (lauroyl macrogol-32 glycerides), Labrasol (caprylocaproyl macrogol-8 glycerides), and HCO-60 (polyoxyethylated hydrogenerated castor oil) were used in preparing the IFN-α patch preparations, an in vitro release study showed that the time when half of the formulated IFN-α is released from the patches were 3.4 ± 0.1 min for HCO-60, 7.8 ± 0.1 min for Gelucire44/14, and 11.4 ± 0.1 min for Labrasol preparations. An in vivo absorption study showed that Gelucire44/14 preparation showed a higher C_{max}, 7.66 ± 0.82 IU/mL, and AUC, 12.85 ± 1.49 IU h/mL, than Labrasol (6.51 ± 0.89 and 8.30 ± 1.34 IU h/mL) and HCO-60 (6.02 ± 1.14, 7.53 ± 1.84 IU h/mL) preparations, respectively. By comparing the AUC obtained after s.c. injection of the same dose of IFN-α with rats, bioavailability was estimated to be 7.8% in the Gelucire44/14 preparation.

Growth Hormone

Growth hormone (GH) is an endocrine hormone produced and stored in the anterior pituitary gland, which is secreted into the blood circulation in a pulsation pattern. Deficiency of GH results in abnormally poor growth. This disease state, namely hypopituitary dwarfism, has been recognized for several years. By the end of 1950s, it was found that a patient with hypopituitary dwarfism given injections of extracts of human pituitary tissue grew remarkably well. However, the supply of human GH (hGH) was extremely limited, because the only source of hGH was from cadaver pituitaries. Specific criteria were established for identifying patients who were clearly GH-deficient and who stood the best chance of benefiting from therapy. If identified, a child would receive intramuscular injections of these pituitary extracts three times per week. The dosing levels were limited and the continuing therapy was always threatened by shortages of material. In addition to being in thin supply, the problem of purifying the material provided a further challenge. As with any therapeutic drug that is derived from human tissue, contaminants of other protein hormones as well as those of viral origin had to be removed. However, more recently, the availability of synthesized hGH, produced through recombinant DNA technology, greatly reduced these concerns and provided a plentiful supply of hormone. As part of the process for proving the safety and efficacy of the use of hGH in humans, pharmacokinetic studies have been conducted in a number of species including mice, rats, monkeys, and humans.

Pharmacokinetics of Growth Hormone in Animals

In 1982, Sigel et al. studied that the disappearance rates of hGH and a 20-kDa variant over 10 min after intravenous injection of iodinated material in male and female mice. The half-lives of hGH and the 20-kDa variant in males were 4.1 and 3.9 min, respectively, whereas the half-lives in females were 4.7 and 4.0 min. There were no significant differences in the protein half-lives between male and female mice. In addition, there was no apparent relationship between the half-lives, the dissimilar binding characteristics for the target sites, and growth-promoting activities. In 1988, the pharmacokinetics of biosynthetic human growth hormone (B-hGH) and pit-hGH were compared in rats. Normal and hypophysectomized male and female rats were injected subcutaneously and intramuscularly with 0.1 mg/kg B-hGH and pit-hGH and intravenously with 0.06 mg/kg B-hGH and pit-hGH. A smaller distribution volume and a slower metabolic clearance rate were found for B-hGH compared with pit-hGH. Moreover, a smaller distribution volume and a slower metabolic clearance rate were found for hypophysectomized rats compared with normal rats for both proteins.

The plasma half-lives was estimated to be about 3–7 min in the initial elimination phase and 29 min in the terminal elimination phase. The plasma levels of hGH were higher after subcutaneous compared with intramuscular administration for both proteins. From these results, it was suggested that an extensive local degradation took place at the subcutaneous and intramuscular injection sites. In addition, comparative tissue distribution studies with radioiodinated B-hGH and pit-hGH showed no differences between the growth hormones. The females accumulated relatively more label in the liver than the males, whereas the males accumulated relatively more label in the kidneys.

On the other hand, the total body clearance (CL) of synthetic hGH was studied in eight adult rhesus monkeys, where four monkeys were lean ($<20\%$ body fat) and the other four were obese ($>20\%$ body fat). The monkeys were given a single i.v. bolus injection of hGH (2.5 mg/kg), followed by a constant infusion of hGH (250 mg/hr) for 2.5 h. Venous blood samples were collected before the infusion and every 10 min during the infusion. In both groups, steady state was reached 70 min after the start of the infusion. The mean CL of synthetic hGH was 12.7 ± 1.7 liters/24 h in the lean group and 19.5 ± 2.9 liters/24 h in the obese group ($p < 0.007$). However, the CL values that standardized by body weight were the same in both groups. These observa tions suggest that the CL of hGH is directly proportional to body weight, and the lower plasma GH levels in obesity may be caused by an increase in its CL not compensated for by an appropriate increase in the rate of GH secretion.

As for the metabolism, the metabolic fate of GH in peripheral tissues has not been clearly defined as with other protein hormones. The clearance of GH from the systemic circulation is thought to occur by receptor-mediated uptake at the liver and filtration at the kidney. After intravenous injection of [^{125}I]hGH to female rats, hGH was speciacally taken up by the liver with radioactivity ultimately becoming associated with the lysosomal subfraction. The specific uptake of [^{125}I]hGH into rat liver was associated with accumulation in the Golgi apparatus. Interestingly, in each of these studies, radioactivity in the liver was characterized by TCA solubility and membrane binding as an intact hormone. These findings suggest that receptor-mediated uptake of GH in the liver is not directly linked to hydrolytic inactivation of the hormone.

Pharmacokinetics of Growth Hormone in Humans

In the early phases of product development, data from laboratory animals can sometimes be used to predict the phamacokinetic profile in humans. Dosing levels for initial clinical trials can thus be selected. In the later stages of development, when human data were available, allometeric analysis is useful for evaluating the clinical relevance of pharmacological data collected in laboratory animals. Actually, the phamacokinetic parameters in humans can often be predicted by using pharmacokinetic data collected in laboratory animals by extrapolation by following equations based on body weight. Application of this method assumes that the pharmacokinetics are dose-proportional over the dosage range under condition. The allometric approach uses the following equation: $Y = aW^b$, where Y represents a pharmacokinetic parameter and W represents body weight in kg; constants, a and b represent the allometric constants and the allometric exponent. Using the allometric equations, that pharmacokinetic parameters (total body clearance, initial volume of distribution, and volume of distribution at steady state for rhGH in mice, rats, monkeys, and humans) show a strong association among these pharmacokinetic parameters as a function of body weight. This good interspecies agreement supports the use of pharmacokinetic data collected in laboratory animals to predict the distribution of rhGH and other proteins in humans.

Growth Hormone Formulation

GH is a pituitary hormone responsible for postnatal growth. Like all polypeptide hormones, GH was long thought to be circulating exclusively in the free form rather than being bound to plasma proteins, which was in contrast to some other hormones of hydrophobic nature (e.g., steroids), which required protein binding for solubilization in the aqueous plasma environment. It is a 20–22-kDa polypeptide that exists in several molecular forms. GH acts by binding to GH receptors in multiple tissues; it initiates a cascade of biochemical events, among which the generation of insulin-like growth factor-I (IGF-I) is important for the growth process at the local tissue level. Other important actions of GH are those involved in anabolism, such as intracellular transport of amino acids and other cellular constituents, nitrogen, and protein synthesis.

The biochemical events immediately following GH binding to receptors (intracellular signaling) are only incompletely understood. In 1987, the hepatic GH receptor was cloned and structurally characterized; it is a single-chain glycoprotein with a 620-amino acid backbone, of which 246 are extracellular, 24 form a hydrophobic transmembrane domain, and 350 are intracellular. Like all polypeptide hormones, GH was long thought to be circulating exclusively in the free form rather than being bound to plasma proteins. At the end of 1980s, however, it was found that GH also circulates by binding to specific GH-binding proteins in plasma. At least two GH-binding proteins (GH-BP) have been identified in human plasma; one binds GH with high affinity, the other with lower affinity.

hGH is currently administered by injection daily or three times a week. To improve patient compliance, there have been a lot of research efforts for the development of long-acting formulations of protein drugs. The parenteral delivery route often requires frequent dosing because of the short half-lives of these drugs. A few clinical studies have shown that a continuous infusion of hGH via a pump resulted in growth velocity and insulin-like growth factor-I (IGF-I) levels comparable with those of daily injections. The results indicate that pulsatile hGH release may not be required for clinical efficacy, and the sustained-release formulation may improve patient compliance and efficacy with a suitable pharmacokinetics release profile. For a development of sustained-release formulation of protein drugs, one of the key requirements may be the integrity of the protein drugs within micro- particles during and after formulation processes contrary to small-molecular-weight drugs; proteins have three-dimensional structures to retain their bioactivity. Some stresses (e.g., temperature, pH, or organic solvents) associated with the preparation of sustained-release formulation can cause deamidation, oxidation, denaturation, or aggregation of the protein, which can turn the protein biologically inactive and even immunogenic.

From the end of the 1990s to the early 2000s, rapid development in molecular biology and recent advancement in recombinant technology increased identification and commercialization of potential protein drugs. It is well known that traditional forms of administration for the peptide and protein drugs often rely on their parenteral injection, as the bioavailability of these therapeutic agents is poor when administered nonparenterally. Tremendous efforts by numerous investigators across the world have occured to improve protein formulations and, as a result, a few successful formulations have been developed including sustained-release hGH. At the end of 1990s, a sustained-release system was developed for rhGH using biodegradable microsphere formulations composed of polymers of lactic and glycolic acid (PLGA). Lee et al. reported that long-acting formulations of rhGH were prepared by stabilizing and encapsulating the protein into three different injectable, biodegradable microsphere formulations composed of PLGA.

In this study, the microsphere formulations were compared in juvenile rhesus monkeys by measuring the serum levels of rhGH and two proteins induced by hGH, insulin-like growth factor-I (IGF-I) and IGF binding protein-3 (IGFBP-3) after single s.c. administration. The results showed that PLGA formulations induced a higher level of IGFBP-3 than was induced by injections of the same amount of rhGH in solution. Moreover, Brodbeck et al. evaluated the effects of altering dynamics of PLGA solution depot on the sustained-release delivery of hGH by subcutaneous injection in rats, and obtained about 28 days of long-term sustained-release profiles from the PLGA solution depot of hGH in normal rats at serum levels of 10–200 ng/mL.

In the early 2000s, several other formulations of hGH have been developed. In 2001, Maeda et al. developed a sustained-release collagen film of hGH and evaluated its effect on wound healing in db/db mice. The release profiles of hGH from the collagen films varied with composition and preparation conditions; however, the film prepared by air-drying of the mixture of hGH and collagen solution released hGH continuously over 3 days both in vitro and in vivo. By application of collagen film containing 3 mg of hGH twice at an interval of 6 days to wounds, the area of wounds on day 21 was significantly reduced compared with that of nontreated wounds in mice. In 2002, Kim et al. reported the usefulness of the synthesized HA/Pluronic composite hydrogels [temperature-sensitive hyaluronic acid (HA) hydrogels, which were synthesized by photopolymerization of vinyl group modified HA in combination with acrylate group end-capped poly(ethylene glycol)-poly(propylene glycol)-poly(ethylene glycol) tri-block copolymer.

This HA/Pluronic composite hydrogels gradually collapsed with increasing temperature over the range of 5 to 40°C suggesting that the Pluronic component formed self-associating micelles in the hydrogel structure. The mass erosion occurred much faster at 37°C than at 13°C, indicating that at the higher temperature, the ester linkage between the Pluronic and acrylate group might be more exposed to an aqueous environment and thus be more readily hydrolyzed because of Pluronic micellization. This HA/Pluronic composite hydrogels is applicable for a formulation of rhGH in sustained-release profiles that followed a mass erosion pattern.

More recently, aiming at once-a-week injection, a novel sustained-release formulation of rhGH using sodium hyaluronate (SR-rhGH) was developed for the treatment of children who have growth failure caused by lack of adequate secretion of endogenous GH. SR-rhGH was produced in the form of solid microparticles by spray-drying technology. A single administration of a prototype formulation of SR-rhGH with a ratio of hGH:HA-1:1 to cymomolgus monkeys through a fine 26-gauge needle induced continuous elevation of serum IGF-I level for 6 days, demonstrating the bioactivity of hGH released from the prototype formulation. When the ratio of hGH to HA changed from 1:1 to 1:3, hGH released more slowly in vitro from SR-rhGH with almost complete release of hGH loaded. According to phamacokinetic and pharmacodynamic studies in beagle dogs, sustained release of hGH from the optimized formulation of SR-rhGH continued for a more extended period longer than 72 h with a lower C_{max} than those of prototype formulations. The single administration resulted in an elevation of serum insulin- like growth factor-I (IGF-I) level for 6 days, with a maximum value that was higher than the baseline level by 350 ng/mL, which supported the possibility of SR-rhGH as a once-a-week injection formulation of hGH. The bioavailability of both formulations was comparable with that of hGH daily injection formulation. Finally, toxicity studies revealed no evidence of adverse effect in both cymomolgus monkeys and beagle dogs.

As for a formulation using another administration route, Leitner et al. developed a nasal delivery system of hGH based on the thiomer polycarbophil-cysteine (PCP-Cys) in combination with the permeation mediator glutathione (GSH). Micro particles were prepared by dissolving PCP-Cys/GSH/ hGH (7.5:1:1.5), PCP/ hGH (8.5:1.5), and mannitol/hGH (8.5:1.5) in demineralized water, followed by lyophilization and micronization. PCP-Cys/GSH/hGH and PCP/hGH microparticles showed a comparable size distribution (80% in the range of 4.8 to 23 ìm) and swelled to almost four fold size in phosphate-buffered saline. Both formulations exhibited almost identical sustained drug release profiles. The intranasal administration of the PCP-Cys/GSH/hGH microparticulate formulation resulted in a relative bioavailability of 8.11%, which represents a three fold and a 3.3-fold improvement compared with that of PCP/hGH microparticles and mannitol/hGH powder, respectively. The nasal microparticulate formulation based on PCP-Cys/GSH/hGH might represent a promising novel tool for the systemic delivery of hGH.

Leuprolide

Leuprolide acetate is a synthetic and superpotent agonist of luteinizing hormone- releasing hormone (LHRH) with a biphasic effect on the pituitary. It is a decapeptide hormone that is effective in the treatment of hormone-dependent diseases such as prostate and mammary tumors and endometriosis. It initially stimulates the secretion of both luteinizing hormone (LH) and follicle stimulating hormone (FSH), and on long-term continuous administration it inhibits secretion of LH and FSH, and the concentration of testosterone in men and estrogen in women drop sharply. It is administered pulsatively for adjuvant hormonal therapy and continuously for hormone-related anti-neoplastic therapy comprising prostatic and breast cancer and endometriosis. As leuprolide is a peptide, it is orally inactive and generally given subcutaneously or intramuscularly. Recently, however, several attempts are considered to improve bioavailability and effectiveness of leuprolide as well as a patient's convenience for taking the medicine.

In vitro Permeation Study of Leuprolide

For most polypeptides, oral administration is often limited by enzyme instability in the gastrointestinal tract. Furthermore, because peptides are highly ionized, and thus are mostly hydrophilic, their potential for permeating gastrointestinal absorption barriers is poor. Attempts to understand the degradation and permeation behavior in the intestine are beneficial to improve oral efficacy. Intramuscular and intranasal routes are the common routes of administration. Undoubtedly, the oral route is the most convenient. However, plasma levels of leuprolide after oral administration of an aqueous solution to rats and humans are mostly below the limit of detection (0.2 ng/mL). Therefore, it is important to understand and elucidate the absorption and degradation mechanisms of leuprolide in the intestinal tract. In 2004, Guo et al. reported the transport mechanism of leuprolide across rat intestine, rabbit intestine, and Caco-2 cell monolayer. Using techniques based on everted gut sac and Caco-2 cell monolayer, it was found that flux of leuprolide increased with increasing concentration of drug, showing a passive diffusion pathway. At a low concentration of leuprolide, trypsin inhibitor had a strong enhancement effect on the permeability of drug by protecting enough drug for permeation. Chitosan had no affect on the activity of α-chymotrypsin. In addition, the authors found that the increase in permeation of leuprolide was caused by opening of the tight junctions and interaction with cells. Therefore, the authors concluded that both inhibition of proteolytic enzymes and opening the tight junctions to allow for paracellular transport of leuprolide improved the intestinal absorption.

Clinical Pharmacokinetics of Depot Leuprolide

In 1984, for cancer treatment, a sustained-release intramascular formulation based on biodegradable microspheres had been developed by Saunders et al. and thereafter marketed. This injectable microsphereiscapable of sustaining required drug levels over a period of 1, 3, and 4 months after a single administration. These systems, in addition to improving the patient convenience and compliance, reduce the needed dose to one-quarter to one-eighth of the injected aqueous solution by sustaining therapeutic drug levels at target receptor sites.

More recently, sustained-release depot formulations, in which the hydrophilic leuprolide is entrapped in biodegradable highly lipophilic synthetic polymer microspheres based on polylactic/glycolic acid (PLGA) or poly-lactic acid (PLA), have been developed to avoid daily injections, where leuprolide is released from these depot formulations at a functionally constant daily rate for 1, 3, or 4 months, depending on the polymer type (PLGA for a 1-month depot and PLA for depot of >2 months), with doses ranging between 3.75 and 30 mg. The mean peak plasma leuprolide concentrations of 13.1, 20.8–21.8, 47.4, 54.5, and 53 μg/L occur within 1–3 h of depot subcutaneous administration of 3.75, 7.5, 11.25, 15, and 30 mg, respectively, compared with 32–35 μg/L at 36–60 min after a subcutaneous injection of 1 mg of a nondepot formulation. Sustained drug release from the PLGA microspheres maintains plasma concentrations between 0.4 and 1.4 mg/L over 28 days after single 3.75-, 7.5-, or 15-mg depot injections. The mean areas under the concentration-time curve are simiiar for subcutaneous or intravenous injection of short-acting leuprolide 1 mg; a significant dose-related increase in the AUC from 0 to 35 days is noted after depot injection of leuprolide 3.75, 7.5, and 15 mg. The mean volume of distribution of leuprolide is 37 L after a single subcutaneous injection of 1 mg, and 36, 33, and 27 L after depot administration of 3.75, 7.5, and 15 mg, respectively.

The total body clearance is 9.1 L/h and the elimination half-life is 3.6 h after a subcutaneous 1-mg injection; corresponding values after intravenous injection are 8.3 L/h and 2.9 h. A 3-month depot PLA formulation of leuprolide 11.25 mg ensures a mean plasma peak concentration of around 20 μg/L at 3 h after subcutaneous injection, and continuous drug concentrations of 0.43 to 0.19 μg/L from day 7 until before the next injection. In addition, an implant administration of these sustained-release systems of leuprolide provided a lasting delivery of leuprolide for 1 year. Serum leuprolide concentrations remained at a steady mean of 0.93 mg/L until week 52, suggesting zero-order drug release from the implant.

Transdermal Iontophoretic Delivery of Leuprolide

As for another route of administration of leuprolide, Kochhar et al. demonstrated an application of transdermal delivery of leuprolide using heat-separated human epidermal membrane from cadaver skin of multiple donors. The author used an iontophoresis technique to deliver the drug and examined the effect of constant voltage or constant current application. When the heat-separated human epidermal membrane was subjected to constant voltage within the range of 250 to 1000 mV during the iontophoretic phase, iontophoretic enhancement of leuprolide permeation at pH 7.2 was greater than at 4.5. A developed model to account for iontophoretic enhancement yielded that, first, the porosity increased with the applied voltage to as much as three times the original at 1000 mV. Second, the lipid pathway scontributed approximately 20% to the total permeation during the passive phase. Third, the electro-osmotic flow contributed significantly to the enhancement and its direction was from anode to cathode at pH 7.2 and the opposite at pH 4.5.

The magnitude of the electro-osmotic flow was at pH 4.5 somewhat lower than at pH 7.2. Repeated iontophoretic applications of 250 mV on the same skin specimen resulted in the same enhancement every time and did not cause any barrier alterations when applied for 1 h every 24 h, which was not the case if the duration between the two iontophoretic applications was only 3 h. In contrast, keeping the current densities at 0.5 to 2.3 $\mu A/cm^2$, the permeation rate of leuprolide increased linearly with the current density for the universal buffer and at pH 7.2 was almost double that at pH 4.5 despite the greater ionic valence of the drug at pH 4.5 compared with pH 7.2. The drug transference number at both pH values was approximately 0.5%. Replacement of the universal buffer with polymaleic acid yielded higher drug permeation rates and increased its transference number at a comparable pH. Transference number of the drug with polymaleic acid appeared to increase with current density. From these in vitro investigations, the authors concluded that the fluxes obtained for both electrolyte systems with the present experimental arrangement could be extrapolated to deliver therapeutically relevant doses of the drug.

DESMOPRESSIN

Desmopressin (the vasopressin analog 1-deamino-8-D-arginine vasopressin, dDAVP), a potent synthetic peptide hormone of the natural pituitary hormone vasopressin, is used chiefly for treatment of enuretic disorders, such as central idiopathic or secondary diabetes insipidus and nocturia and nocturnal enuresis in young children. Desmopressin has also proven to be useful in the treatment of bleeding diseases by activating and mobilizing factor VIII and von Willebrand's factor reserves in hemophilia A and von Willebrand–Jurgens syndrome. The 1100-Da molecule, which is typically taken in doses of 1–20 μg, shows variable and low oral and nasal bioavailability (0.1% and 3.4%, respectively). Although injectable formulations demonstrate better bioavailability, they are poorly suited for routine use in young children. For the treatment of these disorders, desmopressin (Desmopressin) in usually administered intranasally by use of sprays or drops. This route of desmopressin administration was shown to be more efficacious than the oral route, because bypassing the gastrointestinal tract increases the absolute bioavailability from less than 1% to approximately 5%.

A more acceptable route of administration with potentially good bioavailability could be offered by transdermal delivery. It is well documented that the stratum comeum, the outermost layer of the skin, constitutes an impermeable barrier to hydrophilic or high-molecular-weight drugs. These molecules can only be delivered into or through the skin if the barrier function of the stratum corneum is disrupted by any of a number of available methods. In this field, ultrasound and iontophoresis, which are known to enhance transdermal delivery of small molecules, have also been proposed for use with peptides and macromolecules.

Pharmacokinetics of Desmopressin in Humans

As a basic study, Rembratt et al. investigated the pharmacokinetic and pharmacodynamic profiles of desmopressin after oral and intravenous ad-mini-stration in men with a high incidence of nocturia. Based on an open-randomized and four-way crossover design, desmopressin was administered orally (0.2 mg) and intravenously (2 μg) at daytime and nighttime. The concentration-time curve after 2 μg intravenous desmopressin was best fitted by a biexponential equation. The mean (95% CI) AUC at night was 302 (272–335) pg h/mL and in the day was 281 (253–312) pg h/mL. No statistically significant differences were detected between night and day except for terminal half-life, which was 3.1 h at night and 2.8 h in the daytime ($p = 0.02$). Peak plasma concentration (C_{max}) was 6.2 (5.1–7.5) pg/mL at night and 6.6 (5.5–7.9) pg/mL in the daytime, respectively. Median time to reach C_{max} (t_{max}) was 1.5 (range 1.0–4.1) h at night and 1.5 (range 0.5–0.3) h in the day, and the oral bioavailability was 0.08%. The pharmacodynamic effects of oral and intravenous desmopressin given in the daytime were similar during the first 6 h after dosing.

The nighttime dosing and daytime intravenous dose resulted in antidiuresis throughout the measuring period, whereas the effect of the daytime peroral dose receded after 6 h. The authors concluded that the terminal half-life was longer at night than in the daytime, but the difference is considered too small to be of clinical importance. Moreover, they also concluded that, despite low bioavailability, the pharmacodynamic effects of oral desmopressin were similar in magnitude to those after intravenous dose at night and during the first 6 h after daytime administration.

More precisely, d'Agay-Abensour et al. investigated the absolute bioavailability of an aqueous solution of desmopressin from different regions of the gastrointestinal tract (stomach, duodenum, jejunum, ileum, colon, rectum) in 6 healthy male volunteers aged 24 to 35 years. For intravenous administration, the subjects received 4 μg of desmopressin. For intestinal administration, 400 μg of desmopressin was directly applied to six distinct sites in the GI tract via two- or four-channel tubes with or without a distal occlusive balloon. After intravenous administration, the elimination half-life, total body clearance, amount excreted in urine, and renal clearance of desmopressin were 60.0 min, 1.7 mL/min/kg, 2.0 μg, and 0.8 mL/min/kg, respectively. The mean bioavailability of desmopressin after gastric, duodenal, jejunal, distal ileal, proximal colonic, and rectal application was 0.19%, 0.24%, 0.19%, 0.03%, 0.04%, and 0.04%, respectively. Thus, absorption was significantly higher in the three upper GI regions in comparison with the three lower regions.

Renal and Biliary Excretion and Sex Differences in Desmopressin Pharmacokinetics

Agerso et al. investigated the differences in pharmacokinetic profiles of desmopressin between healthy subjects and renally impaired patients after intravenous administration. Overall, 18 renal impairment and 6 healthy volunteers were enrolled in the study. Each subject received a single intravenous dose of 2-μg desmopressin, and blood and urine samples were collected for 24 h, where plasma concentrations and the amounts of desmopressin excreted in the urine were analyzed simultaneously by means of a technique of mixed effects modeling. Their results showed that both renal and nonrenal clearances of desmopressin were found to vary with the creatinine clearance (CrCL). A decrease of 1.67% in the CrCL was found to cause a 1.74% decrease in the renal clearance and a 0.95% decrease in the nonrenal clearance.

The fall in renal failure caused the amount of desmopressin excreted in urine to decrease from 47% in healthy subjects to 21% in the patients with severe renal impairment. The mean total body clearance of desmopressin in healthy subjects and patients with severe renal impairment was 10 L/h and 2.9 L/h, respectively. Correspondingly, the mean terminal half-life was 5.7 h in healthy subjects and 10 h in patients with severe renal impairment. The authors concluded that great caution should be taken when deciding on an efficient dosage regimen if patients with moderately or severely impaired renal function are to be treated with desmopressin at all, despite the drug appearing to be safe and well tolerated by patients with impaired renal function.

The pharmacokinetic profiles of desmopressin in the liver were also investigated. Lundin et al. demonsted the biliary excretion of drug after intrajugular venous, intraportal venous, and intraduodenal venous administration in conscious pigs. In all cases of administration routes, the biliary excretion was less than 1% of the administered dose with the plasma/bile concentration ratio of less than 1.0. A significant first-pass effect was found when the liver was exposed to a high intra-portal dose of desmopressin. The uptake study of [^{3}H] desmopressin by incubating with liver tissue slices showed that desmopressin was rapidly removed from the incubation medium, indicating desmopressin was markedly metabolized in the liver.

As another parameter to alter the pharmacodynamic profile of desmopressin, a sex difference is most important. In 2004, Odeberg et al. demonstrated that there was a sex difference in a human pharmacokinetic (PK) and pharmacodynamic (PD) study, where desmopressin was administered intravenously as a single dose (for the PK study, a 2-μg dose; for the PD study, a 0.2-μg dose), and parameters for urine flow and urine osmolality were estimated. The pharmacokinetics of desmopressin after a fixed bolus injection were influenced neither by piroxicam nor by sex of subjects. However, the pharmacodynamics of desmopressin showed a sex difference where females exhibited a more pronounced antidiuretic effect than males, which was statistically significant when the effects were submaximal (>4.5 h after dose). The sex differences were diminished after pretreatment with an NSAID, piroxicam, indicating a prostaglandin PGE_2-mediated mechanism.

Desmopressin Formulation

Usually, desmopressin is administered intranasally by use of sprays or drops. This administration route of desmopressin was considered to be more efficacious than the oral route, because bypassing the gastrointestinal tract increases the absolute bioavailability from less than 1% to approximately 5%. However, nasal application of desmopressin is accompanied by high intersubject and intrasubject variability in plasma pharmacokinetics. Therefore, there have been several pharmaceutical research efforts to improve nasal delivery of desmopressin.

In 1987, Lethagen et al. demonstrated a comparison study, which was made of intranasal administration of 300-μg desmopressin by spray, with intravenous administration of 0.2-, 0.3-, and 0.4-μg/kg desmopressin in 10 healthy volunteers, where the effect of desmopressin was measured on the antihemophilia factor, factor VIII (F VIII), and on plasminogen activator release. Plasma levels of desmopressin showed a clear dose response with the maximum levels at 0.4 μg/kg intravenous dose. The affect of the spray approximated the 0.2-μg/kg response. However, the maximum response in both F VIII complex and plasminogen activator release was obtained after a 0.3-μg/kg i.v. dose. The response at a 0.4-μg/kg i.v. dose was not significantly different from the response at a 0.3-μg/kg dose, indicating that maximum stimulation was reached with 0.3 μg/kg. There was no correlation between plasma levels of F VIII and desmopressin, indicating that the biological response to the drug is subject to saturation kinetics.

The reproducibility of the effect of the spray dose on F VIII was 21% (c.v.) and 27% for the intraindividual and inter-individual variation, respectively, and compared favorably with intravenous administration. Therefore, they concluded that intranasal desmopressin (300 μg) is as effective as 0.2 μg/kg intravenously and provides an accurate, reproducible, and convenient alternative to parenteral administration. Moreover, in 1988, Harris et al. reported the effects of concentration and dose volume on the nasal bioavailability and biological response to desmopressin in humans. A nasal formulation of 300 μg of desmopressin was administered using a premetered spray device in doses of either 1 × 50-, 2 × 50-, or 1 × 100-μL actuations to both nostrils. Intravenous administration of 0.2 μg/kg was also given as a reference for bioavailability calculations.

The biological response was determined by measuring circulating levels of F VIII. Peak plasma levels of desmopressin were greatest after the 2 × 50-μL dose, followed by the 1 × 50- and 1 × 100-μL doses. The bioavailability of desmopressin from the 2 × 50-μL dose was 20%, which was significantly greater than the 11% after the 1 × 50-μL ($p < 0.01$) and 9% after the 1 × 100-μL ($p < 0.001$) doses. The biological response was clearly enhanced after the 2 × 50-μL dose compared with the 1 × 50- and 1 × 100-μL doses. The interindividual response in F VIII levels to nasal desmopressin ranged from 20% (CV) to 30%, which compared favorably with the 36% variation after intravenous administration. These results show that by optimizing concentration, volume, and splay apparatus, a significant enhancement can be obtained in bioavailability and clinical efficacy of desmopressin.

More recently, as a new apparatus for desmopressin delivery, Cormir et al. reported the usefulness of a coated microneedle array patch system (Macronux technology) to deliver desmopressin through the skin. Although it is available in injectable, intranasal, and oral formulations, intranasal and oral administration result in low and variable bioavailability. However, administering desmopressin transdermally using Macronux technology, which uses a microneedle array to overcome the skin barrier, is markedly useful to improve the bioavailability of desmopressin. In their reports, the tips of microneedles in 2-cm^2 arrays were covered with a solid coating of various amounts of desmopressin and applied to the skin of hairless guinea pigs for 5 or 15 min.

Pharmacologically relevant amounts of desmopressin were delivered after 5 min. Bioavailability was as high as 85% and showed acceptable variability (30%). Immunoreactive serum desmopressin reached peak levels after a T_{max} of 60 min. Elimination kinetics for serum desmopressin was similar after other transdermal and intravenous delivery, suggesting the absence of a skin depot. These results suggest that transdermal delivery of desmopressin by Macroflux technology is a safe and efficient alternative to currently available routes of administration.

Antibodies

Antibodies serve two important functions: They bind and modulate antigens and they bind complement and immune effector cells, such as natural killer cells and monocytes. Recently, targeted therapies using monoclonal anti-bodies (mAbs) have gained increased therapeutic application. Overall, 19 mAbs are currently approved by FDA to treat various disease states, such as oncology, inflammation, infectious disease, and cardiovascular disease. All approved mAbs are of the IgG class. Each IgG molecule contains two identical heavy chains and two identical light chains, 13 of which are intact mAbs, three are conjugated, and one is an mAb fragment (Fab). A feature of mAb therapeutics is the high specificity conferred by the antibody interaction with a specific region on the targeted antigen.

The antigen-binding site is formed by the intertwining of the light-chain variable domain (V_L) and the heavy-chain variable domain (V_H). Each V domain contains three short stretches of peptide known as the complementarily determining regions (CDRs); the CDRs are the prominent determinants of antigen-binding affinity and specificity. The light chain contains one constant domain, CL. The heavy chain contains three constant domains, C_H1, C_H2, and C_H3. The C_H2 and C_H3 domains allow interactions of the IgG molecule with various components of the immune system by either binding C1q, which activates the complement cascade and elicits complement-dependent cytotoxicity, or by binding to Fcγ receptors on immune effector cells, which elicits antibody-dependent cellular cytotoxicity.

These same variable and constant domains of the molecule also affect IgG catabolism and elimination. In addition to their contributions to mAb pharmacological activities, the FcyRs could also regulate elimination and pharmacokinetics of mAbs. Other factors, such as mAb structure and engineering, host factors, concurrent medications, and immunogenicity, can alter the pharmacokinetic and pharmacodynamic profiles. Hence, understanding the factors that affect the pharmacokinetics of mAb is of high importance for effective therapeutic application.

Pharmacodynamics and Pharmacokinetics of mAbs

mAbs can exert their pharmacological effects via several different mechanisms, such as neutralizing antigen function, activating receptors by mimicking endogenous receptor ligands, delivering toxins to specific cells (targeted delivery), and eliciting effector functions in conjunction with antigen modulation. Under some circumstances, where antigen expression is high in crucial organs (e.g., heart, lung, and vasculature), the effector function might not be desirable and could be deleterious; however, in other instances, such as applications in hematological malignancies, effector functions might be a significant part of the mechanism of action and maximizing the antibody effector functions might be highly desirable. Clearance of antibodies through the cells of the reticuloendothelial system (RES) can be regulated through the interaction with various Fc receptors. FcRns are expressed on phagocytic cells of the RES and protect IgG from rapid clearance.

Similarly, cells of the RES express various types of Fcγ receptors. Interactions of IgG antibodies with this subset of receptors could potentially impact antibody clearance. As discussed, polymorphism in Fcγ receptors impacted the therapeutic response to rituximab. Although the favorable clinical outcome was attributed to a more efficient Fcγ RIIIa-dependent cytotoxicity, it is not clear if polymorphism in Fcγ receptors could have any potential impact on antibody clearance. Polymorphism in Fcγ RIIIa was shown to impact in vivo clearance of red blood cells (RBC) coated with an anti-D IgG3 antibody in humans. The faster clearance was attributed to a more efficient elimination of opsonized RBC by phagocytic cells in the spleen of the subjects homozygous for Fcγ RIIIa-F/F158. These results are consistent with previous data demonstrating the impaired clearance of IgG-sensitized RBC in the presence of an anti-Fcγ RIIIa antibody. In addition, downregulation of Fcγ receptor on cells of monocyte lineage by immunomodulatory drugs, such as methotrexate (MTX), might potentially impact the clearance of mAbs such as adalimumab.

As the site on IgG that is responsible for binding to FcRn has been mapped and well characterized, the trend in the field of antibody engineering is to mutate the FcRn-binding site. Therefore, an increased FcRn binding provides altering the pharmacokinetics of mAbs. In 2002, Dall'Acqua et al. found that major improvement in FcRn binding occurred when mutations were introduced at positions 252, 254, 256, 433, 434, and 436, which are at the interface of the Fc-FcRn-binding region. More recently, Hinton et al. discovered two mutations, T250Q and M428L, that caused, respectively, a three fold and seven fold increase in FcRn binding and, when combined together, caused a 28-fold increase in FcRn binding. After intravenous administration of the M428L or T250Q/M428L mutant, about a two fold increase in plasma half-life was observed in rhesus monkeys compared with the parental molecule. As these positions are conserved among different human IgG isotypes, the authors proposed that the beneficial effect of these mutations should hold good for other isotypes as well.

As another way to alter the pharmacokinetics of mAbs, there is a PEGylation technology (the process of conjugating polyethylene glycol chains to the antibody fragments) of mAbs. PEGylation of proteins and liposomes has been a time-tested and successful technique that offered the advantage of reducing immunogenicity, increasing the plasma half-life, increasing solubility, and reducing protease sensitivity. Therefore, the science of antibody PEGylation has two primary aims, which are (1) to preserve the antigen-binding activity completely and (2) to link the PEG molecule to the antibody in a stable manner.

These aims are achieved by performing site-specific PEGylation using maleimide chemistry. Site-specific PEGylation was done by introducing a free cysteine to the end of the hinge region in a Fab or by incorporating the hinge region on the C-terminus of a Fab and scFv. The increase in half-life observed with PEGylated antibody fragments is usually caused by a prolongation of the distribution phase that represents the redistribution of a molecule in the extravascular environment. It, therefore, appears that PEGylation slows the redistribution of the mAbs from the systemic circulation to the interstitial compartment. In the following section, representative mAbs will be described.

Muromonab CD-3 Pharmacokinetics

In 1986, Muromonab CD-3 (OKT-3), which is a monoclonal antibody was first introduced to clinical practice, and the agent has been effective in reversing corticosteroid-resistant acute rejection in renal, liver, and cardiac transplant recipients. OKT-3 is administered only by intravenous injection and has a harmonic half-life of approximately 18 h. It binds specifically to the CD-3 complex, which is involved in antigen recognition and cell stimulation, on the surface of T lymphocytes. Immediately after administration, CD-3-positive T lymphocytes are abruptly removed from the circulation. OKT-3 may be removed by opsonization by the reticuloendothelial system when bound to T lymphocytes, or by human antimurine antibody production.

Basiliximab Pharmacokinetics

Basiliximab (Simulect) is a chimeric monoclonal antibody for immunoprophylaxis against acute rejection in renal transplantation. Basiliximab is a glycoprotein produced by recombinant technology It is used to prevent white blood cells from acute renal transplantation rejection. It specifically binds to and blocks the alpha chain of interleukin-2 receptors (IL-2R alpha), also known ascD25 antigen, on the surface of activated T lymphocytes. In 1997, to identify a single-dose regimen providing IL-2R-saturating serum concentrations in the critical first posttransplant month, Kovarki et al. examined the pharmacokinetic aspects of basiliximab in a multicenter open-label, prospective dose-escalation study. Thirty-two recipients (20 men and 12 women, 47 ± 11 years old, 65 ± 12 kg body weight) of primary mismatched cadaver kidneys were enrolled.

The immunosuppression regimen consisted of steroids and azathioprine from day 0 and cyclosporine from day 10. Basiliximab was infused over 30 min as a single dose (40 mg or 60 mg). Peak concentration and area under the concentration versus time curves increased proportionally with dose. Postinfusion concentrations declined in a biphasic manner with a terminal half-life of 6.5 ± 2.1 days. Widely dispersed correlations were noted between body weight and distribution volume ($r = 0.29$) or between it and total body clearance ($r = 0.45$), suggesting no clinical relevance for weight-adjusted dosing. Moreover, there were no apparent gender-related differences in basiliximab disposition. As serum concentrations in excess of 0.2 μg/mL are sufficient to saturate IL-2R epitopes on circulating T lymphocytes, the authors concluded that 40 mg and 60 mg of infusion dose was sufficient to keep this threshold level for 26 ± 8 days and for 32 ± 11 days, respectively.

Moreover, Kovarki et al. reported the results of a randomized, open-label prospective study with recipients of primary cadaveric liver allografts to characterize the disposition and immunodynamics of basiliximab for immunoprophylaxis of acute rejection. Patients received a total intravenous dose of 4-mg basiliximab in addition to baseline dual immunosuppression consisting of cyclosporine and steroids. The central volume of distribution was 5.6 ± 1.7 L, with a steady-state volume of 7.5 ± 2.5 L. The total body clearance and elimination half-life were 75 ± 24 mL/h and 4.1 ± 2.1 days, respectively. Basiliximab was measurable in drained ascites fluid, and clearance by this route was an average of 20% of total clearance.

Total body clearance correlated positively with the volume of postoperative blood loss ($r = 0.5253$, $p = 0.0101$), suggesting that bleeding may represent an additional route of drug removal. More recently, they conducted a population pharmacokinetic screen to identify demographic-clinical covariates of basiliximab in kidney and liver transplantation. In kidney transplantation (169 basiliximab-treated patients), basiliximab clearance was 36.7 ± 15.2 mL/h, distribution volume 8.0 ± 2.4 L, and half life 7.4 ± 3.0 days.

Body weight (range, 44–131 kg) and age (range, 20–69 years) each contributed to the variability in clearance and volume. However, gender, ethnic group, and the presence of proteinuria had no clinically relevant influences on basiliximab disposition. Receptor-saturating basiliximab concentrations were maintained for 36 ± 14 days (range, 12–91) when patients received 4-mg basiliximab. On the other hand, in liver transplantation (184 basiliximab-treated patients), basiliximab clearance was 55 ± 26 mL/h, the distribution volume was 9.7 ± 4.2 L, and the half-life was 8.7 ± 6.7 days. Patient weight, age, sex, ethnicity, history of alcoholism, hepatitis C seropositivity, and notable post-operative bleeding had no clinically relevant influences on basiliximab disposition; however, the cumulative volume of drained ascites fluid in the first week was positively correlated with the clearance. Receptor-saturating basiliximab concentrations ($\geq$ 0.1 μg/mL) were maintained for 38 $\pm$ 16 days, which was negatively correlated with the cumulative volume of drained ascites fluid in a week. However, there was no apparent relationship between the incidence or day of onset of acute rejection episodes during CD25 saturation and basiliximab concentration in kidney and liver transplants.

Trastuzumab Pharmacokinetics

Trastuzumab (Herceptin) is a monoclonal antibody for human epidermal growth factor receptor 2 (HER2)-positive metastatic breast cancer (MBC). A phase II study by Baselga et al. demonstrated the safety, efficacy, and pharmacokinetics of trastuzumab monotherapy given as first-line treatment once every 3 weeks in women with HER2-positive MBC. Patients received a loading dose of trastuzumab, 8 mg/kg intravenously and then 6 mg/kg at 3-week intervals until disease progression or patient withdrawal. In total, 105 patients received a median of five cycles of therapy. The overall response rate was 19% and the clinical benefit rate was 33%. Median time to progression was 3.4 months. The most common treatment- related adverse events were rigors, pyrexia, headache, nausea, and fatigue. Median baseline left ventricular ejection fraction was 63%.

The mean trough levels of trastuzumab in plasma were lower and the peak levels were higher with 3-weekly trastuzumab compared with weekly treatments. The author concluded that administering higher doses on a three-times-per-week schedule did not compromise the efficacy and safety of trastuzumab in women with HER2-positive MBC, and average exposure was similar to that observed with weekly therapy. In addition, a population pharmacokinetic analysis was performed by Bruno et al. to investigate precise aspects of trastuzumab pharmacokinetics. A nonlinear mixed-effect model was applied for the pharmacokinetic data from phase I, II, and III studies of 476 patients.

The phase I study enrolled patients with advanced solid tumors. The phase II and III studies enrolled patients with HER2-positive MBC. Patients in the pivotal phase II and III studies were treated with a 4-mg/kg loading dose of trastuzumab followed by 2 mg/kg weekly for up to 840 days. A two-compartment linear pharmacokinetic model best described the data and accounted for the long-term accumulation observed after weekly administration of trastuzumab. Population estimates for total body clearance, volume of distribution of the central compartment, and terminal half-life of trastuzumab were 0.225 L/day, 2.95 L, and 28.5 days, respectively. Interpatient variabilities in the total body clearance and volume of distribution were 43% and 29%, respectively. The number of metastatic sites, plasma level of extracellular domain of the HER2 receptor, and patient weight were significant baseline covariates for total body clearance, volume of distribution, or both. However, these covariate effects on trastuzumab exposure were modest and not clinically important in comparison with the large interpatient variability of CL. Concomitant chemotherapy (anthracycline plus cyclophosphamide, or paclitaxel) did not appear to influence clearance.

Infliximab Pharmacokinetics

Infliximab (Remicade) is a chimeric monoclonal antibody against tumor necrosis factor (TNF)-alpha that has shown efficacy in Crohn's disease and rheumatoid arthritis with a disease-modifying activity and rapid onset of action. It is administered intravenously, generally in a schedule with initial infusions at 0, 2, and 6 weeks, followed by administration once every 8 weeks. Infliximab is effective in the treatment of patients with moderately to severely active Crohn's disease with an inadequate response to other treatment options or those with fistulizing disease. In combination with methotrexate, infliximab reduced signs and symptoms and delayed disease progression in patients with active, methotrexate-refractory rheumatoid arthritis and in those with early disease. However, direct pharmacokinetic trials of infliximab in healthy volunteers or patients are not yet available. Infliximab is predominantly distributed to the vascular compartment and eliminated with a $t_{1/2}$beta between 10 and 14 days. No accumulation was observed when it was administered at intervals of 4 or 8 weeks Methotrexate may reduce the clearance of infliximab from serum.

Rituximab Pharmacokinetics

Rituximab (Rituxan) is a B-cell-depleting anti-CD20 chimeric IgG κ monoclonal antibody being investigated for the treatment of rheumatoid arthritis and is approved for the treatment of B-cell lymphoma. Kim et al. investigated pharmacokinetic profiles of rituximab in rabbits following intravitreal administration. After intravitreal injections of 1-mg rituximab, the elimination half-life of rituximab, estimated based on the two compartments, was 4.7 days. Fitting the data to a two-compartment model yielded a clearance from the aqueous humor of 1.2 μL/min. The clearance was less than the reported rate of aqueous humor outflow, indicating that elimination by this route could have been sufficient to account for the disappearance of the drug from the eye.

The duration of time over which sustained levels of rituximab were achieved suggests that intravitreal administration warrants further investigation as an approach to treating vitreous and anterior chamber infiltrates in patients with primary intraocular lymphoma. In addition, a population pharmacokinetic analysis of rituximab using a total of 102 patients by Ng et al. demonstrated that body surface area and gender were the most significant covariates for both a total body clearance and a volume of distribution in central compartment. Body surface area alone only explained about 19.7% of the total interindividual variability of the total body clearance. In a simulation study, body surface area-based dosing normalized drug exposure over a wide range of body surface area but did not seem to improve the predictability of rituximab AUC in rheumatoid arthritis patients. Therefore, no rationale for body surface area-based dosing for rituximab in rheumatoid arthritis patients was found.

Palivizumab Pharmacokinetics

Respiratory syncytial virus (RSV) infection represents a major cause of pediatric respiratory hospitalizations. RSV is the most common cause of lower respiratory tract infection in infants. Palivizumab (Synagis) is a humanized monoclonal antibody to the fusion protein of RSV, and is active in animal models for prevention of pulmonary RSV replication. Based on a phase I/II multicenter, randomized, double-blind, placebo-controlled, dose escalation trial by Subramanian et al. in premature infants or infants with bronchopulmonary dysplasia, it was found that the mean half-life of 20 days was comparable with that of other immunoglobulin G preparations. Mean trough serum concentrations 30 days after infusion were 6.8, 36.1, and 60.6 μg/mL for the 3-, 10-, and 15-mg/kg dose groups, respectively.

Mean serum concentrations of palivizumab that have been shown to produce a 2-log reduction in pulmonary RSV titer in cotton rats were maintained when 10- or 15-mg/kg palivizumab was given every 30 days to pediatric patients at high risk for serious RSV disease. In addition, based on another phase I/II multicenter, randomized, double-blind, placebo-controlled, dose escalation trial in 99 healthy children hospitalized with acute RSV infection by Saez-Llornes et al., it was found that mean serum concentrations of palivizumab in the 5- and 15-mg/kg groups, respectively, were 61.2 and 303.4 μg/mL at 60 min and 11.2 and 38.4 μg/mL after 30 days. There were no significant differences in clinical outcomes between placebo and palivizumab groups for either dose. A single 15-mg/kg dose achieved serum palivizumab concentrations above the 25–30-μg/mL concentration associated with 2-log reduction of pulmonary RSV titer in the cotton rat model.

Recommendations for Future Study

Recombinant DNA technology has produced many proteins and peptides drugs in large scale, and they are becoming increasingly important as therapeutic agents. The successful development of recombinant proteins depends on the proper characterization of their pharmacokinetics and an understanding of the relationship between drug exposure or dose and the pharmacological response. Although pharmacokinetic characterization of proteins is often complicated because of the absence of a specific assay, difficulties exist in identifying metabolites, endogenous circulating concentrations, and the presence of binding proteins. However, nanobiotechnologically derived formulations for peptide/ protein drugs also show some new challenges.

Numerous methods have been explored for increasing the residence time of proteins in the systemic circulation or oral bioavailability and enhancing the pharmacological effect. Some of the techniques have been employed to include site-specific mutagenesis, polymer modifications, and fusion with immunoglobulins, targeted through the use of liposomes or conjugation to toxins, radionuclides, and other proteins. In the future, these methods should provide adequate formulations of peptide drugs to increase the successful therapeutic efficacy when formulations are administered through the alternative administration routes.

2

BASIC CONCEPTS

Pharmacokinetics is defined as the study of the quantitative relationship between administered doses of a drug and the observed plasma/blood or tissue concentrations. The pharmacokinetic model is a mathematical description of this relationship. Models provide estimates of certain parameters, such as elimination half-life, which provide information about basic drug properties. The models may be used to predict concentration vs. time profiles for different dosing patterns.

The field of pharmacokinetics is concerned with drug absorption, distribution, biotransformation, and excretion or elimination. These processes, in addition to the dose, determine the concentration of drug at the effector or active site and, therefore, the intensity and duration of drug effect. The practice of pharmacokinetics has been used in clinical medicine for many years in order to optimize the efficacy of medications administered to treat disease. Through a consideration of pharmacokinetics, physicians are able to determine the drug of choice, dose, route, frequency of administration, and duration of therapy in order to achieve a specific therapeutic objective. In the same manner, study of the pharmacokinetics of abused drugs aids investigators in addiction medicine, forensic toxicology, and clinical pharmacology in understanding why particular drugs are abused, factors that affect their potential for abuse, and how their use can be detected and monitored over time, and also provides a rational, scientific basis for treatment therapies.

TRANSFER ACROSS BIOLOGICAL MEMBRANES

The processes of absorption, distribution, biotransformation, and elimination of a particular substance involve the transfer or movement of a drug across biological membranes. Therefore, it is important to understand those properties of cell membranes and the intrinsic properties of drugs that affect movement. Although drugs may gain entry into the body by passage through a single layer of cells, such as the intestinal epithelium, or through multiple layers of cells, such as the skin, the blood cell membrane is a common barrier to all drug entry and therefore is the most appropriate membrane for general discussion of cellular membrane structure.

The cellular blood membrane consists of a phospholipid bilayer of 7- to 9-nm thickness with hydrocarbon chains oriented inward and polar head groups oriented outward. Interspersed between the lipid bilayer are proteins, which may span the entire width of the membrane permitting the formation of aqueous pores. These proteins act as receptors in chemical and electrical signaling pathways and also as specific targets for drug actions. The lipids in the cell membrane may move laterally, conferring fluidity at physiological temperatures and relative impermeability to highly polar molecules. The fluidity of plasma membranes is largely determined by the relative abundance of unsaturated fatty acids. Between cell membranes are pores that may permit bulk flow of substances. This is considered to be the main mechanism by which drugs cross the capillary endothelial membranes, except in the central nervous system (CNS), which possesses tight junctions that limit intercellular diffusion.

Physicochemical properties of a drug also affect its movement across cell membranes. These include its molecular size and shape, solubility, degree of ionization, and relative lipid solubility of its ionized and non-ionized forms. Another factor to consider is the extent of protein binding to plasma and tissue components. Although such binding is reversible and usually rapid, only the free unbound form is considered capable of passing through biological membranes.

Drugs cross cell membranes through passive and active or specialized processes. Passive movement across biological membranes is the dominant process in the absorption and distribution of drugs. In passive transfer, hydrophobic molecules cross the cell membrane by simple diffusion along a concentration gradient. In this process there is no expenditure of cellular energy. The magnitude of drug transfer in this manner is dependent on the magnitude of the concentration gradient across the membrane and the lipid:water partition coefficient. Once steady state has been reached, the concentration of free (unbound) drug will be the same on both sides of the membrane.

The exception to this situation is if the drug is capable of ionization under physiological conditions. In this case, concentrations on either side of the cell membrane will be influenced by pH differences across the membrane. Small hydrophilic molecules are thought to cross cell membranes through the aqueous pores. Generally, only unionized forms of a drug cross biological membranes due to their relatively high lipid solubility. The movement of ionized forms is dependent on the pKa of the drug and the pH gradient. The partitioning of weak acids and bases across pH gradients may be predicted by the Henderson–Hasselbalch equation. For example, an orally ingested weakly acidic drug may be largely unionized in the acidic environs of the stomach but ionized to some degree at the neutral pH of the plasma. The pH gradient and difference in the proportions of ionized/nonionized forms of the drug promote the diffusion of the weak acid through the lipid barrier of the stomach into the plasma.

Water moves across cell membranes either by the simple diffusion described above or as the result of osmotic differences across membranes. In the latter case, when water moves in bulk through aqueous pores in cellular membranes due to osmotic forces, any molecule that is small enough to pass through the pores will also be transferred. This movement of solutes is called filtration. Cell membranes throughout the body possess pores of different sizes; for example, the pores in the kidney glomerulus are typically 70 nm, but the channels in most cells are <4 nm.

The movement of some compounds across membranes cannot be explained by simple diffusion or filtration. These are usually high-molecular-weight or very lipid soluble substances. Therefore, specialized processes have been postulated to account for the movement. Active processes typically involve the expenditure of cellular energy to move molecules across biological membranes. Characteristics of active transport include selectivity, competitive inhibition, saturability, and movement across an electrochemical or concentration gradient. The drug complexes with a macromolecular carrier on one side of the membrane, traverses the membrane, and is released on the other side. The carrier then returns to the original surface.

Active transport processes are important in the elimination of xenobiotics. They are involved in the movement of drugs in hepatocytes, renal tubular cells, and neuronal membranes. For example, the liver has four known *active transport* systems, two for organic acids, one for organic bases, and one for neutral organic compounds. A different specialized transport process is termed "*facilitated diffusion*." This transport is similar to the carrier-mediated transport described above except that no active processes are involved. The drug is not moved against an electrochemical or concentration gradient and there is no expenditure of energy. A biochemical example of such transport is the movement of glucose from the gastrointestinal tract through the intestinal epithelium.

Absorption

In order for a drug to exert its pharmacological effect, it must first gain entry into the body, be absorbed into the bloodstream, and transported or distributed to its site of action. This is true except in the case of drugs that exert their effect locally or at the absorption site. The absorption site, or port of entry, is determined by the route of drug administration.

Routes of administration are either enteral or parenteral. The former term denotes all routes pertaining to the alimentary canal. Therefore, sublingual, oral, and rectal are enteral routes of administration. All other routes, such as intravenous, intramuscular, subcutaneous, dermal, vaginal, and intraperitoneal, are parenteral routes.

Absorption describes the rate and extent to which a drug leaves its site of administration and enters the general circulation. Factors that, therefore, affect absorption include the physicochemical properties of the drug that determine transfer across cell membranes as described earlier; formulation or physical state of the drug; site of absorption; concentration of drug; circulation at absorption site; and area of absorbing surface.

Gastrointestinal

Absorption of drug may occur at any point along the tract including the mouth, stomach, intestine, and rectum. Because the majority of drugs are absorbed by passive diffusion, the non-ionized, lipid soluble form of the drug is favored for rapid action. Therefore, according to the Henderson–Hasselbalch equation, the absorption of weak acids should be favored in the stomach and the absorption of weak bases in the alkaline environment of the small intestine. However, other factors such as relative surface area will influence absorption. The stomach is lined by a relatively thick mucus- covered membrane to facilitate its primary function of digestion. In comparison, the epithelium of the small intestine is thin, with villi and microvilli providing a large surface area to facilitate its primary function of absorption of nutrients. Therefore, any factor that increases gastric emptying will tend to increase the rate of drug absorption, regardless of the ionization state of the drug.

The gastrointestinal (GI) tract possesses carrier-mediated transport systems for the transfer of nutrients and electrolytes across the gastric wall. These systems may also carry drugs and other xenobiotics into the organism. For example, lead is absorbed by the calcium transporter. Absorption also depends on the physical characteristics of a drug. For example, a highly lipid soluble drug will not dissolve in the stomach. In addition, solid dosage forms will have little contact with gastric mucosa and the drug will not be absorbed until the solid is dissolved. Further, the particle size affects absorption, since dissolution rate is proportional to particle size. Compounds that increase intestinal permeability or increase the residence time in the intestine by altering intestinal motility will thereby increase absorption of other drugs through that segment of the alimentary canal.

Once a drug has been absorbed through the GI tract, the amount of the compound that reaches the systemic circulation depends on several factors. The drug may be biotransformed by the GI cells or removed by the liver through which it must pass. This loss of drug before gaining access to the systemic circulation is known as the first pass effect.

Although oral ingestion is the most common route of GI absorption, drugs may be administered sublingually. Despite the small surface area for absorption, certain drugs that are non-ionic and highly lipid soluble are effectively absorbed by this route. The drugs nitroglycerin and buprenorphine are administered by this route. The blood supply in the mouth drains into the superior vena cava and, because of this anatomic characteristic, drugs are protected from first pass metabolism by the liver.

Although an uncommon route by which abused drugs are self-administered, rectal administration is used in medical practice when vomiting or other circumstances preclude oral administration.

Approximately 50% of the drug that is absorbed will bypass the liver. The disadvantage of this route for drug absorption is that the process is often incomplete and irregular and some drugs irritate the mucosal lining of the rectum.

Pulmonary

Gases, volatile liquids, and aerosols may be absorbed through the lungs. Access to the circulation by this route is rapid because of the large surface area of the lungs and extensive capillary network in close association with the alveoli. In the case of absorption of gases and volatilizable liquids, the ionization state and lipid solubility of the substance are less important than in GI absorption. This is because diffusion through cell membranes is not the rate-limiting step in the absorption process. The reasons include low volatility of ionized molecules, the extensive capillary network in close association with the alveoli resulting in a short distance for diffusion, and the rapid removal of absorbed substances by the blood. Some substances may not reach the lungs because they are deposited and absorbed in the mucosal lining of the nose.

Drugs may be atomized or volatilized and inhaled as droplets or particulates in air; a common example is the smoking of drugs. The advantages of this route include rapid transport into the blood, avoidance of first pass hepatic metabolism, and avoidance of the medical problems associated with other routes of illicit drug administration. Disadvantages include local irritant effect on the tissues of the nasopharynx and absorption of particulate matter in the nasopharynx and bronchial tree. For a drug to be effectively absorbed it should reach the alveoli. However, absorption of particulate matter is governed by particulate size and water solubility. Particles with diameters >5 μm are usually deposited in the nasopharyngeal region; particles in the 2- to 5-μm range are deposited in the tracheobronchiolar region and particles 1 μm and smaller reach the alveolar sacs.

Dermal

The skin is impermeable to most chemicals. For a drug to be absorbed it must pass first through the epidermal layers or specialized tissue such as hair follicles or sweat and sebaceous glands. Absorption through the outer layer of skin, the stratum corneum, is the rate-limiting step in the dermal absorption of drugs. This outer layer consists of densely packed keratinized cells and is commonly referred to as the "dead" layer of skin because the cells comprising this layer are without nuclei. Drug substances may be absorbed by simple diffusion through this layer. The lower layers of the epidermis, and the dermis, consist of porous nonselective cells that pose little barrier to absorption by passive diffusion. Once a chemical reaches this level, it is then rapidly absorbed into the systemic circulation because of the extensive network of venous and lymphatic capillaries located in the dermis. Drug absorption through the skin depends on the characteristics of the drug and on the condition of the skin. Since the stratum corneum is the main barrier to absorption, damage to this area by sloughing of cells due to abrasion or burning enhances absorption, as does any mechanism that increases cutaneous blood flow. Hydration of the stratum corneum also increases its permeability and therefore enhances absorption of chemicals.

Parenteral injection

Drugs are often absorbed through the GI tract, lungs, and skin but many illicit drugs have historically been self-administered by injection. These routes typically include intravenous, intramuscular, and subcutaneous administration. The intravenous route of administration introduces the drug directly into the venous bloodstream, thereby eliminating the process of absorption altogether. Substances that are locally irritating may be administered intravenously since the blood vessel walls are relatively insensitive. This route permits the rapid introduction of the drug to the systemic circulation and allows high concentrations to be quickly achieved. Intravenous administration may result in unfavorable physiological responses because, once introduced, the drug cannot be removed. This route of administration is dependent on maintaining patent veins and can result in extensive scar tissue formation due to chronic drug administration. Insoluble particulate matter deposited in the blood vessels is another medical problem associated with the intravenous route.

Intramuscular and subcutaneous administration involves absorption from the injection site into the circulation by passive diffusion. The rate of absorption is limited by the size of the capillary bed at the injection site and by the solubility of the drug in the interstitial fluid. If blood flow is increased at the administration site, absorption will be increased. Conversely, if blood pressure is decreased for any reason (such as cardiogenic shock) absorption will be prolonged.

Distribution

After entering circulation, drugs are distributed throughout the body. The extent of distribution is dependent on the physicochemical properties of the drug and physiological factors. Drugs cross cell membranes throughout the body by passive diffusion or specialized transport processes. Small water-soluble molecules and ions cross cell membranes through aqueous pores, whereas lipid- soluble substances diffuse through the membrane lipid bilayer. The rate of distribution of a drug is dependent on blood flow and the rate of diffusion across cell membranes of various tissues and organs. The affinity of a substance for certain tissues also affects the rate of distribution.

Because only unbound drug (the free fraction) is in equilibrium throughout the body, disposition is affected by binding to or dissolving in cellular constituents. While circulating in blood, drugs may be reversibly bound to several plasma proteins. For example, basic compounds often bind to á1-acid glycoprotein; acidic compounds bind to albumin. The extent of plasma protein binding varies among drugs: nicotine is 5% bound, whereas the barbiturate, secobarbital, is 50% bound; and the benzodiazepine, diazepam, is 96% bound. The fraction of drug that is bound is governed by the drug concentration, the drug's affinity for binding sites, and the number of binding sites available for binding. At low drug concentrations, the fraction bound is a function of the number of binding sites and the dissociation constant, a measure of binding affinity. When drug concentrations exceed the dissociation constant, concentration also governs the amount of protein binding. Therefore, published protein binding fractions for drugs only apply over a certain concentration range, usually the therapeutic concentration. Plasma protein binding limits the amount of drug entering tissues. Because plasma protein binding of drugs is relatively non-selective, drugs and endogenous substances compete for binding sites, and drug displacement from binding sites by another substance can contribute to toxicity by increasing the free fraction.

Binding to tissue constituents

In addition to binding to plasma proteins, drugs may bind to tissue constituents. The liver and kidney have a large capacity to act as storage depots for drugs. The mechanisms responsible for transfer of many drugs from the blood appear to be active transport processes. Ligandin, a cytoplasmic liver protein, has a high affinity for many organic acids while metallothionein binds metals in the kidney and liver.

Lipid-soluble drugs are stored in neutral fat by dissolution. Since the fat content of an obese individual may be 50% body weight, it follows that large amounts of drug can be stored in this tissue. Once stored in fat, the concentration of drug is lowered throughout the body, in the blood, and also in target organs. Any activity, such as dieting or starvation, that serves to mobilize fat could potentially increase blood concentrations and hence contribute to an increase in the risk of drug toxicity.

Drugs may also be stored in bone. Drugs diffuse from the extracellular fluid through the hydration shell of the hydroxyapatite crystals of the bone mineral. Lead, fluoride, and other compounds may be deposited and stored in bone. Deposition may not necessarily be detrimental. For example, lead is not toxic to bone tissue. However, chronic fluoride deposition results in the condition known as *skeletal fluorosis*. Generally, storage of compounds in bone is a reversible process. Toxicants may be released from the bone by ion exchange at the crystal surface or by dissolution of the bone during osteoclastic activity. If osteolytic activity is increased, the hydroxyapatite lattice is mobilized, resulting in an increase in blood concentrations of any stored xenobiotics.

Blood–brain barrier

The blood–brain barrier is often viewed as an impenetrable barrier to xenobiotics. However, this is not true and a more realistic representation is as a site that is less permeable to ionized substances and high-molecular-weight compounds than other membranes. Many toxicants do not enter the brain because the capillary endothelial cells are joined by tight junctions with few pores between cells; the capillaries of the CNS are surrounded by glial processes; and the interstitial fluid of the CNS has a low protein concentration. The first two anatomical processes limit the entry of small- to medium-sized water-soluble molecules, whereas the entry of lipid-soluble compounds is limited by the low protein content, which restricts paracellular transport. It is interesting to note that the permeability of the brain to toxicants varies from area to area. For example, the cortex, area postrema, and pineal body are more permeable than other regions. This may be due to differences in blood supply or the nature of the barrier itself. Entrance of drugs into the brain is governed by the same factors that determine transfer across membranes in other parts of the body. Only the unbound fraction is available for transfer, and lipid solubility and the degree of ionization dictate the rate of entry of drugs into the brain. It should be noted that the blood–brain barrier is not fully developed at birth. In animal studies, morphine has been found to be three to ten times more toxic to newborns than adults.

Pregnancy

During pregnancy, drugs may also be distributed from the mother to the fetus by simple diffusion across the placenta. The placenta comprises several cell layers between the maternal and fetal circulations. The number of layers varies between species and state of gestation. The same factors govern placental drug transfer as movement by passive diffusion across other membranes. The placenta plays an additional role in preventing transfer of xenobiotics to the fetus by possessing biotransformation capabilities.

BIOTRANSFORMATION

Lipophilicity, a desirable drug characteristic for absorption and distribution across biological membranes, is a hindrance to elimination. To prevent accumulation of xenobiotics, the body chemically alters lipophilic compounds to more water-soluble products. The sum of all the processes that convert lipophilic substances to more hydrophilic metabolites is termed biotransformation. These biochemical processes are usually enzymatic and are commonly divided into Phase I and Phase II reactions. Phase I reactions generally expose or introduce a polar group to the parent drug, thereby increasing its water solubility. These reactions are oxidative or hydrolytic in nature and include *N*- and *O*-dealkylation, aliphatic and aromatic hydroxylation, *N*- and *S*-oxidation, and deamination. These reactions usually result in loss of pharmacological activity, although there are numerous examples of enhanced activity. Indeed, formation of a Phase I product is desirable in the case of administration of prodrugs.

Phase II reactions are conjugation reactions and involve covalent bonding of functional groups with endogenous compounds. Highly water-soluble conjugates are formed by combination of the drug or metabolite with glucuronic acid, sulfate, glutathione, amino acids, or acetate. Again, these products are generally pharmacologically inactive or less active than the parent compound. An exception is the metabolite morphine-6-glucuronide. In this case, glucuronidation at the 6-position increases the affinity of morphine for binding at the mu receptor and results in equivalent or enhanced pharmacological activity.

The enzymes that catalyze the biotransformation of drugs are found mainly in the liver. This is not surprising considering the primary function of the liver is to handle compounds absorbed from the GI tract. In addition, the liver receives all the blood perfusing the splanchnic area. Therefore, this organ has developed a high capacity to remove substances from blood, and store, transform, and/or release substances into the general circulation. In its primary role of biotransformation, the liver acts as a homogeneous unit, with all parenchymal cells or hepatocytes exhibiting enzymatic activity. In tissues involved in extrahepatic biotransformation processes, typically only one or two cell types are used. Many organs have demonstrated activity toward foreign compounds but the major extrahepatic tissues are those involved in the absorption or excretion of chemicals. These include the kidney, lung, intestine, skin, and testes. The main cells containing biotransformation enzymes in these organs are the proximal tubular cells, clara cells, mucosa lining cells, epithelial cells, and seminiferous tubules, respectively.

Phase I Enzymes

Phase I enzymes are located primarily in the endoplasmic reticulum of cells. These enzymes are membrane bound within a lipoprotein matrix and are referred to as microsomal enzymes. This is in reference to the subcellular fraction isolated by differential centrifugation of a liver homogenate. The two most important enzyme systems involved in Phase I biotransformation reactions are the cytochrome P450 system and the mixed function amine oxidase.

With the advances in recombinant DNA technology, eight major mammalian gene families of hepatic and extrahepatic cytochrome P450 have been identified. A comprehensive discussion of the cytochrome P450 system is beyond the scope of this chapter and the reader is referred to a number of reviews. Briefly, this system comprises two coupled enzymes: NADPH-cytochrome P450 reductase and a heme-containing enzyme, cytochrome P450. Numerous oxidative pathways for xenobiotics exist, both in humans and other animals. Much drug oxidation is performed by a group of enzymes known as CYPs (from CYtochrome P450, the 450 being derived from the cytochrome's maximal absorbance of light at 450 nm). The cytochrome P450s or CYPs are categorized according to amino acid sequence homology. CYPs that have less than 40% homology are placed in a different family (e.g., 1, 2, 3, and so on). CYPs that are 40 to 55% identical are assigned to different subfamilies (e.g., 1A, 1B, 1C, and so on). P450 enzymes that are more than 55% identical are classified as members of the same subfamily (e.g., 2B 1, 2B2, 2B3). The P450 enzymes are expressed in numerous tissues, but are especially prevalent in the liver.

This complex is associated with another cytochrome, cytochrome b with a reductase enzyme. In reactions catalyzed by cytochrome P450, the substrate combines with the oxidized form of cytochrome P450 (Fe^{3+}) to form a complex. This complex accepts an electron from NADPH, which reduces the iron in the cytochrome P450 heme moiety to Fe^{2+}. This reduced substrate–cytochrome P450 complex then combines with molecular oxygen, which in turn accepts another electron from NADPH. In some cases, the second electron is provided by NADH via cytochrome b5. Both electrons are transferred to molecular oxygen, resulting in a highly reactive and unstable species. One atom of the unstable oxygen molecule is transferred to the substrate and the other is reduced to water. The substrate then dissociates as a result, regenerating the oxidized form of cytochrome P450.

Phase II Enzymes

Many of the Phase II enzymes are located in the cytosol or supernatant fraction after differential centrifugation of a liver homogenate. These reactions are biosynthetic and therefore require energy. This is accomplished by transforming the substrate or cofactors to high-energy intermediates. One of the major Phase II reactions is glucuronidation. The resultant glucuronides are eliminated in the bile or urine. The enzyme uridine diphosphate (UDP) glucuronosyltransferase is located in the endoplasmic reticulum. This enzyme catalyzes the reaction between UDP–glucuronic acid and the functional group of the substrate. The location of this enzyme means that it has direct access to the products of Phase I enzymatic reactions. Another important conjugation reaction in humans is sulfation of hydroxyl groups. The sulfotransferases are a group of soluble enzymes, classified as aryl, hydroxysteroid, estrone, and bile salt sulfotransferases. Their primary function is the transfer of inorganic sulfate to the hydroxyl moiety of phenol or aliphatic alcohols.

Another important family of enzymes is the glutathione-*S*-transferases, which are located in both the cytoplasm and endoplasmic reticulum of cells. The activity of the cytosolic transferase is 5 to 40 times greater than the endoplasmic enzyme. These transferase enzymes catalyze the reaction between the sulfhydryl group of the tripeptide glutathione with substances containing electrophilic carbon atoms. The glutathione conjugates are cleaved to cysteine derivatives, primarily in the kidney. These derivatives are then acetylated resulting in mercapturic acid conjugates, which are excreted in the urine.

Many factors affect the rate at which a drug is biotransformed. One of the important factors is obviously the concentration of the drug at the site of action of biotransforming enzymes. Physicochemical properties of the drug, such as lipophilicity, are important, in addition to dose and route of administration. Certain physiological, pharmacological, and environmental factors may also affect the rate of biotransformation of a compound. Numerous variables affect biotransformation including sex, age, genetic polymorphisms, time of day or circadian rhythms, nutritional status, enzyme induction or inhibition, hepatic injury, and disease states.

Elimination

Drugs are excreted or eliminated from the body as parent compounds or metabolites. The organs involved in excretion, with the exception of the lungs, eliminate water-soluble compounds more readily than lipophilic substances. The lungs are important for the elimination of anesthetic gases and vapors. The processes of biotransformation generally produce more polar compounds for excretion. The most important excretory organ is the kidney. Substances in the feces are mainly unabsorbed drugs administered orally or compounds excreted into the bile and not reabsorbed. Drugs may also be excreted in breast milk and, even though the amounts are small, they represent an important pathway because the recipient of any drugs by this route is the nursing infant.

For a comprehensive discussion of renal excretion of drugs, the reader is referred to Weiner and Mudge. Excretion of drugs and their metabolites involves three processes, namely, glomerular filtration, passive tubular reabsorption, and active tubular secretion. The amount of a drug that enters the tubular lumen of the kidney is dependent on the glomerular filtration rate and the fraction of drug that is plasma protein bound. In the proximal renal tubule organic anions and cations are added to the filtrate by active transport processes. Glucuronide drug metabolites are secreted in this way by the carrier-mediated system for naturally occurring organic acids. In the proximal and distal tubules of the kidney, the non-ionized forms of weak acids and bases are passively reabsorbed. The necessary concentration gradient is created by the reabsorption of water with sodium. The passive reabsorption of ionized forms is pH dependent because the tubular cells are less permeable to these moieties. Therefore, in the treatment of drug poisoning, the excretion of some drugs can be increased by alkalinization or acidification of the urine.

Under normal physiological conditions, excretion of drugs in the sweat, saliva, and by the lacrimal glands is quantitatively insignificant. Elimination by these routes is dependent on pH and diffusion of the unionized lipid-soluble form of the drug through the epithelial cells of the glands. Drugs excreted in saliva enter the mouth and may be reabsorbed and swallowed. Drugs have also been detected in hair and skin, and although quantitatively unimportant, these routes may be useful in drug detection and therefore have forensic significance.

Pharmacokinetic Parameters

Pharmacokinetics assumes that a relationship exists between the concentration of drug in an accessible site, such as the blood, and the pharmacological or toxic response. The concentration of drug in the systemic circulation is related to the concentration of drug at the site of action. Pharmacokinetics attempts to quantify the relationship between dose and drug disposition and provide the framework, through modeling, to interpret measured concentrations in biological fluids. Several pharmacokinetic parameters are utilized to explain various pharmacokinetic processes. It is often changes in these parameters, through disease, genetic abnormalities, or drug interactions, that necessitate modifications of dosage regimens for therapeutic agents. The most important parameters are clearance, the ability of the body to eliminate drug, volume of distribution, a measure of the apparent volume of the body available to occupy the drug, bioavailability, the proportion of drug absorbed into the systemic circulation, and half-life, a measure of the rate of drug elimination from the blood. These concepts are discussed below.

Clearance

Clearance is defined as the proportionality factor that relates the rate of drug elimination to the blood or plasma drug concentration:

$$\text{Clearance} = \text{Rate of elimination/Concentration}$$

In the above equation, the concentration term refers to drug concentration at steady state. The units of clearance are volume per unit time and, therefore, this parameter measures the volume of biological fluid, such as blood, that would have to have drug removed to account for drug elimination. Therefore, clearance is not a measure of the amount of drug removed.

The concept of clearance is useful in pharmacokinetics because clearance is usually constant over a wide range of concentrations, provided that elimination processes are not saturated. Saturation of biotransformation and excretory processes may occur in overdose and toxicokinetic effects should be considered. If a constant fraction of drug is eliminated per unit time, the elimination follows first-order kinetics. However, if a constant amount of drug is eliminated per unit time, the elimination is described by zero-order kinetics. Some drugs, for example, ethanol, exhibit zero-order kinetics at "normal" or non-intoxicating concentrations. However, for any drug that exhibits first-order kinetics at therapeutic or nontoxic concentrations, once the mechanisms for elimination become saturated, the kinetics become zero order and clearance becomes variable.

Clearance may also be viewed as the loss of drug from an organ of elimination such as the liver or kidney. This approach enables evaluation of the effects of a variety of physiological factors such as changes in blood flow, plasma protein binding, and enzyme activity. Therefore, total systemic clearance is determined by adding the clearance (CL) values for each elimination organ or tissue:

$$CL_{systemic} = CL_{renal} + CL_{hepatic} + CL_{lung} + CL_{other}$$

Clearance from an individual organ is a product of blood flow and the extraction ratio. The extraction ratio is derived from the concentration of drug in the blood entering the organ and the concentration of drug in the blood leaving the organ. If the extraction ratio is 0, no drug is removed. If it is 1, then all the drug entering the organ is removed from the blood. Therefore, the clearance of an organ may be determined from the following equation:

$$CL_{organ} = Q(C_A - C_V/C_A) = Q \times E$$

where

Q = blood flow

C_A = arterial drug concentration

C_V = venous drug concentration

E = extraction ratio

Volume of Distribution

The plasma drug concentration reached after distribution is complete is a result of the dose and the extent of uptake by tissues. The extent of distribution can be described by relating the amount of drug in the body to the concentration. This parameter is known as the volume of distribution. This volume does not indicate a defined physiological dimension but the volume of fluid required to contain all the drug in the body at the same concentration as in the plasma or blood. Therefore, it is often called the apparent volume of distribution (V) and is determined at steady state when distribution equilibrium has been reached between drug in plasma and tissues.

$$V = \text{Amount in body/Plasma drug concentration}$$

The volume of distribution depends on the pKa of the drug, the degree of plasma protein and tissue binding, and the lipophilicity of the drug. As would be expected, drugs that distribute widely throughout the body have large volumes of distribution (for example, the V_d of fluphenazine, which is a widely distributed drug, is 11; the V_d for ketoconozole is only 0.7, indicating that very little drug leaves the circulation). In the equation above, the body is considered one homogeneous unit and therefore exhibits a one-compartment model. In this model, drug administration occurs in the central compartment, and distribution is instantaneous throughout the body. For most drugs, the simple one-compartment model does not describe the time course of drug in the body adequately and drug distribution and elimination are more completely described in multiple exponential terms using multicompartmental models. In these models, the volume of distribution, V_{area}, is calculated as the ratio of clearance to the rate of decline of the concentration during the elimination phase:

$$V_{area} = CL/k$$

where k = rate constant.

Bioavailability

The bioavailability of a drug refers to the fraction of the dose that reaches the systemic circulation. This parameter is dependent on the rate and extent of absorption at the site of drug administration. Obviously, it follows that drugs administered intravenously do not undergo absorption, but immediately gain access to the systemic circulation and are considered 100% bioavailable. In the case of oral administration, if the hepatic extraction ratio is known, it is possible to predict the maximum bioavailability of drug by this route assuming first-order processes, according to the following equation:

$$F_{max} = 1 - E = 1 - (CL_{hepatic}/Q_{hepatic})$$

The bioavailability of a drug by various routes may also be determined by comparing the area under the curve (AUC) obtained from the plasma concentration vs. time curve after intravenous and other routes of administration:

$$\text{Bioavailability} = AUC_{oral}/AUC_{IV}$$

Half-Life

The half-life is the time it takes for the plasma drug concentration to decrease by 50%. Half-life is usually determined from the log-terminal phase of the elimination curve. However, it is important to remember that this parameter is a derived term and is dependent on the clearance and volume of distribution of the drug. Therefore, as CL and V change with disease, drug interactions, and age, so a change in the half-life should be expected. The half-life is typically calculated from the following equation:

$$t_{1/2} = 0.693/k$$

where $t_{1/2}$ = half life and

k = elimination rate constant.

Because k = CL/V, the interrelationship between these parameters is clearly evident.

DOSAGE REGIMENS

Pharmacokinetic principles, in addition to clinical factors such as the state of the patient, are utilized in determining dosage regimens. Factors that relate to the safety and efficacy of the drug, such as activity–toxicity relationships (therapeutic window and side effects), and pharmaceutical factors, such as dosage form and route of administration, must be considered.

The goal of a therapeutic regimen is to achieve therapeutic concentrations of a drug continuously or intermittently. The latter is useful if tolerance to the drug develops, or if the therapeutic effects of the drug persist and increase in intensity even with rapid drug disappearance. Adjustments to the dosage regimen are made to maintain therapeutically effective drug concentrations and minimize undesirable effects. Optimization of drug therapy is typically determined empirically, that is, changing the dose based on response of the individual. However, there is often better correlation between blood or plasma concentration or amount of drug in the body than the dose administered. Therefore, pharmacokinetic data are useful in the design of dosage regimens. In theory, data following a single dose may be used to estimate plasma concentrations following any dosing design.

For drugs whose effects are difficult to measure, or whose therapeutic index is low, a target- level or steady-state plasma concentration is desirable. A dose is computed to achieve this level, drug concentrations are measured, and the dose is adjusted accordingly. To apply this strategy, the therapeutic range should be determined. For many drugs the lower limit of this range appears to be the concentration that produces 50% maximal response. The upper limit is determined by drug toxicity and is commonly determined by the concentration at which 5 to 10% of patients experience a toxic effect. The target concentration is then chosen at the middle of the therapeutic range.

Loading Doses

The loading dose is one or a series of doses that are administered at the beginning of therapy. The objective is to reach the target concentration rapidly. The loading dose can be estimated using the following formula:

$$\text{Loading Dose} = \text{Target } C_p \times V_{ss}/F$$

where C_p = concentration in plasma, V_{ss} = volume of distribution at steady state, and F = fractional bioavailability of the dose.

A loading dose is desirable if the time to achieve steady state is long compared to the need for the condition being treated. One disadvantage of a loading dose is the acute exposure to high concentrations of the drug, which may result in toxic effects in sensitive individuals.

Dosing Rate

In the majority of clinical situations, drugs are administered as a series of repeated doses or as a continuous infusion in order to maintain a steady-state concentration. Therefore, a maintenance dose must be calculated such that the rate of input is equal to the rate of drug loss. This may be determined using the following formula:

$$\text{Dosing Rate} = \text{Target} \times \text{CL}/F$$

where CL = clearance and F = fractional bioavailability of the dose.

It is obvious from the above that in order to design an appropriate dosage regimen, several pharmacokinetic factors, including CL, F, V_{ss}, and half-life, must be known in addition to an understanding of the principles of absorption and distribution of the drug in question. The clinician must also be aware of variations in these factors in a particular patient. One should note that even "normal" individuals exhibit variations in these parameters. For example, one standard deviation on clearance values may be 50%. These unpredicted variations in pharmacokinetic parameters may result in a wide range of drug concentrations. This is unacceptable in most cases especially for those drugs with a low therapeutic index. Therefore, C_p should be measured and estimates of CL, *F*, and V_{ss} calculated directly.

THERAPEUTIC DRUG MONITORING

Blood or plasma drug concentrations at steady state are typically measured to refine estimates of CL/*F* for the individual. Updated estimates are then used to adjust maintenance doses to reach the desired target concentration. Drug concentrations can be misleading if the relevant pharmacokinetics (and toxicokinetics) are not considered. In addition, individual variability in drug response, due to multiple drug use, disease, genetic differences, and tolerance, must be considered. Pharmacokinetic characteristics of drugs may differ with development and age. Therefore, drug effects may vary considerably among infants, children, and adults. For example, water constitutes 80% of the weight of a newborn, whereas in adults it constitutes approximately 60%. These differences affect distribution of drugs throughout the body.

Plasma

Measurement of drug concentrations in plasma is the cornerstone of therapeutic drug monitoring (TDM), but it is not without pitfalls. In many instances, clinical response does not correlate with plasma drug concentrations. Other considerations may be as follows.

Time delays

It often takes time for a response to reflect a given plasma concentration due to the individual kinetics of the drug. Until this equilibrium is reached, correlation between response and concentration is difficult and may lead to misinterpretation of the clinical picture. Delay may be due to lack of equilibration between plasma and target organ as the drug distributes throughout the body. In addition, delay may be because the response measured is an indirect measure of drug effect, e.g., a change in blood pressure is an indirect measure of either change in peripheral resistance or cardiac output or both.

Active metabolites

Poor correlation may be found between response and plasma concentration of parent drug if active metabolites are present and not measured. Formation of active metabolites may be a function of the route of drug administration because oral ingestion generally produces an initial surge of metabolites due to the first-pass effect of the liver compared with drugs administered intravenously.

Exposure duration

Some drugs exhibit unusual concentration/response relationships, which minimizes the utility of TDM. In these cases, clinical response correlates more with duration of dosing than the actual dose or resultant plasma concentrations.

Tolerance

The effectiveness of a drug may diminish with continual use. Tolerance denotes a decreased pharmacological responsiveness to a drug. This is demonstrated by several drugs of abuse including ethanol and heroin. The degree of tolerance varies but is never complete. For example, tolerance to the effects of morphine quickly develops, but the user is not totally unresponsive to the pharmacological effects. To compensate for the development of tolerance, the dose is increased. Tolerance may develop slowly, such as in the case of tolerance to the CNS effects of ethanol, or can occur acutely (tachyphylaxis) as in the case of nicotine. In these cases, a correlation may be found between plasma drug concentration and the intensity of response at a given moment, but the relationship is not consistent and varies with time.

Saliva

In recent years, saliva has been utilized for TDM. The advantage is that collection is noninvasive and painless and so it has been used as a specimen of choice in pediatric TDM. Due to the low protein content of saliva, it is considered to represent the unbound or free fraction of drug in plasma. Since this is the fraction considered available for transfer across membranes and therefore responsible for pharmacological activity, its usefulness is easy to understand. Saliva collection methods are known to influence drug concentrations, but if these are compensated for and a standardized procedure utilized, correlation between plasma and saliva drug concentrations may be demonstrated for several drugs (e.g., phenytoin). Inconsistent results have been found for some drugs such as phenobarbital, so additional studies are needed to clearly define the limitations of testing saliva for TDM.

3

Effects of Food and Fasting

Patient compliance may be improved when drug administration is tied to meal timing and intake. However, depending on the drug, the composition and the size of the meal, and the time of food intake relative to dose administration, the pharmacokinetic properties of the drug may be altered. These perturbations in the pharmacokinetics of a drug as mediated by food may cause a wide range of effects including increased drug absorption, prolonged time to peak concentrations, increased variability in drug exposure, decreased drug absorption, or inhibition of metabolism and elimination processes. Many times, these changes may adversely influence the safety and efficacy of the drug substance or product and they are highly undesirable. For new chemical entities that have been approved for marketing, the label alerts the patient and the physician by including a statement under Dosage and Administration on the extent of alterations in peak concentrations (C_{max}) and area under the plasma concentration vs. time curve (AUC), potential clinical significance and directions on time of dose administration relative to time of meal intake. The Food and Drug Administration (FDA) has issued a draft biopharmaceutics guidance for industry entitled "Food-Effect Bioavailability and Fed Bioequivalence Studies: Study Design, Data Analysis, and Labeling" in October 2001. However, a final guidance has not yet been issued to date.

A number of intrinsic and extrinsic factors influence the pharmacokinetics of a drug in both the fasted and the fed states. These include anatomical, pathological, and physiological factors as well as the physical and chemical properties of the drug, formulation, or excipients. Because of the inherent complexities in perturbations that food may cause in the pharmacokinetics, safety, and efficacy of a drug, food-effect assessments in early drug development are typically performed proactively by pharmaceutical companies to facilitate design of pivotal clinical efficacy studies and, eventually, the drug product label. This article will highlight the factors influencing the pharmacokinetics of the drug in the fasting and the fed conditions as well as the importance of performing food-effect studies in early drug development. This article will also provide a pharmaceutical industry perspective on the models that are presently available to predict the presence and the extent of food-mediated alterations in absorption, metabolism, and clearance as they relate to a drug development program. Although food intake can affect the pharmacokinetics of a drug for a number of routes of administration, the emphasis of this article will be on drugs administered via the oral route of administration.

Effects of Food in the Pharmacokinetics of a Drug

Food has a myriad of effects on the pharmacokinetic behavior of a drug substance regardless of therapeutic class. Key variables include the meal itself, the composition of the meal, the drug, the formulation, the concomitant medications, the time of day, and the disease pathology. Such differences

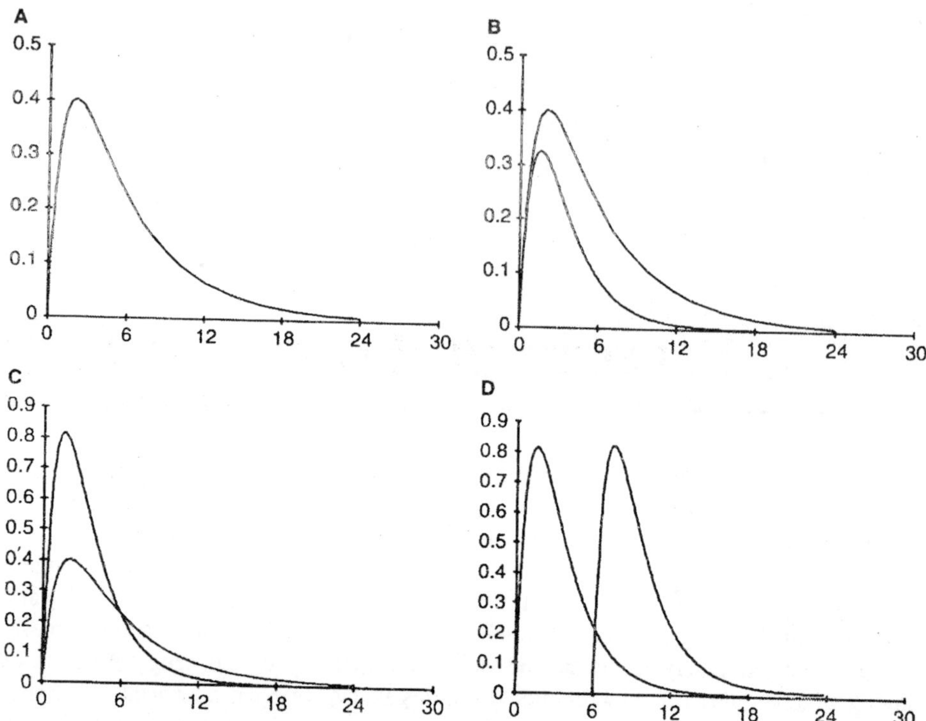

Fig. 3.1. A–Representative plasma concentration vs. time profile of a drug A after oral dosing in the fasted state. B–Food decreases exposure (C_{max} and AUC) of drug A. C–Food increases exposure (C_{max}) of drug A. D–Food delays exposure but does not decrease or increase exposure (C_{max} or AUC) of drug A.

are often as a result of altered physiological influences mediated by food. Examples of these physiological effects include the degree to which the gastric emptying rate is reduced, the variations in the degree to which digestive enzymes are secreted, the dynamics of an altered pH and the consequences for ionized drugs in the gastrointestinal (GI) tract, the biliary excretion, and the stimulation of hepatic and/or splanchic blood flow. Other important influences include physical interaction between the elements of food and the drug itself, which can interfere with absorption of a drug or merely act as a barrier to absorption from gut mucosa. The discussion below is primarily centered on how this knowledge can be integrated into rational drug development. Examples are drawn from case studies of drugs in drug development, the issues of identifying food effects early in the development, timing, design, and conduct of such studies as well as the issues and opportunities in this specific area of drug development.

Human Food-effect Studies and Available Pharmacokinetic Methodologies

The variation in the size and intake of food, the type of food, ethnicity, the caloric value, the fat content, the time gap between meals, and the intergastric volume can influence the physiological environment wherein the drug may find itself upon administration. All of these factors may result in alterations in the bioavailability of a given drug such as stimulation of biliary secretion and splanchnic blood flow, changes in GI pH, or delay in gastric emptying. In order to capture these perturbations in bioavailability, the FDA recommends a high-fat and high-calorie meal for testing the effect of a meal on drug pharmacokinetics. Historically, this meal has been considered a "*worst case scenario*" for a drug–food interaction study. For new chemical entities submitted for approval in the United States, well-controlled pharmacokinetic studies are performed using this "*standard high-fat meal*" as the fed condition. One may argue that the above definition of standard high-fat meal is probably not representative of a standard breakfast in the United States or other parts of the world. Exceptions include vegetarian or vegan meals, low-fat/low-calorie meals for diabetics as recommended by the American Diabetic Association (ADA), and meals that are specific for each ethnic group. All of these differences compounded by genetic predisposition to pharmacokinetics may profoundly impact the pharmacokinetics of a drug and its prescribing habit. Nonetheless, keeping the type (or lack) of meal as a constant, one can eludicate the effect of other variables (formulation, time of meal intake relative to dose, etc.) on pharmacokinetics keeping in mind that the meal should be reflective of one that is used (recommended) during patient therapy.

There are two types of food-effect studies that are often performed in humans. These studies are designed to provide dosing recommendation with meals or to provide a mechanistic investigation on the effect of food on the pharmacokinetics of drugs. Examples of the former include studies done in conformity with the FDA guidance on food-effect studies or called "*standard assessments*." Examples of the latter include exploratory mechanistic studies to investigate gastric emptying using tools, such as gamma-scintiography, or modulating gastric pH using ranitidine coadministration, with the aim to provide/elucidate underlying reasons for observed food effects.

Standard Food–Effect Assessments— Regulatory and Product-Labeling Considerations

The draft FDA guidance entitled "Food-Effect Bioavailability and Fed Bioequivalence Studies: Study Design, Data Analysis, and Labeling" provides sponsors with information on the design of appropriate studies to assess impact of food-mediated alterations in pharmacokinetics and to provide suitable dosing guidelines on drug product label. The guidance provides useful strategies for biowaivers if the drug in question belongs to a particular Biopharmaceutics Classification System (BCS) category. For example, for highly soluble and highly permeable drugs (i.e., BCS Class I), food effects should be inconsequential (between test and reference products) due to the inherent properties of the drug. The premise is that the compound is minimally influenced by food as a result of pH- or site-independent absorption and lack of dissolution differences.

A suitable study design for definitively assessing the influence of food on the pharmacokinetics of a drug or drug product includes performing a single-dose, randomized, balanced, two-period, two-treatment (fed vs. fasted) crossover study, with an adequate washout period between treatments. The number of subjects in the study should provide adequate statistical power for capturing small differences in exposure variables [peak concentrations (C_{max}), T_{max}, and area under the plasma concentration vs. time curve (AUC)]. The guidance also asks for using the highest strength of the formulation to be evaluated in such studies. For the fasting treatment, at least a 10-hr fast prior to dosing is recommended: "Following an overnight fast of at least 10 hours, subject should take the drug product. No food should be allowed for at least 4 hours post- dose. Water can be allowed at libitum after 2 hours. Scheduled standardized meals should be served throughout the remaining study period." The issue is not the "number" of hours of predose fast time, but the stomach volume. If it contains <50 mL (fasting state depends on the volume present in the upper region of the stomach), the stomach is in an interdigestive state. It is generally recommended to have a postdose fast time of about 4 h. For the fed treatment, the regulatory guidance indicates a standard high-fat meal composed of two eggs fried in butter, two strips of bacon, two slices of toast with butter, 4 oz of hash brown potatoes, and 8 oz of whole milk. The caloric breakdown of this meal translates into approximately 150 cal from protein, 250 cal from carbohydrate, and 600 cal from fat. Standard pharmacokinetic calculations are performed using non-compartmental methods, e.g., C_{max}, AUC, T_{max}, etc. The guidance provides directions on how the data are applied to claim label attributes; for example, the degree to which 90% confidence intervals for the ratio of geometric means between fasted and fed legs are contained relative to the bounds of 80–125% for AUC or C_{max}.

One issue that routinely arises is how to provide the FDA-recommended high-fat meal at non-U.S. investigative sites, where this meal is not readily accessible. Simple substitution of locally available food (e.g., sausage for bacon) that maintains the caloric breakdown of the FDA-recommended high-fat meal has been an acceptable approach.

A second type of study involves applying food as a covariate in population pharmacokinetic models.

This is an emerging area of interest that is gaining regulatory concurrence. The advantages of using multilevel population pharmacokinetic models include the determination of the extent of both interindividual and intraindividual variability, the use of a limited sparse sampling approach, and the use of multiple covariates within a large Phase III trial setting. This strategy allows the simultaneous analysis of relevant covariate relationships (negative vs. positive correlation, proportional correlation, etc.) influencing the key pharmacokinetic parameters as a function of body surface area, age, weight, sex, hematological or biochemical indices, creatinine clearance, and, more importantly, any delays in drug absorption as mediated by food intake. Such analyses can be performed using tools, such as NONMEM, with standard conditional estimation methods (first order, first-order conditional estimate, or first-order conditional estimate with interaction, etc.). This allows for estimation of typical values for key pharmacokinetic parameters, *V*/*F*, *CL*/*F*, absorption rate constant, or lag time. Shepard et al. used a sequential approach with an indicator variable to assess the effect of food on the parameter of interest. Their model included $K_a = \theta_1(1 - Q) + \theta_2 Q$, where Q was an indicator variable with a value of 0 (fasted) or 1 (fed), and θ_1 and θ_2 were the parameters of interest, with $K_a = \theta_1$ for fasted treatment and $K_a = \theta_2$ for fed treatment.

A number of recent examples in the literature describe the powerful use of population pharmacokinetic strategies to maximize information pertaining to food–effect behavior. These include a combination of non-compartmental and population pharmacokinetic analyses to answer a scientific question. For example, Zhou et al. used non-compartmental analysis to determine the extent of decrease in bioavailability of a drug mediated by food and then showed, using deconvolution and subsequent population pharmacokinetic analysis to assess the impact of meal timing on absorption, that the reduction in biovailability under fed conditions was related to a reduction in the extent of absorption and not to a reduction in the rate of absorption. The use of the population pharmacokinetic approach in a multicenter trial in patients to assess food effect using sparse sampling and several categorical and continuous covariates is a more common application of this strategy. However, it is not clear that a population pharmacokinetic approach definitively addresses a food interaction without a traditional Phase I study.

Scintigraphic Assessments

The technique of gamma scintigraphy has been used to evaluate biopharmaceutic properties of drug substances administered orally in the fed and the fasted states to evaluate food effects. Specifically, the procedure allows for studying GI transit of radiolabeled drug formulations in the fed state. With this method, one can understand the physiological processes by which the GI tract manages food and how the stomach empties meals of varying chemical composition. Such type of studies may also reveal the potential sites of absorption of an investigational product throughout the GI tract and how this is impacted in the fed state. This information is particularly useful when designing modified-release formulations. Technitium (^{99m}Tc) is a widely used nuclide in radiopharmaceuticals because of its optimal energy, short half-life, and small radiation dose needed.

Models for Assessing Impact of Food on the Pharmacokinetics of a Drug Substance

In Vitro Models

Biorelevant dissolution models have been described in the literature as a means to predict food-effect behavior on the absorption of drugs. Reppas et al. have suggested several dissolution media that simulate fasted and fed conditions in the human body. They used milk (3.5% fat) and United States Pharmacopeia (USP)-simulated gastric fluid with and without pepsin as dissolution media representing the fed and the fasted states in the stomach, respectively. Dressman and Reppas have showed that such biorelevant media have distinct advantages over compendial media in the prediction of food effects for poorly water-soluble drugs. An example of how dissolution tests may be used to predict the in vivo effect of food on drug absorption is highlighted for a BCS class II (highly permeable, poorly water-soluble drug) drug, danazol. Fig. 3.2A shows the dissolution profile of danazol in different media, namely, water, simulated intestinal fluid (SIF), FaSSIF, and FeSSIF. FaSSIF represents the fasted state in small intestine and FeSSIF represents fed state in small intestine. From these dissolution tests, it is clear that there is enhanced dissolution in the simulated fed state relative to the simulated fasted condition. Not surprisingly, the extent of this in vitro increase is similar to the extent of increase in danazol exposure in human subjects observed in the fed state as shown in Fig. 3.2B. The mechanism of food effect is related to increased solubilization mediated by bile salts for this steroid drug. This strategy appears to be predictive of drugs that belong to the BCS Class II category and may not be generally applicable to drugs belonging to other categories.

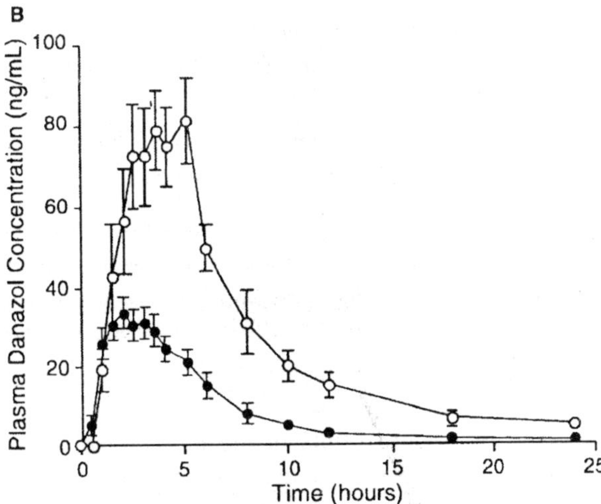

Fig. 3.2. A–In vitro dissolution profile for Danazol. B–In vivo plasma concentration vs.time profile for Danazol.

In Vivo Models

A number of animal models have been used to describe the fasting and the fed pharmacokinetics of drugs with the aim of predicting human performance. These include mice, rats, rabbits, guinea pigs, dogs, pigs, monkeys, to name a common few. The discussion below will address the relative merits and demerits of rodents, dogs, and pigs as predictive models for humans. It should be kept in mind that animal models may be helpful in assessing large and overt food interactions in oral bioavailability. However, relatively small differences that may be ultimately important in human studies and therapeutics will probably not be detected.

Rodents

Rodents (mice, rats, guinea pigs) are generally not preferred as models for assessing food effects for various reasons, namely, differences in GI anatomy and physiology, difficulties in administering "human" food, and lack of implementing a crossover design assessment. Other potential caveats include differences in the pharmacokinetic and the metabolism behavior in rodents as compared to humans and non-human primates that may negate assessment in this species. Metabolic profiling of the investigational product in a panel of animal models will reveal the suitability of a particular species as a predictor of human pharmacokinetic behavior. Furthermore, the extent of serial sampling is also constrained in smaller rodents such as mice. However, rodents are one of the two species commonly and typically used as a toxicology species in drug development; it is of importance to assess the impact of food not necessarily from the point of view of predicting human food effect but more so in ensuring adequate exposure multiples are obtained for toxicokinetic purposes. Few authors have explored rat as a model for predicting food-effect behavior.

Dogs

Pentagastrin-pretreated dogs have been shown to be useful in screening biopharmaceutic properties of new formulations. Coupled with the features that a cross-over study design can be easily applied and human food easily administered to these animals, the dog remains one of the commonly used models in assessing the pharmacokinetics of drugs. The disadvantages of using a dog model include dissimilar GI physiology and, hence, differences in pharmacokinetic behavior (for the pentagastrin-untreated dogs), need for modulation of GI physiology using pentagastrin and other physiological agents, and dissimilar drug metabolism/ transport between dogs and humans for some compounds. Additionally, dogs are relatively more sensitive to physiological effects of certain pharmaceutical excipients commonly employed in solubilization of poorly water-soluble drugs (e.g., Polysorbate 80 and resultant orthostatic hypotension).

Although gastric emptying time is relatively similar between dogs and humans in the fasted state, the intestinal transit time is almost twice as long in humans. These apparent differences can be offset by administering pentagastrin pretreatment which allows the gastric acidity, the emptying time, and the small intestinal transit time to closely approximate human conditions, i.e., approximately pH 2, 0.7 and 4 hr, respectively. Another approach to synchronize the gastric environment in dogs to closely mimic humans includes a combined treatment of intramuscular pentagastrin with intravenous atropine sulfate.

Pentagastrin is an analog of gastrin that reproducibly stimulates gastric acid secretion and is usually administered intramuscularly prior to biopharmaceutic experimentation in doses of approximately 6–10 μg/kg. Conflicting results in the literature of drugs studied in these pretreated dogs have negated the extensive use of this model. For example, pentagastrin-pretreated dogs were more predictive of the human bioavailability of didanosine than the untreated dogs. In contrast, data from Kanerva et al. suggest that the pentagastrin-pretreated dog was unable to reliably predict the absorption of deramciclane, an acid-labile drug.

A typical design of a food-effect study in dogs is as follows. Beagle dogs (usually n = 6–8) are administered a pharmacological dose of a drug formulation (hard gelatin capsule or tablet) in a randomized or non-randomized crossover design. Treatment legs may include dosing after an overnight fast (fasted state) and dosing with a low-fat meal, a high-fat meal, or other specialized meals (fed state). The composition of meals that have been administered to dogs can be highly variable. For example, Paulson et al. administered low-, medium-, and high-fat diets. The low- fat diet was composed of one slice of toasted white bread spread with 0.5 oz of jelly, 8 oz of skim milk, and 6 oz of orange juice. The medium-fat diet was composed of one slice of toasted white bread with 0.5 oz each of peanut butter and jelly, 1 oz of dry cereal (cornflakes), 8 oz of skim milk, 6 oz of orange juice, and one banana. The high-fat diet was composed of two slices of toasted white bread spread with 1.2 oz of butter, two eggs fried in butter, two slices of cooked bacon, 2 oz of hash brown potatoes fried in butter, and 8 oz of whole milk. These diets were homogenized then administered either in a bowl or with a syringe to the dogs. A suitable washout period separated the treatment legs. Blood samples are collected at predetermined intervals predrug and postdrug administration and pharmacokinetic behavior assessed with and without food.

Pigs and minipigs

The digestive tract of a minipig is anatomically and physiologically similar to that of the human adult digestive tract. In fact, the weanling minipig model has a GI tract that is closely similar to children between the age of 2 and 5 years. Specifically, the similarities exist for the gastric villi, the regulation and the composition of gastric secretions, the transit times as well as in the digestive and the absorptive behaviors. Regardless of these advantages, the use of the minipig in pharmacokinetic assessments has been relatively uncommon. One example of an application to the assessment of food effects in minis- wine is the study on the effect of various fat-content diets on the bioavailability of theophylline following a 400-mg single-dose Theo-24. The observed similarities in the pharmacokinetics of theophylline in pigs and humans led Koritz et al. to suggest swine as a predictive model for the assessment of theophylline bioequivalence in humans.

Food-Effect Assessment in Drug Development: Key Considerations

Timing of Food-Effect Studies

There are generally two types of clinical pharmacokinetic/pharmacodynamic (PK/PD) studies that may be performed during drug development. One is a "pilot" study to obtain preliminary exploratory assessment used for facilitating internal decision making for the progression of a compound and the other is a more formal statistically powered "pivotal" study to provide dosing recommendation for purposes of the drug product label. The key difference is that the pilot study is often powered for large differences and the pivotal study is powered for small differences for a priori defined endpoint. The pilot study, which usually uses a developmental formulation and a guess of the therapeutic dose, can also provide valuable information for developing a well-designed pivotal study. Label-driven food-effect assessments are performed in later stages of drug development, particularly when the "market" formulation is available and the therapeutic dose is known from Phase III efficacy studies. Appropriate recommendations for performing such studies are available in the Guidance for Industry issued by the FDA in the United States.

The exploratory assessment of food on the pharmacokinetics of new chemical entities in the drug development chain of events varies largely within companies. This is also driven by marketing considerations, competitive advantage, flexibility for dosing options, and the therapeutic index of the drug if known. Several authors have suggested inclusion of an exploratory assessment early in the drug development program because appropriate formulation development may be initiated for drugs exhibiting undesirable food effects. A caveat for this approach is the large number of food-effect studies that may need to be performed if multiple changes are made for the formulation and/or the excipients within them. If multiple- formulation switches occur in a program, it may be worthwhile to delay the food-effect assessment to discount the formulation as a variable.

A convenient method to examine food effects is the inclusion of a food-effect assessment as part of the first-in-man study once the maximum tolerated dose (MTD) is identified. Depending on the drug bioavailability characteristics in animals, physicochemical properties of the drug and preliminary data on whether the drug exhibits dissolution rate-limited absorption behavior, a dose that is 1/2 to 1/4 of the MTD, may initially be used for the preliminary food-effect assessment. This method potentially avoids undesirably high exposures of the drug when adequate safety data are not available. Dose selection will also depend on the predicted therapeutically relevant dose range, the linearity in pharmacokinetic behavior, and the sensitivity of the bioanalytical assay. Typically, the FIM study design includes non-randomized, non-crossover, single-ascending doses in eight subjects (six active, two placebo), where doses are escalated until an MTD is reached and dosing typically performed after an overnight fast. For example, in the food-effect leg, 0.25–0.5 $\times$ MTD cohorts return for a second dose after a washout period wherein dose is administered with a standard high-fat meal. This allows within- subject comparison of exposure with and without food, but does not account for period effects. Hence, it is not unusual to obtain inconclusive results with this design. To lend rigor in the scientific assessment of food effect, it may be more desirable to have the food-effect assessment done as part of the first-in-man (FIM) study using a randomized crossover design in eight active subjects. In general, however, it is recommended to perform specific well-designed food-effect studies with adequate power for large differences to capture meaningful deviations in exposure.

Single vs. Multiple Dosing—Dose Selection

The selection of the appropriate dose in assessing the effect of food on the pharmacokinetics of a drug is an important consideration. Dose selection may be based on several criteria, namely, therapeutically relevant concentrations (if known), safety margin, linear pharmacokinetics, etc. It is generally required to evaluate a single dose of a drug for such an assessment. However, depending on non-linear pharmacokinetic behavior and the degree of accumulation (or induction) upon multiple dosing, a multiple dose may be a better option. A multiple-dose study may also be more meaningful if the primary or secondary objective is to evaluate the effect of food on the safety or the pharmacodynamics of a drug, where single-dose administration may not be sufficient to induce meaningful perturbations in pharmacodynamics. An example of this approach is in the multiple-dose administration of the "statin" group of antihyperlipidemic agents for assessing the effect of food on the lipid-lowering efficacy [i.e., LDL-cholesterol (LDL-C) levels] given the slow turnover rate of LDL-C.

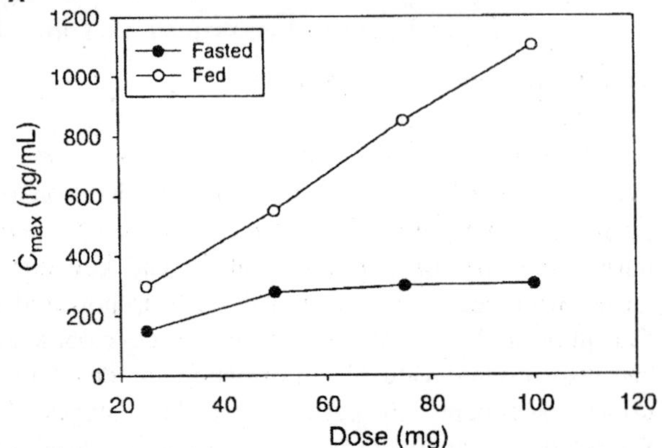

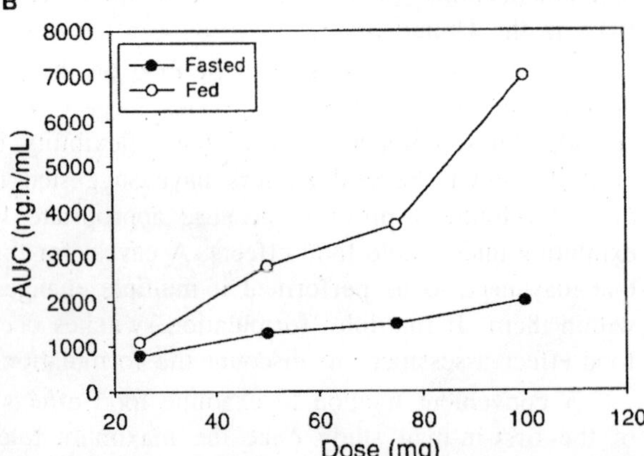

Fig. 3.3. A–Relationship between dose and C_{max} for acitrein. B–Relationship between dose and AUC for acitretin.

Dose selection based on pharmacokinetic profile

The oral absorption of certain highly permeable, poorly water-soluble drugs with low oral bioavailability in the fasted state may be profoundly influenced by the intake of fatty meal. Dose selection for such drugs can be challenging and important. For example, acitretin is a retinoid indicated for the treatment of psoriasis. Depending on the dose of acitretin used, food appears to increase the absorption in a varying manner. In the fasted state, both the C_{max} and the AUC reach a plateau at 50-mg dose with minor, if any, increases in exposure at doses higher than 50 mg. In contrast, the drug exhibits almost dose-proportional increases in C_{max} and AUC over the entire tested dose range up to 100 mg, when the drug is administered with a high-fat meal. When acitretin is given with food, there is also a decrease in inter subject variability in exposure parameters. These results have important implications for investigational agents exhibiting dissolution rate-limited absorption during drug development as this presents an opportunity for key formulation development to increase bioavailability if safety is not an issue and if formulation options are available. This example also illustrates the need for an early assessment of a food interaction study. In acitretin, the patients in the Phase III pivotal studies were instructed to take their daily acitretin dose with the main meal of the day based on this information.

Dose selection based on PK/PD relationship

A second more germane consideration is dose selection based on PK/PD relationships. Depending on the reference point on a PK/PD chart, food may have little or profound effect on either PK, PD, or both. For example, drug A shows profound reductions in C_{max} and AUC, but blood pressure reduction is relatively unaffected by food; it is conceivable that the drug PD is at the maximal effect where large differences in PK leads to minor changes in PD. On the other hand, if the dose of drug B was selected such that its PD is at 50% of maximal effect, then there is much larger PD differences for observed differences in drug exposure.

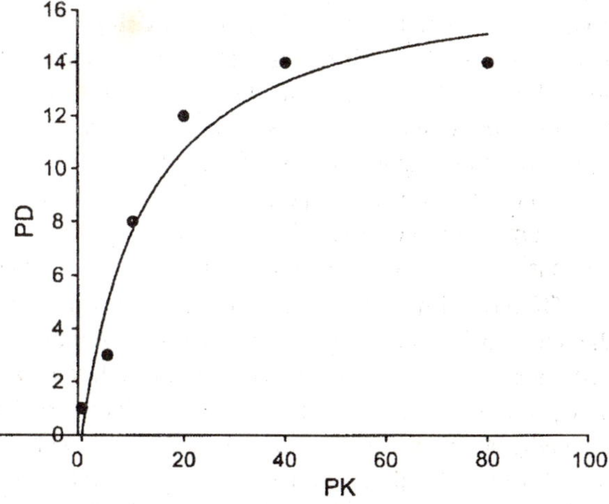

Fig. 3.4. Representative illustration of PK/PD relationship for a hypothetical drug.

An example of the former case (drug A behavior) is illustrated in the effect of food on the PK and the PD of pravastatin, a representative statin in the treatment of hyperlipidemia. Although a low-fat, low-cholesterol meal altered the pharmacokinetics of 20-mg pravastatin significantly, no adverse impact on pharmacodynamics (lipid-lowering efficacy) was observed. Concomitant intake of meals reduced pravastatin C_{max} by 49% and AUC by 31%, the change in LDL-C-lowering efficacy was minimal (-37% with meal vs. -36% 1-hr premeal). The authors recommend administering pravastatin without regard to meals. It is worth noting here that the LDL-C-lowering efficacy of pravastatin plateaus at ca. –32% (20 mg) to ca. –37% (80 mg) changes from baseline; at –37%, the PD is already at the flat portion of the sigmoidal PK–PD curve. Consequently, even with a change in PK approximating 50%, there is minimal impact on PD. It is unlikely that the PD would be influenced significantly by food for compounds whose PD is at this flat portion of the PK–PD curve than would be the case if the dose selected represented a PD of 0.5 times maximal effect, where there is a much larger variability for PD differences with variability in PK.

Type of Meals

Another key consideration when performing food- effect studies is the type of meal utilized for assessing effect of food on the pharmacokinetics of a drug. Because of differing ethnicities, geographical regions, and variations in the eating behavior of human beings across the world, it is conceivable that the "standard" breakfast, lunch, and dinner will vary extensively. Then it becomes increasingly difficult to assess the true significance of food and its impact on PK/PD and to develop dosing recommendations that are systematically applied to a drug that is prescribed globally.

In order to provide a systematic basis for capturing food-mediated alterations in the pharmacokinetics of drugs, the FDA draft guidance recommends a standard high-fat meal as being composed of "2 eggs fried in butter, 2 strips of bacon, 2 slices of toast with butter, 4 ounces of hash brown potatoes, 8 ounces of whole milk." Differences in pharmacokinetic behavior may be expected depending on the type of breakfast utilized; for example, an English breakfast is different in composition and caloric value to an American breakfast or a special diet in adherence with ADA recommendations. To derive meaningful data across these varying types of meals, meals are often categorized in terms of carbohydrate, protein, and fat content as "high-fat," "low-fat," "high-protein," or "high- carbohydrate" diet. An alternate categorization is based on the caloric value of the meal itself, as "low calorie" or "high calorie."

The influence of differing breakfast compositions and the influence of a solid vs. a liquid (whole milk) meal were investigated by Colburn et al. for etretinate. The drug was administered in the fasted state or in the fed state with a standard high-fat breakfast, a standard high-carbohydrate breakfast, and whole milk (16 oz). Etretinate concentrations in plasma were greater when given with a high-fat meal and whole milk compared to the fasted state or when given with a high-carbohydrate meal. Meals with differing fat contents can also influence drug absorption and disposition by influencing physiology. It is known that higher levels of fat may inhibit gastric emptying. Moreover, the GI transit times are different for solid and liquid meals and this may impact the pharmacokinetics of a drug. The lack of consistency in the scientific literature on the type of meal used in the investigation prohibits data comparisons across populations unless such differing compositions are used in a single study.

Of more importance in relation to the influence of food on absorption is the rate of blood flow in the capillary system. Food may cause an increase in splanchnic blood flow leading to alterations in drug absorption, depending on the ingredients present in the food that is ingested. Closely tied into this principle is the extent to which a given drug is extracted by first-pass metabolism when traversing through the liver via the portal circulation. Both the type and the size of meal can influence splanchnic blood flow. Using a non-invasive technique for the assessment of hepatic haemodynamics using radiocolloid imaging, Walmsley et al. assessed the influence of meal on hepatic, mesenteric, and splenic arterial effective blood flows. They showed that both the total effective liver blood flow and the mesenteric arterial effective flow increased by 28–69% after eating. It is known that long-chain fatty acids stimulate human intestinal blood flow.

It has become increasingly evident that several ingredients in food or components of a meal can influence drug metabolism and clearance via inhibition of cytochrome P450 isozymes or modulation of drug transporters such as *p*-glycoprotein. These ingredients include vegetables and fruit products and components such as St. John's wort, garlic, grapefruit juice, certain type of orange juices, apple juice, red, black, or white pepper. Red wine and green tea also have ingredients that can alter the metabolism/ clearance of a drug. In order to differentiate these influences from those arising from the altered GI physiology, the drug development program may need to include separate food and metabolism–transporter interaction studies to assess the overall impact on dosing recommendations.

Time of Meal Consumption Relative to Dose

The time of meal consumption relative to dose has important implications for compounds whose pharmacokinetics are severely impacted by food. The extent of food-mediated alterations in pharmacokinetics are influenced by the time interval between ingestion of food and intake of drug. Notably, as the time elapsed between meal ingestion and drug intake becomes longer, the less severe the effect of food on the pharmacokinetics of a drug would presumably be. Consider the following example. If one were to fix the meal intake as a constant and to vary the time of intake of a meal, then differences in the rate and the extent of drug absorption may be observed. The treatments were: (A) 10-hr fast; (B) drug intake 1 hr before breakfast; (C) drug intake immediately following consumption of the breakfast; and (D) drug intake 1.5 hr after beginning consumption of the breakfast. As expected, tacrolimus absorption was the highest in the fasted state. The lowest impact on bioavailability was when taking the drug 1 hr prior to a meal; the highest impact was when tacrolimus was ingested immediately after a meal (treatments C and D).

Marathe et al. have investigated the effect of food on the pharmacokinetics of avitriptan in a systematic manner as part of the avitriptan drug development program. In the first study, they showed that concomitant ingestion of food significantly reduced avitriptan bioavailability. Specifically, mean C_{max} and AUC were reduced 70% and 45%, respectively, while Tmax was delayed from 45 min to 2 hr when avitriptan was administered as a 50 mg capsule 5 min after a standard high-fat meal. Because avitriptan was developed as a treatment for migraine, this dramatic food effect has important implications for the developability of the drug for this indication. In the second study, Marathe et al. designed a meal-timing study where avitriptan was administered after an overnight fast and at 0.5, 1, 2, and 4 hr after intake of a standard high-fat meal. There was a meaningful relationship between avitriptan bioavailability as a function of time interval between dose and meal intake with the impact of food decreasing over time. Mean C_{max} decreased by 61%, 58%, 50%, and 35% after 0.5-, 1, 2-, and 4-hr postmeal, respectively; mean AUC decreased by 35%, 31%, 34%, and 19% after 0.5-, 1, 2-, and 4-hr postmeal, respectively. Median T_{max} values were 0.5 hr (fasted), 1.5 hr (0.5- and 1-hr postmeal), 1.25 hr (2-hr postmeal), and 0.75 hr (4-hr postmeal). In a later study by the same authors, scintigraphic analysis showed that avitriptan was rapidly absorbed from the upper small intestine after emptying from the stomach. Gastric emptying was slow and continuous in the fed state leading to extended absorption. The authors also attributed the high intrasubject variability in Cmax and AUC to variability in gastric emptying under fasted and fed conditions.

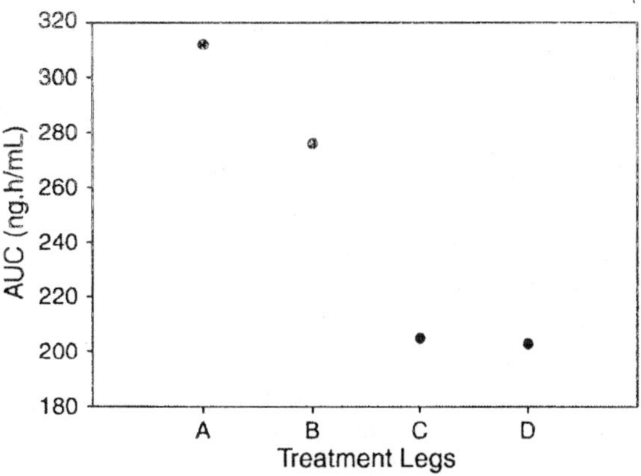

Fig. 3.5. Relationship of time of meal and drug AUC.

A similar study was reported by Laitinen et al. on the effect of time of meal on the bioavailability of the bisphosphonate drug clodronate. Exposure (AUC) was the highest when clodronate was administered 2-hr premeal, followed by a 1-hr premeal (91% of 2-hr premeal AUC), a 0.5-hr premeal (69% of 2-hr pre- meal AUC), with meal (10% of 2-hr premeal AUC), and a 2-hr postmeal (34% of 2-hr premeal AUC). Although the 2-hr premeal does not present a "true" fasting state, there was a measurable difference between these short time intervals premeal and postmeal leading the investigators to conclude that clodronate be administered at least 0.5 hr prior to breakfast. The closeness of this prescribed time of drug intake to the meal ensures some balance of patient compliance with minimally acceptable compromise on the impact on drug absorption.

For a drug with a wide therapeutic margin, such variations in drug absorption relative to timing of a meal may be inconsequential in terms of clinical relevance; however, the same cannot be said for a drug with narrow therapeutic margin.

Type of Formulation

The type of formulation used, the excipients contained in the formulation as well as the particle size of the drug substance all may influence drug absorption and, thus, confound the observed food-effect behavior for a given drug. For example, a highly water-soluble drug may be formulated in a tablet that contains a poorly water-soluble polymer excipient that influences release of the drug from the matrix and subsequent dissolution properties of the tablet. Certain hydrophilic polymers, such as hydroxypropylmethyl-cellulose, have been implicated in dose dumping of modified- or controlled-release formulations in the presence of food. The use of varying excipients within formulations are often the cause of conflicting data for observed food effects. Whereas some excipients, such as mannitol, influence drug absorption by altering transit times, others, such as PEG-300, Cremophor EL, and Polysorbate 80, inhibit p-glycoprotein and other drug transporters.

In a drug development program, it is sometimes necessary to change the formulation depending on drug development time-lines and availability of drug substances to meet the needs of clinical pharmacology and PK/PD studies in a timely manner. For example, the formulation may change from an aqueous suspension in the first-in-man study to a capsule formulation in proof-of-concept study to, eventually, a market formulation that would be a tablet formulation. Each time such formulation changes are made, a new food-effect study may need to be performed to assess the influence of the altered formulation on the observed food effect to design the Phase III study in an optimal manner. To minimize the number of food-effect studies performed due to formulation changes, it is essential to maintain consistent formulation strategy across the drug development phase. Inclusion of excipients should occur based on informed input from a variety of functional areas including pharmaceutical sciences, clinical pharmacology, clinical PK/PD, and drug safety. A pivotal food-effect study needs to be performed using the same formulation used in Phase III pivotal efficacy trials or the market formulation so that appropriate dosing recommendations with regard to meals are provided.

Site of Drug Absorption

Absorption of drugs from the GI tract differs extensively depending on the intrinsic properties of the drug. For example, a drug may be absorbed from the upper GI tract or throughout the GI tract. This will have important implications for food effects as well as for other applications such as developing modified-release formulations or demonstrating bioequivalence of a test formulation vs. the reference formulation. For a drug that has an absorption window of the upper GI tract, a delay in T_{max} as mediated by food may lead to suboptimal absorption. It is very clear that food can have significant pharmacokinetic and pharmacodynamic consequences for drug substances. Although not discussed in this article, food can also have deleterious effects on efficacy and safety of a product. A growing body of literature now points at many pharmaceutical excipients that are typically used in drug development cycle to influence drug disposition by modulating metabolism and efflux properties of drugs. Whether the information on food effects is derived for internal company decision making and developability considerations or for dosing recommendations with the final market formulation, understanding the myriad and often complex actions mediated by food is critical in drug development. A rationale selection of available choices within the context of a well-designed and adequately powered clinical study will provide important clues for the drug development scientist to: (1) enable well-designed late-stage clinical efficacy trials; (2) optimize the formulations for early- and midstage developmental compounds; and (3) provide prescribing options to the physician for optimal patient compliance on soon-to-be-marketed products.

4

PHARMACOKINETIC MODELING

Pharmacokinetics is the study of absorption, distribution, metabolism, and excretion of a drug over a time course. Measurement of a drug in the body is usually limited to the blood or plasma. Pharmacokinetic data analysis consists of examining plasma concentration–time data and estimating pharmacokinetic parameters that describe drug disposition. Methods used for pharmacokinetic analysis include noncompartmental analysis or pharmacokinetic modeling. Noncompartmental analysis does not depend on fitting mathematical models to the drug disposition data. Compartmental analysis is the most often used pharmacokinetic modeling approach. This chapter discusses various aspects of compartmental modeling.

SAMPLING STRATEGIES

In Phase I studies, the number of blood specimens taken and their timing must allow for the accurate description of the plasma disposition of the drug in individual subjects and for the estimation of individual pharmacokinetic parameter values. Because at the time of Phase I drug testing, the disposition of a drug in humans is usually unknown, it is necessary to employ an intensive (frequent) and extensive (prolonged) blood sampling scheme. To maximize the chances that all the phases of drug disposition are identified and measured, the following steps are undertaken: (1) sample intensively during drug administration and immediately following the discontinuation of drug administration; (2) sample at time points as far out after drug administration as is feasible; and (3) utilize highly sensitive assay methods. Intensive and extensive sampling schemes provide enough plasma concentration data to select among alternative models that best describe all the plasma disposition phases of the drug (e.g., biexponential vs triexponential behavior) and allow for the detection and characterization of unexpected dispositional phenomena, such as enterohepatic recirculation.

In later stages of drug development, limited-sampling strategies are employed to allow estimation of pharmacokinetic parameters using a small number of plasma samples. This is possible only when the pharmacokinetic behavior of an agent is known. One approach to designing a limited-sampling strategy is by combining D-optimality with a Bayesian algorithm. D-optimality uses optimal design theory to select a limited number of sampling times. A Bayesian algorithm then combines information from the limited sampling scheme with prior information about the population pharmacokinetic parameter values (e.g., the average value and variance) to then estimate pharmacokinetic parameters for individual patients. A linear regression approach is another method to design limited sampling schemes. This latter method generally allows for estimation of only a single pharmacokinetic parameter such as clearance or area under the concentration–time curve (AUC).

Disadvantages of the linear regression approach include the requirement for consistent timing of infusion duration and blood sampling. All data points must be obtained; all conditions are required for calculation of the pharmacokinetic parameter. The Bayesian algorithm is usually more robust and flexible and allows the description of the full pharmacokinetic profile and estimation of more than one pharmacokinetic parameter. The development of a limited-sampling strategy using a Bayesian algorithm may be approached in the following manner. First, a population pharmacokinetic model is developed and average values for each pharmacokinetic parameter and the variance about the pharmacokinetic parameter are determined. Next, the concentration–time data sets to be used for developing a limited sampling scheme are randomly divided into two equal subsets, a training data set and a validation data set. Using the sample module of the software program ADAPT II (which employs D-optimality), a limited sampling scheme is defined for the training data set. The validation data set is then used to validate the limited-sampling scheme. Individual plasma concentrations, at the selected time points, are fitted using a Bayesian algorithm as implemented in ADAPT II, where the Bayesian priors and covariance matrix are derived from the population pharmacokinetic model. Reference pharmacokinetic parameters for individual patients in the validation set are determined using the full pharmacokinetic profile and maximum likelihood estimation. The predictive performance of the limited-sampling strategy is evaluated by calculating the bias and precision of the Bayesian parameter estimates.

Noncompartmental Analysis

Noncompartmental analysis, which is based on the statistical moment theory, is routinely performed to calculate pharmacokinetic parameters quickly and easily. Noncompartmental analysis does not require the assumption of a specific compartmental model for drug disposition, which for some drugs can be a complex and time-consuming process. An underlying assumption with noncompartmental analysis is pharmacokinetic linearity, in which the pharmacokinetic parameter values do not vary with dose and/ or time. This assumption applies to all parameters describing drug absorption, distribution, metabolism, and elimination.

Compartmental Analysis

Compartmental analysis is useful to describe drug disposition, estimate pharmacokinetic parameters, and predict plasma concentrations utilizing various schedules and doses of administration. During compartmental analysis, plasma disposition curves are fit by equations that describe the time course of plasma drug concentrations for the given mode of drug input. For example, the following equations describe a drug administered as an intravenous bolus that exhibits a mono- (Eq. 1) or bi-exponential (Eq. 2) decline:

$$C_t = C_0 e^{-Kt} \qquad \ldots(1)$$

$$C_t = Ae^{-\alpha t} + Be^{-\beta t} \qquad \ldots(2)$$

where C_t represents the concentration at a particular time, C_0 is the concentration at time zero, A and B are macro-rate constants, K is the apparent first-order elimination rate constant, and α and β are macro-elimination rate constants. For a drug exhibiting a biexponential decline (Eq. 2), α and β

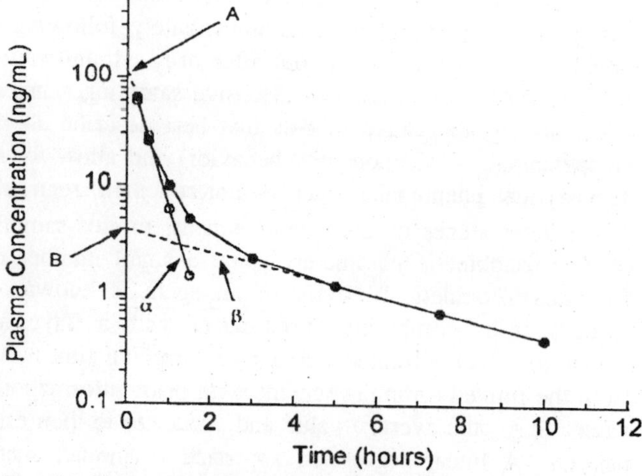

Fig. 4.1. Plasma concentration-time profile for a drug administered as an intravenous bolus dose and exhibiting a biexponential or two-compartment behaviour.

correspond to the initial and terminal slopes, respectively. The method of residuals can be applied to the concentration–time data to estimate A and B, which are zero-time intercepts for each disposition phase.

Plasma disposition curves can also be fit by equations that incorporate microconstants. For an open linear two-compartment model, the microconstants include the central volume of distribution (V_c), the elimination rate constant (k_{10}), and the intercompartment rate constants (k_{12}, k_{21}). The microconstants are also known as the structural parameters of the model. Micro-constants can be estimated from macro- constants and vice-versa by the following equations:

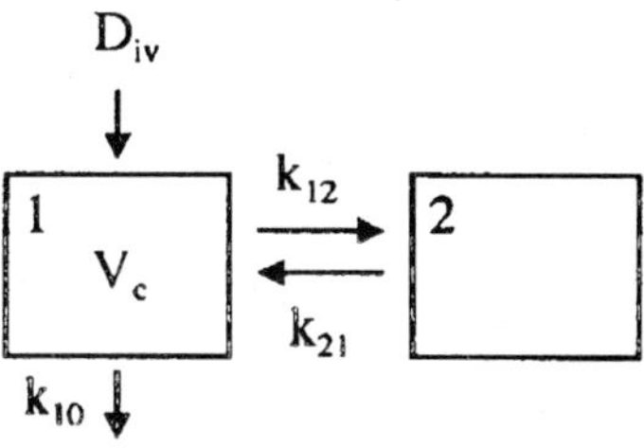

Fig. 4.2. Two-compartment model parameterized with micro-constants.

$$A = \frac{D_{iv}}{V_c} \times \frac{(\alpha - k_{21})}{(\alpha - \beta)} \qquad \ldots(3)$$

$$B = \frac{D_{iv}}{V_c} \times \frac{(\beta - k_{21})}{(\beta - \alpha)} \qquad \ldots(4)$$

$$\alpha = \frac{k_{21} \times k_{10}}{\beta} \qquad \ldots(5)$$

$$\beta = \frac{1}{2} \times \left[(k_{12} + k_{21} + k_{10}) - \sqrt{(k_{12} + k_{21} + k_{10})^2 - (4 \times k_{21} \times k_{10})} \right] \qquad \ldots(6)$$

$$k_{10} = \frac{\alpha \times \beta}{k_{21}} \qquad \ldots(7)$$

$$k_{12} = (\alpha + \beta) - (k_{21} - k_{10}) \qquad \ldots(8)$$

$$k_{21} = \frac{(A \times \beta) + (B \times \alpha)}{A + B} \qquad \ldots(9)$$

$$V_c = \frac{D_{iv}}{A + B} \qquad \ldots(10)$$

The following secondary parameters can be calculated from the model-estimated parameters using the equations listed below:

Half-life during the alpha (initial) disposition phase ($t_{1/2}$, α):

$$t_{1/2,\alpha} = \frac{\alpha}{0.693} \qquad \ldots(11)$$

Half-life during the beta (terminal) disposition phase ($t_{1/2}$,β)

$$t_{1/2,\beta} = \frac{0.693}{\beta} \qquad \ldots(12)$$

Systemic clearance (Cl_s):

$$Cl_s = V_c \times k_{10} \qquad \ldots(13)$$

$$Cl_s = \frac{D_{iv}}{AUC} \qquad \ldots(14)$$

Area under the concentration–time curve (AUC):

$$AUC = \frac{A}{\alpha} + \frac{B}{\beta} \qquad \ldots(15)$$

$$AUC = \frac{D_{iv}}{Cl_s} \qquad ...(16)$$

Area under the first moment curve (AUMC)

$$AUMC = \frac{A}{\alpha^2} + \frac{B}{\beta^2} \qquad ...(17)$$

Mean residence time (MRT):

$$MRT = \frac{AUMC}{AUC} \qquad ...(18)$$

Volume of distribution at steady state (V_{ss}):

$$V_{ss} = Cl_s \times MRT = \frac{D_{iv} \times AUMC}{AUC^2} \qquad ...(19)$$

Volume of distribution during the terminal disposition phase (V_β):

$$V_\beta = \frac{Cl_s}{\beta} \qquad ...(20)$$

Bioavailability (*F*) can be estimated when a drug is given by both intravenous and an extravascular route (e.g., orally, subcutaneously, intramuscularly) route using eq. (21).

$$F = \frac{D_{iv} \times AUC_{oral}}{D_{oral} \times AUC_{iv}} \qquad ...(21)$$

In addition, bioavailability can be estimated as a structural parameter of a pharmacokinetic model with simultaneous fit of the oral and intravenous plasma concentrations. This approach was applied to data for 5-fluorouracil (5-FU) given intravenously and orally with the oral dihydropyrimidine dehydrogenase inhibitor eniluracil. As demonstrated for carboxyamidotriazole (CAI), relative bioavailability can be estimated as a structural parameter with simultaneous fit of plasma concentrations achieved following different oral formulations.

When fitting a model to the concentration–time data, the model should fit the data to some degree of precision and accuracy, demonstrate no bias, and follow the rule of parsimony. Generally, a coefficient of variation of up to 50% for clearance and half-life is deemed acceptable for most compounds. A large coefficient of variation for pharmacokinetic parameters may be due to insufficient (e.g., not extensive enough) or improper (e.g., poor time selection) sampling schema. Bias is determined by the inspection of the residual plot and determining whether the model consistently over- or underpredicts the actual concentration. When choosing between several models, the rule of parsimony is followed in that the simplest model that can adequately describe the data should be chosen. A model is validated when it has been demonstrated that extrapolation (e.g., single-dose to multiple-dose or a change in the dose or infusion duration) is accurate and if study conditions are adjusted (e.g., renal function changes) that the model accommodates the changes and maintains the robustness. The limitations of compartmental modeling potentially include the inability of a drug to be described by a single model (e.g., a two-compartment model at lower doses vs a three-compartment model at higher doses) and the oversimplification of body processes (e.g., multiple false assumptions regarding drug distribution). Some of the limitations are due to (1) sampling limited to plasma; (2) variability in the pharmacokinetics between patients; (3) lack of sensitive analytical techniques; (4) drug–drug and drug–formulation vehicle interactions. An advantage of compartmental analysis is that pharmacokinetic linearity is not assumed and can be incorporated into a model during any of the pharmacokinetic processes (e.g., drug absorption, distribution, metabolism, and elimination).

Nonlinear Pharmacokinetic Modeling

Nonlinear pharmacokinetic behavior can be a substantial source of variability in drug exposure and response. Linearity is evaluated by examining dose and time dependence. Dose dependence is assessed by normalizing plasma concentration–time profiles for dose and examining relationships between dose and exposure parameters such as maximum concentration (C_{max}), steady-state concentration (C_{ss}), and the area under the concentration–time curve (AUC). The average value for each exposure parameter is examined and a determination is made if they increase proportionally with increasing dose. Relationships between dose and clearance, half-life, and volume of distribution are also assessed.

Time dependence is evaluated when a drug is given by prolonged infusion or on multiple dosing schedules. During prolonged infusions, a change in C_{ss} over time suggests a change in drug clearance. With repetitive dosing schedules, an increase in pretreatment trough levels over time (in the absence of expected achievement of steady state based on the drugs half-life and dosing schedule) or a change in a pharmacokinetic parameter value suggests a change in drug clearance. For example, changes in AUC or half-life following the first and subsequent doses may suggest that clearance is changing with time. If apparent nonlinearity is not felt to reflect the dosing schedule, assay sensitivity, or interpatient variability, sources for true nonlinearity should be evaluated. Sources for dose- or time-dependent pharmacokinetics following oral or intravenous administration may include saturable gut wall transport or first-pass hepatic metabolism, saturable plasma protein and tissue binding, concentration-dependent renal excretion, capacity-limited metabolism, and enzyme induction or inhibition. In addition, formulation effects may affect the apparent nonlinear behavior of a drug. Nonlinear pharmacokinetic models are employed to describe drug disposition. This model was fit to docetaxel concentrations to explain an apparent nonlinear pharmacokinetic behavior of docetaxel administered at doses of 115 mg/m^2.

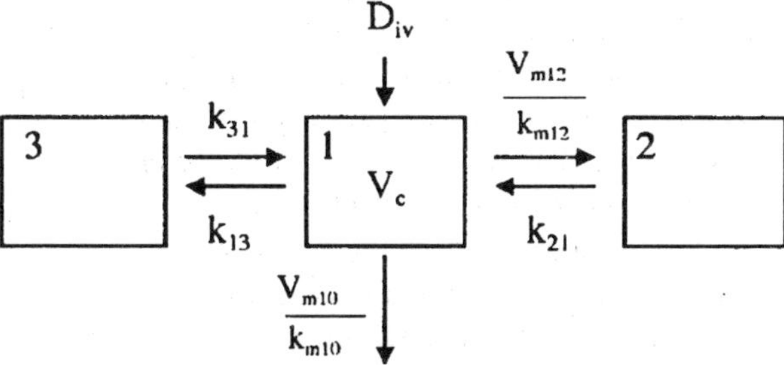

Fig. 4.3. Nonlinear three-compartment pharmacokinetic model that was fitted to docetaxel concentration-time profiles.

Parameter Estimation and Model Assessment

After the appropriate model has been identified (e.g., the model describes the concentration vs time data), pharmacokinetic parameters are calculated using pharmacokinetic modeling software (e.g., ADAPT II, WinNonlin, or other commercially available programs. The goodness of fit of the pharmacokinetic model is based on visual inspection of the observed and fitted concentration–time curve, minimization of the weighted sum of squares, examination of the dispersion of the weighted residuals, and inspection of the standard error, coefficients of variation (CV), and confidence intervals (CI) of each estimated pharmacokinetic parameters. In addition, discrimination between compartmental pharmacokinetic models is guided by minimization of the weighted least-squares, residuals, Akaike information criterion, Schwarz criteria, and the *F*-test.

A main assumption made in pharmacokinetics is that the observations are independent and are measured with homoscedastic, random error. Because the error is normally heteroscedastic or evenly distributed, methods to correct the error are done with weighting and will normally correct the bias. Commonly used algorithms include the generalized least-squares regression, maximum likelihood, maximum *a posteriori* Bayesian (MAP-Bayesian), or weighted least-squares regression. The weighted least-squares regression approach finds the parameter values that will minimize the residuals. This can be accomplished with fixed variances of $1/y$ or $1/y^2$. The maximum likelihood approach determines the parameter values and variance parameters that most likely give rise to the observed value by maximizing this probability. The generalized least-squares regression is a combination of both the weighted least-squares regression and maximum likelihood approaches in a stepwise fashion. At first the variance parameters are fixed while the parameter values are optimized using weighted least-squares regression; then, the parameter values are fixed while the variance parameters are optimized using maximum likelihood; this stepwise approach occurs until the both the parameter values and variance parameters are stable. Finally, the MAP-Bayesian approach is used with sparse data sets or when there is large variance. MAP-Bayesian is a common approach in population pharmacokinetics. In this technique, the parameter values are determined by minimizing actual residuals for that patient and the difference between that patient's parameter values and the population's parameter values. Once the parameters are determined, one should verify that the true global minimum is found and not the local minimum. This is done by overestimating the parameters in the opposite direction from the initial parameter values and verifying that the same final parameter value is achieved upon convergence.

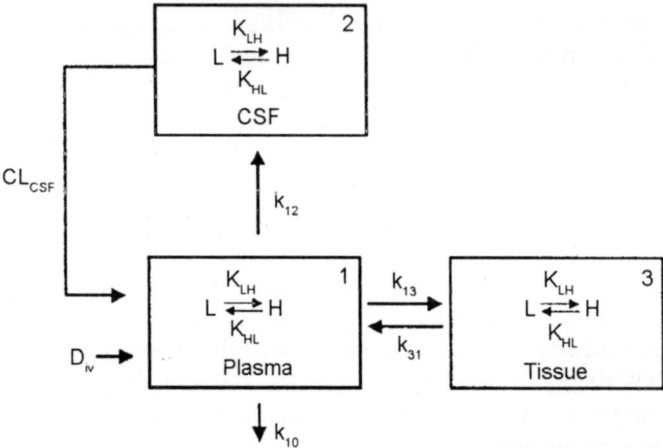

Fig. 4.4. Three-compartment model for topotecan lactone and total concentrations in the plasma and CSF.

The modeling of concentration–time profiles sometimes involves samples from sites other than or in addition to plasma. This may require the development of pharmacokinetic models that are more elaborate than standard compartmental pharmacokinetic models. A three-compartment open model that simultaneously described topotecan lactone and total concentrations in the plasma and cerebrospinal fluid has been described. However, one must always apply the rule of parsimony when distinguishing the model that best fits the data.

Metabolite Kinetics

Many anticancer agents are extensively metabolized to inactive or active metabolites. Pharmacokinetic parameters for a drug metabolite are usually estimated using noncompartmental methods. The AUC ratio of metabolite to parent drug on a molar basis is then calculated to determine relative exposure of metabolite compared to parent compound. Pharmacokinetic parameters can also be estimated using compartmental models that describe the drug metabolite disposition. For example, the plasma disposition of temozolomide and its metabolites were characterized using a one-compartment linear model that had first-order absorption, first-order metabolite formation and elimination, and a peripheral distribution compartment for the metabolite, 4-amino-5-imidazole-carboxamide. An alternative model for temozolomide has been described that incorporates clearance of parent drug via both chemical breakdown to 5-(3-methyltriazen-1-

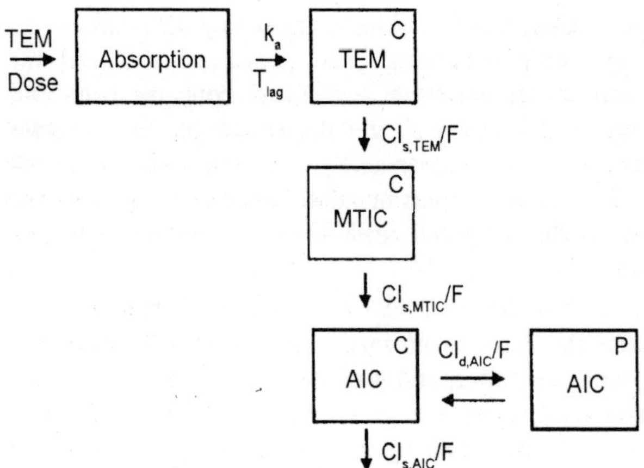

Fig. 4.5. Compartmental model for TEM, MTIC, and AIC concentrations in plasma.

yl)imidazole-4-carboxamide and renal clearance. Pharmacokinetic modeling is a useful tool to be able to describe and predict concentration-time data.

The sampling strategy is the most important first step to describing adequately the pharmacokinetics of a compound. If inadequate sampling occurs, various phenomena may be missed (e.g., a prolong elimination phase). Although noncompartmental analysis does provide a quick and easy determination of the pharmacokinetic parameters, it is based on the assumption that the pharmacokinetics is linear. This assumption can be remedied by analyzing the concentration–time profile with compartmental analysis. Various pharmacokinetic programs are commercially available that can aid in compartmental analysis of data. Compartmental analysis can involve a simple linear two-compartment model or more complicated models that incorporate nonlinear processes. As early clinical trials incorporate more pharmacokinetic and pharmacodynamic endpoints, the role of pharmacokinetic modeling will continue to grow.

Physiologically Based Pharmacokinetic Models

Although technical advances in drug discovery are identifying an increasing number of biologically active compounds, many of these are still eliminated during the selection and development phases. Historically, a high proportion of these failures have been due to poor pharmacokinetic properties. To reduce this failure rate, candidate compounds are now being screened for ADME properties (absorption, distribution, metabolism, excretion) and the derived parameters are then being used to predict their human pharmacokinetic profiles. These predicted profiles not only help to select the best candidates for development but can also provide a starting dose for the first clinical studies. Such predictions can, therefore, drastically reduce the time and expense of drug research and development. Furthermore, because ADME issues are considered during the selection process, fewer compounds are now dropping out of development because of pharmacokinetic reasons.

The approaches used to predict human pharmacokinetics tend to fall into two categories: empirical interspecies scaling and physiologically based pharmacokinetic (PBPK) modeling. With the recent developments of in silico and in vitro tools together with a marked increase in computing power, PBPK modeling is rapidly becoming a powerful tool for predicting human pharmacokinetics. The present chapter reviews recent developments in physiologically based methods for predicting human pharmacokinetics. First, some general background information is given on these methods. A number of applications in drug research are also described, together with some strategic issues that may be considered when applying such simulation tools.

Disposition models

Physiologically based pharmacokinetic models divide the body into compartments, including the eliminating organs, e.g., kidney and liver, and noneliminating tissue compartments, e.g., fat, muscle, and brain, which are connected by the circulatory system. The models use physiological and species-specific parameters such as blood flow rates and tissue volumes to describe the pharmacokinetic processes. These physiological parameters are coupled with physicochemical, biochemical and compound specific parameters (e.g., tissue/blood partition coefficients and metabolic clearance) to predict the plasma and tissue concentration vs. time profiles of a compound in an in vivo animal or human system.

Once a model has been developed, the concentrations in the various tissues can be determined by using the following mass balance (Eqn. 22):

drug concentration in tissue =
rate of drug distribution into tissue
– rate of drug distribution out
– rate of drug elimination within the tissue ...(22)

Depending on the drug and tissue, the distribution can be perfusion rate or diffusion rate limited. Perfusion rate limited kinetics tend to occur with relatively low-molecular-weight, hydrophobic drugs which have no problem crossing the lipid barrier of the cell wall. In this case, the process limiting the penetration of the drug into the cells is the rate at which it is delivered to the tissue, i.e., blood flow is the limiting process. By contrast diffusion rate limited kinetics occur with more-polar and/or larger drugs that do not freely dissolve in the lipid of the cell membrane and, therefore, have difficulty in penetrating into the cell. In this case, the diffusion of drug across the membrane, which is independent of blood flow, becomes the limiting process.

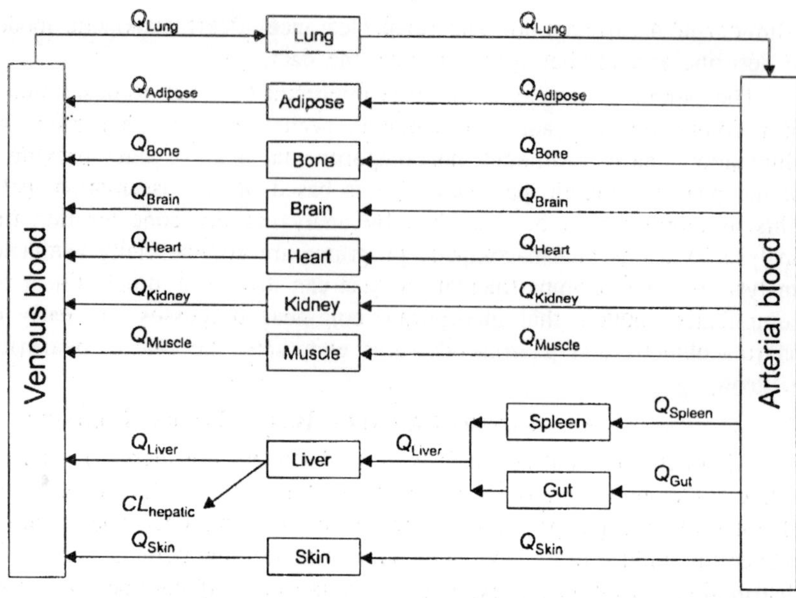

Fig. 4.6. Examples of a physiologically based pharmacokinetic (PBPK) model.

For perfusion limitation, the rate of change of drug concentration in a tissue, where no elimination occurs, can be described in Eqn. 23:

$$V\frac{dC}{dt} = Q\left(C_{in} \frac{C_{in}}{K_p}\right) \qquad \ldots(23)$$

where V is the physical volume of the tissue, C the drug concentration in tissue, Q the blood flow to the tissue, C_{in} the drug concentration entering the tissue, and K_p the partition of the drug between tissue and blood.

When diffusion rate limitation occurs, diffusion to and from the extra- cellular space must be taken into account (*Eqn.* 24):

$$V_e\frac{dC_e}{dt} = Q(C_{in} - C_e) - P(C_e - C_i) \qquad \ldots(24)$$

where P is the membrane permeability coefficient, C_e the free extra- cellular drug concentration, C_i the free intracellular drug concentration, and V_e the anatomical extracellular volume.

With organs such as liver, where elimination can occur, the rate of elimination must be included in the mass balance equation. The rate of elimination is described in Eqn. 25:

$$\text{Rate of elimination} = CL_{int}Ct \qquad \ldots(25)$$

where CL_{int} is the intrinsic clearance of the drug from that organ, and C_t the concentration in tissue. In some instances, C_t may also be replaced by C_{vt}(concentration in the venous blood leaving the tissue equivalent to C_{in}/K_p). A comparative validation is still needed to find out which of these terms (C_t or C_{vt}) is most relevant for the in vivo situation. This term can then be inserted into the mass balance equation, such as that for the perfusion limitation (Eqn. 26):

$$V\frac{dC}{dt} = Q\left(C_{in} - \frac{C_{in}}{K_p}\right) - CL_{\text{int}}C_t \qquad \ldots(26)$$

As the above equations indicate, a considerable amount of information is required to construct physiologically based pharmacokinetic models. Thus, estimates of tissue/blood partitioning and intrinsic clearance are required for each drug. Recently, tissue composition models have been developed which allow the tissue/blood partition coefficients to be estimated either in silico or to be measured experimentally as physicochemical descriptors. These approaches have dramatically reduced the amount of experimentation needed to support the use of flow models, considerably extending their utility. Such approaches to predict tissue distribution are discussed elsewhere.

Absorption Models

Oral absorption is determined by complex mechanisms, which are governed by physiology and biochemical processes (e.g., pH in the gastrointestinal tract (GIT), gastric emptying, intestinal transit, active transport, and gastrointestinal metabolism), drug-specific properties (e.g., lipophilicity, pK_a, solubility, particle size, permeability, metabolic stability) and formulation factors (e.g., release kinetics, dissolution kinetics). These are some of the main determinants which could be important parts of an absorption model. The interplay of parameters describing these processes determines the rate and extent of absorption.

The available simulation tools to predict oral absorption in animals and humans have been recently reviewed. Different absorption models have been developed and in part described in the literature. These GIT models are developed to a degree that they are commercially available as software tools. In brief, these models are physiologically based transit models segmenting the GIT into different compartments, where the kinetics of transit, dissolution, and uptake are described by sets of differential equations. The simulation models for oral absorption use a variety of measured or calculated in vitro input data such as permeability, solubility, pK_a, and dose.

Utility of Physiologically Based PK Models

A number of publications illustrate the potential of this approach, both for predicting human pharmacokinetics and for mechanistic purposes. The utility of physiologically based pharmacokinetic models to drug development and rational drug discovery candidate selection was also reviewed recently. The following advantages of the mechanistic PBPK modeling framework can be considered: (a) They predict plasma (blood) and tissue PK of drug candidates prior to in vivo experiments; (b) They support a better mechanistic understanding of PK properties and help the development of more-rationale PK–PD relationships from tissue kinetic data predicted, thus facilitating a more-rational decision during clinical candidate selection. And (c) they allow the extrapolation across species, routes of administration, and dose levels. Two of these applications are discussed below.

Applications of Physiologically Based PK Models

Generic Simulations During Drug Discovery

During drug discovery, considerable resources are required to assess the pharmacokinetic properties of potential clinical candidates in vivo in animals, and there is interest in optimizing the use of such testing by applying simulation techniques.

Physiologically based models have the potential to do this by predicting pharmacokinetics based on in vitro and in silico input data. Such approaches may help to rank compounds based on their predicted profiles, provide the project teams with a balanced view on the properties of potential drug candidates, and help to select the optimal molecules for further in vivo experiments. However, before such tools are routinely used and accepted, there is a need for extensive validation.

Our in-house developed PBPK model has been applied in a generic mode to predict plasma profiles after i.v. and p.o. dosing to the rat in a number of discovery projects. The predictions were made on the basis of a minimum of measured data, namely calculated log *P*, calculated pK_a values, calculated protein binding, and intrinsic clearance determined in hepatocytes. The results support the use of the generic PBPK approach at the early stages of drug discovery. Even when based on a minimum of data, the models are able to give reasonable initial estimates of the expected pharmacokinetics of novel compounds. The generic PBPK approach based upon minimal input data is better able to rank the PK properties of compounds across different chemical classes than within a close series. In addition, a good prediction of in vivo solubility still represents a major challenge for the prediction of the oral absorption profile of low-soluble compounds. At this time, it is recommended that generic PBPK models should only be applied for lead optimization after verification of the simulations with in vivo PK for a few compounds of a given chemical class. Such verification will help to identify invalid model assumptions or important missing processes, where additional data is needed, and will allow an assessment of the prediction error expected.

Prediction of Pharmacokinetics in Humans

To reduce failures related to pharmacokinetic (PK) issues in the drug development process and to find out about the suitability of compounds for an intended dosing regimen, it is important to predict human PK as early as possible. Empirical methods (e.g., allometric scaling) have been traditionally used for this purpose. Although in some cases, these methods give good predictions, their physiological basis and predictive value is questionable. Recently, mechanistic physiologically based PK (PBPK) models have been developed. These models are mathematically more complex, and until recently their use in drug development has been limited. Recently, empirical and PBPK approaches were compared for the prediction of human PK using 19 Roche compounds having reached clinical development, covering a broad range of physicochemical properties. Predicted values (PK parameters, plasma concentrations) were compared to observed values to assess the accuracy of the prediction methods.

The PBPK approach gave more-realistic predictions than the classical empirical methods for all 19 compounds. A greater proportion of the predicted parameters (e.g., C_{max}, AUC, $t_{1/2}$) and plasma concentrations were within twofold error of the observed values. For example, 76% and 42% of the compounds had a predicted AUC within twofold error of the observed value using PBPK and the *Dedrick* approach, respectively. Any poor prediction was generally a result of biliary elimination and/or enterohepatic recirculation processes that were not incorporated into the model.

In addition to improved prediction accuracy, PBPK approaches offer more potential in the early stages of the drug development process, including a reduction in the quantity of animal in vivo input data required, as well as greater insights into the mechanistic understanding of the compound characteristics, ultimately resulting in an improved selection process. The use of both empirical methods and physiologically based models to predict human pharmacokinetic profiles can help to select the best candidates for drug development. They can also help to select doses for the first clinical studies.

Allometric scaling explores the mathematical relationships between pharmacokinetic parameters from various animal species, and these can then be used to predict the corresponding values in other species, including human. Such methods are also built to some extent on physiological principles. They are relatively easy to apply but resource demanding for the collection of in vivo data in animals. Nevertheless, their application has led to useful predictions of individual pharmacokinetic parameters (e.g., clearance, fraction absorbed, volume of distribution).

Physiologically based models (PBPK) can be used to explore, and help to explain, the mechanisms that lie behind species differences in pharmacokinetics and drug metabolism. Such models can provide a rational basis for interspecies scaling of individual parameters which can then be integrated to provide quantitative and time-dependent estimates of both the plasma and tissue concentrations in humans. Furthermore, being mechanistically based, they can be used diagnostically to generate information on new compounds and to understand the sensitivity of the in vivo profile to compound properties. Despite this great potential, the use of PBPK models in drug discovery and development has been relatively limited. However, recent developments of in silico and in vitro models, which can provide estimates of these input parameters, have dramatically reduced the amount of experimental work required. Another reason for the limited use of PBPK models relates to their mathematical complexity, so that a high level of expertise is needed to develop such models. Again, recent improvements in the availability of well-validated and user-friendly software packages should remove this barrier. In the very near future, therefore, the use of physiologically based models is likely to increase dramatically in the prediction of concentration–time profiles and as diagnostic tools to better understand potential development compounds.

Compartmental Modeling

The pharmacokinetic profile of a drug is described by the processes of absorption, distribution, metabolism, and excretion. The disposition of a drug in the body may be further delineated by mathematical modeling. These models are based on the concept that the body may be viewed as a series of compartments in which the drug is distributed. If the compartmental concept is considered literally, then each tissue and organ become an individual compartment. However, in pharmacokinetic modeling, several organs or tissues exhibit similar characteristics in drug deposition and are often considered the same compartment. The pharmacokinetic profiles of many drugs may be explained using one- or two-compartment models, but more complex models exist and, with advances in computer software, the ability to describe drug disposition has increased. The use of models does not mean that the drug distributes into distinct physiological compartments, but that these mathematical models adequately describe the fate of the drug in the human body.

One-Compartment Models

In the one-compartment model the entire body is considered as one unit. The drug is administered into the compartment and distributed throughout the compartment (the body) instantaneously. Similarly, the drug is eliminated directly from the one compartment at a rate measured by k_{el}, the elimination rate constant. The time course of the drug, as measured in the readily accessible blood or plasma, is typically graphed as a log concentration vs. time profile. The dotted line demonstrates the time course after intravenous administration and the solid line demonstrates the time course after oral administration. Since intravenous administration does not have an absorption phase, the time course of drug in the plasma is linear. For oral administration, the drug concentration on the blood is slower to reach a peak due to absorptive processes of the GI tract.

Two-Compartment Models

In this model, the drug is administered into the central compartment and then there is a time lag due to slower distribution into other tissues and organs. These other organs are represented by the peripheral compartment(s). More complex models may be developed if distribution to other organs occurs at different rates that can be mathematically differentiated. In the two-compartment model, equilibrium is reached between the central and peripheral compartments and this marks the end of the distribution phase. The beginning of the distribution phase may be observed graphically by an initial rapid decline after peaking in the drug concentration in the central compartment (represented by the plasma/blood). Rate constants may be estimated for drug movement between the central and peripheral compartments, but drug elimination from the body is assumed to occur from the central compartment.

As mentioned previously, more complex models may be developed including models in which the number of compartments into which the drug distributes is not assumed in the initial modeling.

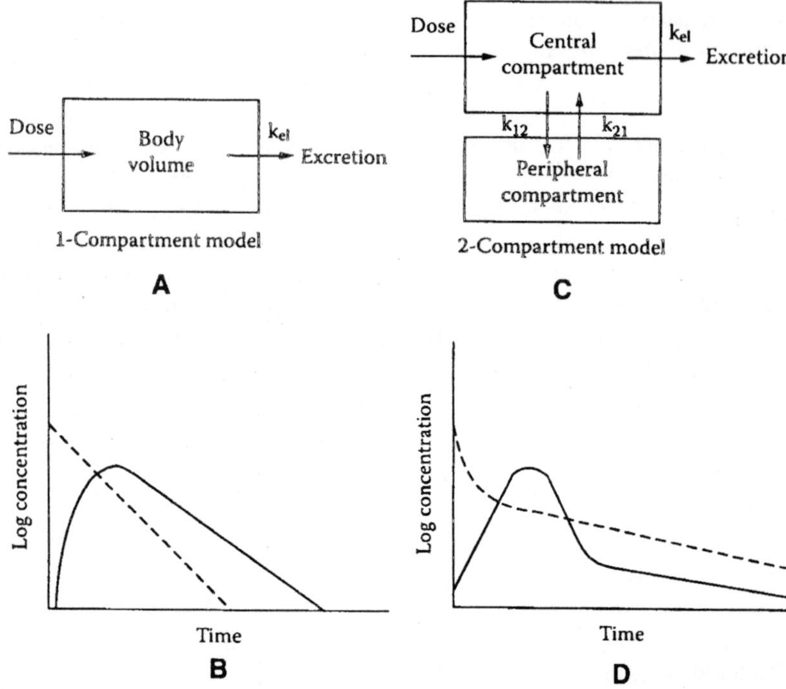

Fig. 4.7. A–Schematic representation of a one-compartment model. B–Log plasma concentration vs. time curve after intravenous (---) and oral (—) administration. C–Schematic representation of a two-compartment model. D–Log plasma concentration vs. time curve after intravenous (---) and oral (—) administration.

Elimination Kinetics

The concept of zero- or first-order kinetics may be utilized to describe any rate process in pharmacokinetics. Therefore, if we are discussing drug absorption, a drug exhibits zero-order kinetics if a constant amount of drug is absorbed regardless of dose. Conversely, a drug exhibits first-order absorption kinetics if the amount absorbed is dependent on dose, i.e., is a fraction of the dose. Similarly, when considering drug excretion, ethanol exhibits zero-order elimination kinetics because a constant amount of drug is excreted per unit time regardless of the drug concentration (unless processes become saturated). Most drugs exhibit first-order elimination kinetics in which a constant fraction of drug is eliminated per unit time.

Zero-order elimination kinetics are described by the following equation:

$$C = C_0 - kt \qquad \ldots(27)$$

where C = drug concentration at time t, C_0 = the concentration at time zero or the initial concentration, and k = the elimination rate constant.

A plot of this equation is linear with a slope, $-k$, and a y-intercept, C_0. The elimination half-life may be calculated from this equation for a drug that exhibits zero-order elimination. When $t = t_{1/2}$, then $C = 1/2\ C_0$ the initial or peak concentration. This results in the following equation:

$$t_{1/2} = 1/2\ C_0/k \qquad \ldots(28)$$

This equation has a concentration term, C_0, indicating that the half-life is variable and dependent on drug concentration. Changes in pharmacokinetic parameters that occur as a function of dose or drug concentration are referred to as nonlinear pharmacokinetic processes. Nonlinearity is usually due to saturation of protein binding, hepatic metabolism, or active renal transport of the drug.

First-order elimination kinetics are described by the equation:

$$C = C_0 e^{-kt} \qquad \ldots(29)$$

Taking the natural logarithm of this equation and plotting it semilogarithmically results in a linear graph with a slope of $-k$, and a y-intercept of ln C_0. Again, to determine the half-life, $1/2\ C_0$ is substituted into the equation to give:

$$1/2\ C_0 = C_0 e^{-kt1/2} \quad ...(30)$$

Taking natural logs and solving for $t_{1/2}$:

$$t_{1/2} = 0.693/k \quad ...(31)$$

It is important to note that the elimination half-life is a derived term, and any process that changes k will change the half-life of the drug. Factors that may affect pharmacokinetic parameters are discussed elsewhere, but in this example may include disease states, changes in urinary pH, changes in plasma protein binding, and coadministration of other drugs.

Physiological Models

An alternative method of building a pharmacokinetic profile of a drug in the body is to utilize anatomic and physiological informaion. Such a model does not make assumptions about body compartments or first-order processes for drug absorption and elimination. The first step in such modeling is to decide whether drug distribution into a particular tissue is perfusion rate or membrane transport limited. These decisions are based on the physicochemical characteristics of the drug and physiological conditions in addition to reference to any experimental data. In order to write a mass balance equation, blood flow, Q, and the volume, V, of the organ or tissue of interest is needed and may be obtained from the literature. The other parameters, venous drug concentration, C_v, and the partition coefficient, R, are determined experimentally. A simple mass balance equation may be written as:

$$V_t \times dC_t/dt = Q_t \times [C_v - C_t/Rt] \quad ...(32)$$

where t = tissue.

Mass balance equations may be constructed for each organ or tissue considered and algebraic equations added to account for growth, changes in tissue weight ratios, and other physiological parameters. The advantage of this modeling over the more traditional compartmental method is provision of a time course of drug distribution to any organ or tissue, and this model allows estimation of the effects of changing physiological parameters on tissue concentrations. Disadvantages include the need for complex mathematical equations and the lack of data on the physiological parameters necessary to construct the differential equations.

Pharmacokinetic–Pharmacodynamic Correlations

Pharmacodynamics (PD) may be defined as the quantitative relationship between the measured plasma or tissue concentration of the active moiety and the magnitude of the observed pharmacological effect(s). The study of pharmacokinetics (PK) has been defined previously. A PK/PD model is a mathematical description of the relationship. Knowledge of the model and model parameter estimates permits prediction of concentration vs. time and effect vs. time profiles for different dosing regimens. Different drugs are characterized by different PK and PD models and by differences in model parameters such as volume of distribution and receptor affinity. Understanding the PK/PD model permits comparison of the pharmacological properties for different drugs. For a specific compound, there may be significant variation in model parameters between individuals. PK/PD modeling allows assessment of the contribution of the variability in model parameters to the overall variability in drug response. To fully understand the significance of PK/PD modeling, it is important to note that the observed effect vs. time profile for a particular individual is determined by several factors. These include: (1) drug input dose, rate, and route of administration; (2) intrinsic PK drug properties; and (3) intrinsic PD drug properties. Modeling allows estimation of PK/PD parameters. Further, PK/PD modeling provides dose–response curves for the onset, magnitude, and duration of effects that can be utilized to optimize dose and dosing regimens. Models have been described for reversible and irreversible drug effects and for a range of drug classes including analgesics, benzodiazepines, and anticonvulsants.

5

POPULATION PHARMACOKINETICS

Population pharmacokinetics (PPK) is an area of clinical pharmacology, which aims at the quantitative assessment of between and within individual variability in drug absorption, distribution, metabolism, and excretion. The purpose of PPK is to provide quantitative guidelines for dosage individualization/ optimization. Ideally, the clinician could select an appropriate dose and dose interval once a patient has been adequately characterized by history, physical examination, and clinical laboratory tests. However, all predictive techniques are essentially imperfect. Therefore, a dosage regimen predicted for an individual may differ to some degree from the optimum regimen. Sources of variation that contribute to differences between expectation and outcome are usually categorized as interindividual and residual in nature. Even though expected parameter values can be calculated for an individual patient based on previous research and experience, the parameter values of a particular patient at hand may differ from the expected values because of interindividual variability. Residual variation includes intraindividual variability (random changes in a patient's parameter values over time), interoccasion variability (change in a patient's parameter from one occasion (period) to another), drug concentration measurement error, and model misspecification errors arising because all mathematical calculations for predicting parameter values are oversimplifications of reality. Interindividual variability in pharmacokinetics is viewed by many incorrectly as a nuisance factor that has to be overcome, often through complex study designs and control schemes, and reduced through restrictive study inclusion criteria. The subjects of pharmacokinetic studies are usually healthy volunteers or highly selected patients. Traditionally, the average behavior of a group (i.e., the mean plasma concentration-time profile) has been the main focus of interest. Study design and selection of volunteers that are rigidly standardized so that they are as homogeneous as possible are typical features of pharmacokinetic investigations. These studies are, therefore, often performed under artificial conditions that do not represent the intended clinical use of the drug. In contrast to traditional pharmacokinetic evaluation, the population approach to pharmacokinetic evaluation encompasses some or all of the following features:

1. It seeks to obtain relevant pharmacokinetic information in patients who are representative of the target population to be treated with the drug.
2. It recognizes variability such as intersubject, intrasubject, interoccasion variability as an important feature that should be identified and measured during drug development or evaluation.
3. It seeks to explain variability by identifying factors of demographic, pathophysiological, environmental, or drug-related origin that may influence the pharmacokinetic behavior of a drug.
4. It seeks to quantitatively estimate the magnitude of the unexplained part of the variability in the patient population.

The magnitude of the unexplained (random) variability is important because the efficacy and safety of a drug may decrease as unexplainable variability increases. As the drug levels outside the target range become more likely, the greater the uncompensated variability in the relationship of dosage to steady state drug concentration. In addition to interindividual variability, the degree to which steady state drug concentrations in individuals typically vary about their long-term average is also important. Concentrations appear to vary due to inexplicable day-to-day or week-to-week kinetic (i.e., interoccasion) variability and due to errors in concentration measurement. Estimates of this kind of variability (residual intrasubject, interoccasion variability) are important for therapeutic drug monitoring using the empiric Bayes approach. The knowledge of the relationship between dose, concentration, response, and pathophysiology is essential for designing dosing strategies for rational therapeutics that may not necessarily require therapeutic drug monitoring.

Pharmacokinetic variability is affected by several factors, which can be classified as either intrinsic or extrinsic factors. Intrinsic factors include demographics (gender, body-weight etc.), genetics (e.g., enzyme polymorphism) and physiological or pathophysiological states. Extrinsic factors are mainly environmental such as smoking and diet. Drug to drug interactions, compliance to medication, and several other extrinsic factors also contribute to variability. Resolving the above issues provides a framework for defining optimum dosing strategies in a population, a subpopulation, or for the individual patient. Recognizing the importance of resolving these issues in drug development has led to a surge in recent years in the application of PPK to new drug development and the regulatory process. A comprehensive guide to the PPK approach is now available from the US Food and Drug Administration.

Advantages of PPK

There are some potential advantages to PPK when compared with the traditional approach to studying drug pharmacokinetics. Unlike the traditional studies in which subjects are sampled intensively, the population approach to studying the pharmacokinetics of a drug involves sparse sampling. It allows pharmacokinetic studies to be conducted in special populations such as neonates, elderly, AIDS, and cancer patients where the number of samples to be obtained per subject are limited because of ethical and medical concerns. Sparse sampling also helps to lower the cost of the bioanalytical component in drug development programs.

The sparse sampling approach for characterizing PPK yields better estimates of intersubject variability than the traditional approaches that yield positively biased estimates of this measure of dispersion. A combination of robust (accurate and precise) estimates of intersubject variability and the mean parameter value for a drug is useful for selecting a starting dose for drug therapy in a patient, and allows Bayesian feedback analysis to be performed for dosage individualization.

Population pharmacokinetic analysis provides not only an opportunity to estimate variability, but also to explain it. Variability is usually characterized in terms of fixed and random effects. The fixed effects are the population average values of pharmacokinetic parameters, which may in turn be a function of patient characteristics discussed above. The random effects quantify the amount of pharmacokinetic variability, which is not explained by the fixed effects, i.e., inter-subject variability, interoccasion variability, intraindividual, and residual variability. Karlsson and Sheiner have demonstrated that the lack of separation of interoccasion variability from residual intrasubject variability produced bias in estimation of population pharmacokinetic parameters.

Disadvantages of PPK

A disadvantage of this approach is that it requires highly skilled pharmacokineticists (pharmacometricians). The methodology is resource-intensive and can be time-consuming. In the sections that follow, we discuss the statistical theory of PPK, review several methods and software programs to be used to estimate PPK parameters, address the design and analysis of PPK studies and some applications of PPK to pharmaceutical technology.

Models and Methods

Models

Individual model

The pharmacokinetic model for estimating individual pharmacokinetic parameters can be written as

$$y_j^m = f_i(\phi_j, x_j) \quad \text{...(1)}$$

where y_j^m is the model predicted vector of values of y_j, when the pharmacokinetic parameters take the value ϕ_j, and where f_j stands for the functional relationship (i.e., pharmacokinetic model) between the predictions and the ϕ_j. x_j is a also a function of known quantities (dose D and time t_j). Assuming measurement errors to be zero, model would be rewritten as follows:

$$y_j = f_j(\phi_j, x_j) \quad \text{...(2)}$$

assuming that the model-predicted values, y_j^m, are equal to the measured values y_j. In practice, however, the observations must be related to individual true parameters ϕ_j through a somewhat more elaborate model:

$$y_j = f_j(\phi_j, x_j) + \varepsilon_j \quad \text{...(3)}$$

where the vector ε_j is a sample of the measurement noise E_j.

Maximum likelihood (ML) estimation can be performed if the statistics of the measurement noise E_j are known. This estimate is the value of the parameters for which the observation of the vector, y_j, is the most probable. If we assume the probability density function (pdf) of E_j to be normal, with zero mean and uniform variance, ML estimation reduces to ordinary least squares estimation. An estimate, ϕ_j^*, of the true *j*th individual parameters ϕ_j can be obtained through optimization of some objective function, $O_j(\theta_j)$. Model is assumed to be a natural choice if each measurement is assumed to be equally precise for all values of y_j. This is usually the case in concentration-effect modeling. Considering the multiplicative log-normal error model, the observed concentration y is given by:

$$y_j = f_j(\phi_j, x_j) * e^{\varepsilon_j} \quad \text{...(4)}$$

where ε_j is assumed to follow a log-normal distribution with median 1 and constant coefficient of variation CV. The variance of the prediction of the deviations is proportional to the square of the predicted response. The log-normal error model is often appropriate if measurements can only be positive and if they become less precise when the measured value increases. This is often true of pharmacokinetic models. However, other error models may be used in practice such as a combination of the additive and log-normal error model to improve prediction at the lower limit of assay precision where variance may be assumed constant, and the power function model, where the variance of the deviations is assumed proportional to some power (which is to be estimated) of the predicted response.

When the estimation procedure is clearly specified, an approximate covariance matrix of the estimate, S_j, can also be calculated. This matrix reflects the degree of precision of the estimate, and depends on the experimental design, parameters, and the noise statistics. A well-designed experiment with small random fluctuations will lead to precise estimations ("small" covariance), while a small number of uninformative data and/or a high level of noise will produce unreliable estimates ("large" covariance).

Population model

Unlike the individual model discussed above, a more elaborate statistical model is required to deal with sparse pharmacokinetic data. In formulating the model, it is recognized that overall variability in the measured (response) data in a sample of individuals reflects both measurement error and intersubject variability. The observed response (e.g., concentration) in an individual within the framework of population (regression) non-linear random mixed-effect models can be described as:

$$y_{ij} = f_{ij}\ (\varphi_{ij}, x_{ij}) + \varepsilon_{ij} \qquad \ldots(5)$$

where y_{ij} for $i = 1, \ldots, n_j$ are the observed data (e.g., blood or urinary levels at time points x_{ij}) of the jth subject. Model is defined for all $j = 1, \ldots, N$, where N is the number of subjects in the sample. f_{ij} is a specified function for predicting the response in the jth subject (e.g., one or several exponentials). φ_j and ε_{ij} are as previously described. From the notations, it is clear that the population model is indeed a collection of models for individual observations. Various doses and/or dosage regimens and/ or administration routes are generally used in patient drug therapy and clinical trials. Also, diverse administration schedules (single-dose and multiple dosing) might be used and several responses (e.g., plasma and urinary drug levels) might be measured. Correspondingly, in drug-related "*population applications*," the functions f_{ij} will differ across individuals. Contrarily, it is realistic to assume that the set of underlying structural parameters (in this case, pharmacokinetic parameters) is qualitatively the same for all individuals and that the parameters vary quantitatively among individuals. Mathematically this can be written as

$$\phi_j = g(\theta, z_j) + \eta_j \qquad \ldots(6)$$

where g is a known function that describes the expected value of ϕ_j as a function of known individual specific covariates z_j, such as weight, age, disease state, concomitant medication, etc. and the vector of population parameters θ. Covariates are assumed constant within an individual, for simplicity. However, time- varying covariates can also be incorporated in the model by permitting individual pharmacokinetic parameters to depend on i as well as j. η_j represents the random variation of the individual parameter vectors around the population prediction. The η_j is usually assumed to be independent across individuals (i.e., η_j, η_l are independent for $j \neq 1$). The individual ϕ_j is assumed to arise from some (multivariate) probability $F(\theta)$.

In the mixed-effects context, the collection of population parameters is composed of a "population-typical value" (generally the mean) and of a "population-variability value" (generally the variance-covariance matrix). The mean and variance are the first two "moments" of a probability distribution. They build a minimal set of hyperparameters or "population characteristics" for it, which is sufficient (in a statistical sense) when F is taken as normal or log-normal.

Thus, a pharmacokinetic model that describes the time-course of the drug in the body in a specific individual, a model describing the relationship between patient characteristics and the pharmacokinetic model parameters, a variance model for residual random variability, and a population model for intersubject random variability, which describes the unexplained random variability of the model parameters in the population of subjects studied are essential for describing a population pharmacokinetic model.

Data Type

Two types of data can be used in population analysis: experimental data and observational (or population) pharmacokinetic data, which are sparse in nature. Experimental (EP) data arise from traditional pharmacokinetic studies characterized by controlled conditions of drug dosing and extensive blood sampling. EP data are usually analyzed per subject for the estimation of individual parameters that are later used for the estimation of population parameters. Population pharmacokinetic data are collected, most often, as a supplement in a study designed and carried out for another purpose, or during routine clinical care where the data is of the observational type. A detailed contrast of these two types of data and their collection procedures has been given by Sheiner and Beal. Observational data are characterized by minimal control and few design restrictions: the dosing history is subject-specific; the amount of pharmacokinetic data collected from each subject varies, the timing of blood sampling in relation to drug administration differs, and the number of samples per patient, one to six, is typically small. Unlike EP data, PPK data do not lend themselves to the estimation of individual subject pharmacokinetic parameters because of sparseness. Population pharmacokinetic parameters can only be estimated from the data using some of the global methods discussed below.

Methods for Estimating Population Pharmacokinetic Parameters

Over the past two and half decades, a variety of methods have been proposed for the characterization of PPK of drugs. A discussion of some of the methods followed with a presentation of their performance will be the focus of this section. Some of the methods will be discussed in detail, while others will not be, because of their infrequent use. The goals of the analysis and the data- type determine the method selected for the analysis.

Naive average data approach

The above applies to studies in which the drug administration and the sampling schedules are identical for all subjects. The analysis consists of computing the average value of the data for each sampling time followed by fitting a model $y^m = f(\phi)$ to the mean-data n-vector $\bar{y} = (\bar{y}_1, \ldots, \bar{y}_n)'$ and estimating the best-fit parameter values ϕ^*. The latter notation (ϕ^*) is used to distinguish it from individual estimates, denoted by $\hat{\phi}$.

The Naive average data (NAD) approach is attractive because of its simplicity. One unique fitting is sufficient for obtaining estimates of parameters describing the mean response. ϕ^* components are quite often interpreted as "mean" parameter values. Correspondingly, $\hat{\mu}_{NAD}$ will be used for ϕ^* in the latter. The method is widely applicable in EP studies with standardized designs, and examples of these include bioavailability, bioequivalence, and dose- proportionality studies. Because of smoothing effect of averaging, mean data generally look nicer than individual data, and better fitting often results when compared with individual data.

Several drawbacks of this approach must be pointed out. The use of NAD to establish a pharmacokinetic model may be misleading. Data averaging can, quite often, produce a distorted picture of the response. Averaging of monoexponential data from two subjects with very different half-lives has been shown to produce a mean curve that exhibits an apparent biexponential decay. Sometimes the opposite situation is the case. The smoothing effect of the averaging will tend to obscure peculiarities that can be seen in individual data. The existence of secondary peaks in the plasma level, time-course of individuals, may be undetectable in the average curve if the rebounds occur at different time-points.

NAD also performs poorly in terms of parameter estimation. The reference to individual data disappears after data averaging. All sources of variability are confounded. The average concentration curve derived with the NAD approach does not necessarily follow the individual model function. A wrong model may be obtained. Undefined statistical uncertainties and large "unknown" animal variations might smooth the average response curve in an unpredictable manner. Thus, the NAD estimate $\hat{\mu}_{NAD}$ should not, as a general rule, be regarded as a valuable estimate of the expected value of pharmacokinetic parameters. This rule holds even if the true model, that is, the one that adequately describes the individual data, has been used for the fitting.

The essential parametric non-linearity of pharmacokinetic models is responsible for this. Exceptions to this rule occur when the signal-to-noise ratio is small. This is the case when variability contributes less to the spread in observations than other sources of fluctuation (interoccasion variability, measurement error, and model misspecification). This situation might be seen when concentrations are measured in standardized laboratory animals. The quality of estimates may be improved by using averaging methods other than straightforward arithmetic mean. These ad hoc solutions do not fundamentally solve the problems described above. Moreover, no estimate of pure interindividual variability can be obtained with the NAD approach because it tends to mask variability rather than reveal it. Thus, the NAD approach is not a reliable method for pharmacokinetic data analysis.

Naive pooled data approach

Sheiner and Beal proposed the Naive pooled data (NPD) approach for the method in which all data from all individuals are considered as arising from one unique individual. Unlike the NAD approach, the NPD approach is far more general. It can easily deal with experimental data, non-standard data, and routine pharmacokinetic data. After a unique fitting of all data at once, parameter estimates are obtainable. It may perform well when variations between subjects are small. This is occasionally the case in a group of homogeneous laboratory animals from a given strain, but it is rarely true for humans. The drawbacks of NPD are the same as those of NAD, as has been repeatedly pointed out. The NPD approach tends to confound individual differences and diverse sources of variability in a manner different from the NAD approach, but with similar negative consequences. In addition, estimate of the dispersion of parameters in the population is not provided.

Extrapolation of mean outcomes on the basis of the set of estimates obtained should be done with caution. These problems notwithstanding, it has been shown by Shafer and his coworkers that for several drugs used in anesthesia, a pooled analysis approach provided population mean parameters that, when prospectively tested, accurately predicted drug concentrations after drug administration by a computer-controlled infusion pump.

The data, in all circumstances, originated from well-controlled experiments with extensive sampling. That is, the data were of the EP type. Moreover, the NPD analysis provided similar population mean parameter estimates when compared to several other population analysis methods. These findings are in contrast with an earlier simulation study that showed that the NPD approach provided biased estimates of the population mean parameters even when a well-balanced experimental study design was used. The discrepancy may be due to the large amount of interindividual variability present or inappropriate weighting scheme used in the latter study.

Imbalance and confounding correlations present in a data set pose serious problems for the NPD approach. These features are prevalent in observational data and make the NPD approach inappropriate for this type of data. When the design of the study correlates with the outcome, confounding correlations occur. Confounding correlations is usually prevented with randomization. This, however, is not guaranteed with observational data. Thus, the NPD approach is not a reliable method for analysis of PPK data.

Two-stage approach

With this approach, individual parameters are estimated in the first stage by separately fitting each subject's data and combined in the second stage to obtain population parameter estimates. The salient features of the methods that constitute the two-stage approach will be discussed briefly.

Standard two-stage method

Population characteristics of each parameter are estimated as the empirical mean (arithmetic or geometric) and variance of the individual estimates ϕ_j. Standard two-stage (STS) has been recommended as a very simple and valuable approach for pooling individual estimates of pharmacokinetic parameters derived from experimental pharmacokinetic studies. The advantage of the STS approach is its simplicity, but the validity of its results should not be overemphasized. It has been shown from simulation studies that the STS approach tends to overestimate parameter dispersion.

Global two-stage method

An extensive description of the method is provided by Steimer et al. The global two-stage (GTS) approach has been shown, through simulation, to provide unbiased estimates of the population mean parameters and their variance–covariance, whereas the estimates of the variances were upwardly biased if the STS approach was used. These simulations were done under the ideal situation that the residual error was normally distributed with a known variance. However, it is a well-known fact that the asymptotic covariance matrix used in the calculations is approximate and under less ideal conditions, the approximation can be poor.

Iterative two-stage method

A computationally "heavier" two-stage method that relies on repeated fittings of individual data iterative two-stage (IT2S) has been described. The IT2S approach can be implemented with rich data, sparse data, or a mixture of both. The method may be implemented with programs supporting Bayesian estimation and least squares regression or with the IT2S routine, which has been implemented in the USC*PACK collection of programs. Mentre and Geomeni proposed a similar method based on an expectation-maximization (EM)-like algorithm, and is implemented in the software P-PHARM.

Bayesian two-stage method

Proposed by Racine-Poon, this method uses the estimates of the individual parameters ϕ_j and asymptotic variance matrix V_j obtained from the individual fits, with very weak assumptions about the prior distribution of the population parameters to calculate a posterior density function from which ϕ and Ω can be obtained. In an iterative method suggested by Dempster, Laird, and Rubin, the EM algorithm is used to calculate the posterior density function. Simulation studies showed that the Bayesian Two-stage Approach provides good parameter estimates. An increasingly used Bayesian software for PPK data analysis is WinBayesian inference Using Gibbs Sampling (WinBUGS), which involves implementation of the Markov chain Monte Carlo (MCMC) method.

Non-linear mixed-effects model approach

The first attempt at estimating interindividual pharmacokinetic variability without neglecting the difficulties (data imbalance, sparse data, subject-specific dosing history, etc.) associated with data from patients undergoing drug therapy was made by Sheiner et al. using the Non-linear Mixed-effects Model Approach. The vector θ of population characteristics is composed of all quantities of the first two moments of the distribution of the parameters: the mean values (fixed effects), and the elements of the variance–covariance matrix that characterize random effects.

The number of samples per subject used for this approach is typically small, ranging from one to six. As does the pooled analysis technique, nonlinear mixed-effects modeling approaches analyze the data of all individuals at once, but take the inter- individual random effects structure into account. This ensures that confounding correlations and imbalance that may occur in observational data are properly accounted for.

Most of the non-linear mixed-effects modeling methods estimate the parameters by means of ML. The probability of the data under the model is written as a function of the model parameters, and parameter estimates are chosen to maximize this probability. This amounts to asserting that the best parameter estimates are those that render the observed data more probable than they would be under any other set of parameters. It is difficult to calculate the likelihood of the data for most pharmacokinetic models because of the nonlinear dependence of the observations on the random parameters η_i and, possibly, ε_{ij}. To deal with these problems, several approximate methods have been proposed. These methods, apart from the approximation, differ widely in their representation of the probability distribution of interindividual random effects.

First-order (NONMEM) method

The first nonlinear mixed-effects modeling program introduced for the analysis of large pharmacokinetic data was NONMEM, developed by Beal and Sheiner. In the NONMEM program, linearization of the model in the random effects is effected by using the first-order Taylor series expansion with respect to the random effect variables η_i and ε_{ij}. This software is the only program in which this type of linearization is used. The jth measurement in the ith subject of the population can be obtained from a variant of Eq. (5) as follows:

$$y_{ij} = f(\phi, x_{ij}, \eta_i) + \varepsilon_{ij} \quad \ldots(7)$$

The first-order Taylor series expansion of the above model with respect to the random variables *ili* and *e*ij around zero is given by

$$y_{ij} = f(\phi, x_{ij}) + G_{ij}(\phi, x_{ij})\eta_i + \varepsilon_{ij} \quad \ldots(8)$$

where

$$G_{ij}(\phi, x_{ij}) = \delta f\,(\theta, x_{ij}\eta_i, \varepsilon_{ij})/\delta\eta_i^T\,|\,\eta_{i=0} \quad \ldots(9)$$

$G_{ij}(\phi, x_{ij})$ is 1 × p matrix of the first derivatives of $f(\theta, x_{ij}, \eta_i, \varepsilon_{ij})$ with respect to η_i, evaluated at η_i equals zero. In Eq. (8), the model is linear in ε_{ij}; therefore, no approximation is made with respect to ε_{ij}. Logarithmic transformation of the data can be done to ensure linearity in ε_{ij}.

The random effect parameters η_i and ε_{ij} are independent (multivariate), normally distributed with zero means and variances Ω and σ^2, respectively. Ω is the $p \times p$ covariance matrix of the p vector η_i. Based on the fact that η_i and ε_{ij} are independent identically, normally distributed, and the linearization of Eq. (8), the expectation and variance–covariance of all observations for the ith individual (first two moments) are given by

$$E_i = f(\theta, x_i) \quad \ldots(10)$$

and

$$C_i = G_i((\theta, x_i)\Omega G_i(\theta, x_i)^T) + \sigma^2 I_{ni} \quad \ldots(11)$$

where $f(\theta, x_i)$ is the vector of model predictions of y_i, $G_i(\theta, x_i)$ represents the $n_i \times p$ matrix of first derivatives of $f(\theta, x_i, \eta_i, \varepsilon_i)$ with respect to η_i evaluated at η_i equals zero, and I_{ni} represents the identity matrix of size n_i. Maximum estimates of the population parameters θ, Ω, and σ^2 can be obtained by minimizing minus twice the logarithm of population likelihood as expressed below

$$-2LL = \sum_{i=1}^{N}\left(\log(\det(C_i)) + (y_i - E_i)^T C_i^{-1}(y_i - E_i)\right) \quad \ldots(12)$$

This approach is called the first order (FO) method in NONMEM. This is the most widely used approach in population pharmacokinetic and pharmacodynamic data analysis, and has been evaluated by simulation. The use of the first-order Taylor series expansion to approximate the non-linear model in η_i and, possibly, ε_{ij} by a linear model in these parameters is the greatest limitation of the FO approach.

The performance of the FO approach for the analysis of observational and experimental data have been evaluated by Sheiner and Beal with the Michaelis-Menten pharmacokinetic model., and the one- and two-compartment models. In all instances, a comparison was made with the NPD and STS approaches for the analysis of the two types of data. The FO approach outperformed the NPD and the STS approaches on both data types. Despite the approximation, the FO approach provides good parameter estimates. If the residual error increases, the STS approach quickly deteriorates, especially with respect to variance parameters. However, the STS still performs reasonably well but the bias and imprecision of the estimates tend to increase with increasing residual error. Estimates of residual variability have been shown to deteriorate with the FO approach when residual error increases.

Deterioration in parameter estimation has been observed in simulation studies in which the value of the intersubject variability was greater than 60% and the residual variability was set at 15%.[47] A series of studies in which observations were randomly deleted from a data-rich set to create a sparse data set, and parameter estimation done using the FO, showed good performance of the FO approach when compared with the results obtained using the full data set. The correspondence of the results in the two situations suggests that the FO approach can be used to estimate parameters using only a few observations per individual. Simulation studies have been performed to show that the FO approach can be used in the limiting case where only one sample is obtained per subject. In this case, there is an upper limit of residual variability (not exceeding 20%) for the production of reliable parameter estimates.

The impact of the linearization approximation of the FO approach for a simple one-compartment model was evaluated by Beal. He compared the performance of this approach with the exact solution to the population likelihood. No difference was observed, which indicated that the approximation used in the FO method was not detrimental to the analysis under the conditions evaluated (interindividual variability was set at 25%, CV%). Other simulation studies, however, have shown that the FO approach has a potential for providing modestly biased estimates. For a one-compartment multidose scenario, White et al. showed that biased estimates are more likely when residual and intersubject variability are very high.

Ette, Sun, and Ludden observed that the biased estimates are obtained at high levels of intersubject variability with a two-compartment multidose situation, although the residual variability did not exceed 15%. The bias may be due to the fact that the first-order Taylor series expansion is not a particularly good approximation of the underlying "real" (log-normal) distribution used to generate the simulated data in these studies. Also, it may be due to the first- order Taylor series expansion being evaluated at η_i equals zero (the population mean estimate of η_i). This may not be a good approximation depending on the magnitude of intersubject variability and the non-linearity of the pharmacokinetic model. During data analysis, this can be compensated for, in part, by including explanatory covariates in the model to reduce the variance of η_i. With a one-compartment model experimental data set, the GTS approach was shown to outperform the FO approach with respect to bias and precision of both the population mean and variance estimates. Similar results were obtained in a study in which the FO approach was compared with the Bayesian two-stage approach.

The NONMEM program implements two alternative estimation methods, the first-order conditional estimation and the Laplacian methods. The first-order conditional estimation (FOCE) method uses a first- order expansion about conditional estimates (empirical Bayes estimates) of interindividual random effects, rather than about zero. In this respect, it is like the conditional first-order method of Lindstrom and Bates. Unlike the latter, which is iterative, a single objective function is minimized, achieving a similar effect as with iteration. The Laplacian method uses second-order expansions about the conditional estimates of the random effects.

Conditional first-order (NLME) method

Proposed by Lindstrom and Bates, this uses a first-order Taylor series expansion about conditional estimates of interindividual random effects. This estimation method is available in S-plus statistical software as the function NLME.

Other non-linear mixed-effects methods

These are less widely used than the above methods and include, but not limited to, alternative first-order (MIXNLIN) by Vonesh and Carter available in the SAS macro and MIXLIN 3.0 of Vonesh, alternative first-order implemented in the SAS macro NLINMIX, non-parametric maximum likelihood (NPML) of Mallet and non-parametric expectation-maximization (NPEM) program of Schumitzky, which performs similar to STS under certain conditions. A semi-non-parametric maximum likelihood (SNP) approach, introduced by Davidian and Gallant, has been discussed in detail but has limited use.

Design and Analysis of Population Studies

Study Design

Unlike the traditional intensive sampling (of individual subjects) pharmacokinetic studies, population pharmacokinetic studies are usually performed under less restrictive design considerations. Thus, most population pharmacokinetic studies reported in the literature have been of the observational type. Recently, efforts have been directed toward the design of prospective population pharmacokinetic studies and the focus here is on this type of studies. This prospective population pharmacokinetic study design will be referred to as experimental population pharmacokinetic study design or full pharmacokinetic screen. With this design approach, blood samples are drawn from subjects at various times (typically one to six time points) following drug administration. This approach permits an estimation of pharmacokinetic parameters of the drug in the study population and an explanation of variability using the non-linear mixed-effects modeling approach.

The full pharmacokinetic screen study can be designed to explore the relationship between the pharmacokinetics of a drug and demographic/pathophysiological features of the target population (with its subgroups) for which the drug is being developed. A full pharmacokinetic screen study requires careful design considerations, and it is helpful to know the qualitative aspects of the model before embarking on a population study.

The objective for performing a population pharmacokinetic study should be taken into consideration in designing such a study. When designing a population pharmacokinetic study, the practical limitations of sampling times, number of samples/subject, and number of subjects should be considered. Also, the sampling of subjects at various periods (study days) should be considered if interoccasion variability is to be estimated. Preliminary information on variability from pilot studies and assay precision make it possible, through simulation, to anticipate certain fatal study designs as well as informative ones. Simulation studies can be used to optimize design features for accurate and precise estimation of population pharmacokinetic parameters.

Optimization of sampling design is critical to efficient experimental design when there are severe limitations on the number of subjects and/or samples/subject, as in pediatrics and the elderly. Such studies need to include enough patients in important subgroups to ensure accurate and precise parameter estimation and the detection of any subgroup differences.

Another approach to optimizing sampling design is through the use of the Fisher information matrix. This is implemented in ADAPT II for individual PK studies with D-optimality as a design criterion. In 1994 Ette, Sun, and Ludden developed a method, the informative block randomized (IBR) design, for designing PPK studies that combines the efficiency of the D-optimality criterion with the robustness afforded by random sampling. Subsequently, Mentre, Mallet, and Baccar proposed the use of the population Fisher information matrix (PFIM) in designing PPK studies. The method has been implemented in S-plus and Mat Lab. The IBR design approach was recently compared with PFIM in a simulation study by Roy and Ette and the two methods were found to perform similarly.

If a population pharmacokinetic study consists of pharmacokinetic observations solely from individuals, each studied on only a single occasion, the interoccasion variability will appear incorrectly in interindividual variability term and not in the intraindividual variability term. This may lead to inappropriate optimism about the ability to control individual therapy within the therapeutic range by using feedback (e.g., therapeutic drug monitoring, or simply adjusting dose according to observed drug effects), and also to a fruitless search for interindividual covariates that might explain the spuriously inflated interindividual variability. It is of utmost importance to avoid this artifact by ensuring that at least a moderate subset of subjects contributing data to a population pharmacokinetic study contribute data from more than one occasion. Indeed if this is done, one may be able to separately estimate the components of intraindividual variability.

Analysis of Population Studies

The nature of the application of a PPK model must be taken into account during the entire modeling process. The intended use of a model should influence the attitude and modeling approaches used by the pharmacometrician at various stages of the modeling process. This would determine what covariates are considered important, which parameters are of primary concern, and the extent of and method of model evaluation (goodness of fit, reliability, and stability assessment) and validation (predictive performance), to arrive at the appropriate PPK model. Model appropriateness can only be established when the problem to be solved by estimating the model is clearly stated, the intended use of the model is clearly stated, the model is developed and validated (if the model is for predictive purposes). Descriptive models do not require validation.

There are many approaches used for PPK model development in the literature. These range from modeling population pharmacokinetic data without exploratory data analysis to approaches that incorporate the latter. Excellent examples of population pharmacokinetic model development, which incorporate exploratory data analysis into population pharmacokinetic model development, can be found in the articles by Ette and Ludden and Mandema, Verotta, and Sheiner Excellent reviews on the validation of PPK models are available in the literature. Thus, validation will not be discussed.

Population pharmacokinetic data analysis can be carried out using three interwoven steps: exploratory data analysis, population pharmacokinetic model development, and model validation. Recently, Ette et al. proposed that population pharmacokinetic modeling in itself is a process of knowledge discovery from a pharmacokinetic dataset. In that sense, knowledge discovery is broader than the narrow definition of knowledge discovery as being the search for relationships and global patterns that exist in large databases, but are hidden among the vast amounts of data.

Knowledge discovery from a population pharmacokinetic dataset incorporates all the steps from data assembly to the development, validation, and utilization of the model in decision-making in drug development and/or clinical practice. Hidden knowledge can be discovered from a population dataset with the use of modern graphical, modeling, and statistical approaches. The use of these techniques for knowledge discovery from a large pharmacokinetic dataset gives the data analyst the liberty to choose statistical methodology appropriate to the problem at hand with the maximization of information extraction, rather than on the basis of mathematical/statistical tractability.

APPLICATION

Some examples of the use of PPK to address biopharmaceutic issues such as drug delivery, absorption, and the extent of availability, and bioequivalence can be found in articles by Hossain et al., Holford, Ambros, and Stoeckel, Kaniwa et al., Graves and Chang Sheiner and Karlsson, Pentikis et al. and Hu et al.

Pentikis et al. evaluated the use of individual and population compartmental methods for bioequivalence determination, and compared these compartmental approaches to the traditional non-compartmental approach. Data from three bioequivalence studies of chlorthalidone were analyzed using PCNONLIN for individual compartmental modeling and NONMEM for population analyses. The authors parameterized the population model to quantify the difference in the absorption rate (KA) and lag time (ALAG) between the reference (R) and test (T) formulations (expressed as test to reference ratio, T/R). Following this, the likelihood profile approach was used to generate 90% confidence intervals for

KA (T/R), bioavailability F (T/R) and ALAG (T/R). Monte Carlo simulations were then used to derive estimates of maximum concentration CMAX (T/R) and area under the curve AUC (T/R) from the population compartmental analyses using 10,000 sets of mean concentration-time profiles. The results from population modeling, individual compartmental modeling, and non-compartmental approaches were compared according to the criteria above and found similar.

The population method provided direct estimates of the test to reference ratios (T/R) of KA and ALAG and thus might be useful for bioequivalence determination in conjunction with the standard method especially for drugs with complex concentration- time profiles. Thus, the population approach can be used to compare the biopharmaceutic performance of drug products. The definitions and statistical theory of PPK, advantages, and disadvantages of PPK have been discussed in this chapter. Models, data type, methods, and software programs for estimating population pharmacokinetic parameters, design, and analysis of population pharmacokinetic studies have been reviewed, as well as its application in biopharmaceutics. The use of population methods continues to increase while there is a shortage of those who can implement the approach.

6

PRECLINICAL PHARMACOKINETICS

The preclinical pharmacokinetics of protein pharmaceuticals is distinctively different from small-molecule drugs. The phase I and phase II metabolizing enzymes, for example, the cytochrome P450 and glucoronosyl transferases, which play dominant roles in the metabolism of small-molecule drugs, are not significantly involved in protein metabolism. Instead, because all protein pharmaceuticals invariably share a common polypeptide backbone, they are susceptible to proteolysis as a clearance mechanism. However, the disposition, pharmacokinetics, and pharmacodynamics of proteins can be modulated by a variety of additional factors, including glycosylation and receptor binding, binding proteins, and neutralizing antibodies.

DISPOSITION OF MACROMOLECULES

Absorption

During drug development, the oral route is often targeted as a preferred route of administration for small molecules. However, the oral route is not usually an option for protein pharmaceuticals. Each organ in the gastrointestinal tract contains a variety of digestive proteases that enable it to break down nutritional proteins to small peptides and amino acids that can be absorbed in the intestine via secondarily active transport mechanisms. These digestive pro teases also cause the extensive hydrolysis of the polypeptide bond in protein drugs in the gastrointestinal tract resulting in poor bioavailability. Protein pharmaceuticals are usually, therefore, administered via injection, such as the intravenous, subcutaneous, or intramuscular routes.

The absorption of protein drugs from extravascular sites is dependent on the size of the molecule. Upon subcutaneous administration, small molecules with molecular weights less than 1 kD predominantly enter the systemic circulation via blood capillaries, whereas subcutaneously administered proteins with molecular weights greater than 16 kD enter the systemic circulation predominantly via the lymphatic system. The extent of the

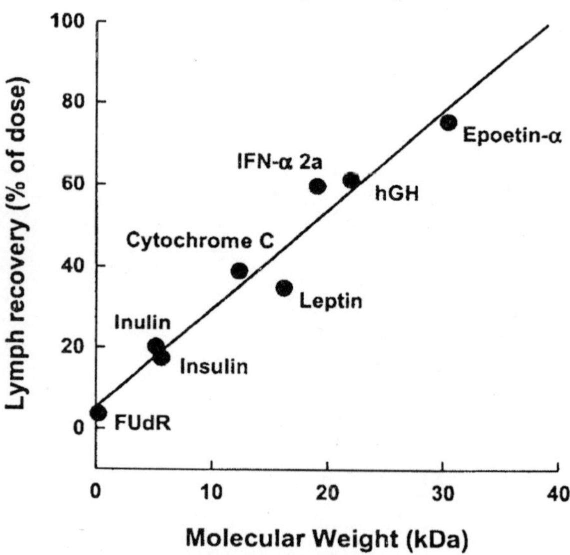

Fig. 6.1. Linear relationship between cumulative lymphatic recovery and molecular weight of various therapeutic peptides and proteins.

lymphatic recovery after subcutaneous administration is a linear function of molecular weight. Nonparenteral routes of administration for protein drugs in general are not extensively used; however, recombinant human deoxyribonuclease I solution (dornase alfa or PULMOZYME) and, more recently, insulin powder by inhalation (EXUBERA) have been approved for clinical use in the United States.

The approval of inhaled insulin may provide the stimulus for greater interest in the inhalation route for other protein drugs in the near future. The lung presents a large surface area for transport and high permeability compared with other barriers. Inhaled insulin is administered as a novel powder formulation that is metered from a propellant-free metered dose inhaler. However, delivery to the lungs, particularly to the alveolar regions deep in the lung, presents several technological challenges and the overall system bioavailability (which is based on the amount of drug loaded into the inhaler device) of inhaled insulin is 9–22% that of the subcutaneous route. The reduced bioavailability is managed by dose adjustment and compared with subcutaneously administered regular insulin, the serum insulin con centrations after inhalation peak earlier (at 7–80 minutes compared with 42–274 minutes for subcutaneous regular insulin) and decay more rapidly; the pharmacodynamics of glucose changes are also correspondingly more rapid. The duration of inhaled insulin action are comparable with regular insulin.

Distribution

The distribution of protein drugs is limited compared with that of small-molecule drugs and is primarily a function of the physico-chemical properties of the macromolecule and the physiological characteristics of the vasculature and cellular membranes. Primary molecular descriptors, such as size, charge, and lipophilicity, will determine or influence the extent of specific and nonspecific protein binding and passage through various types of capillary endothelia. The relatively large size of peptide and protein drugs alone can often account for the limited volume of distribution of these compounds, which is generally restricted to the extracellular space. Following intravenous injection, the initial volume of distribution for most macromolecules is confined approximately to plasma volume (3–8 L), and the total volume at steady state is typically only up to two fold greater.

Active transport and receptor-mediated uptake also may influence the biodistribution of macromolecules. For example, the internalization of monoclonal antibodies into cells may occur via Fcã receptors, found on various immune and hematopoietic cells, or binding to membrane-localized antigens. Thus, active uptake processes can serve to increase the volume of distribution to a large extent relative to that which would be expected based only on physico-chemical properties. Receptor-mediated endocytosis may represent a significant elimination pathway as well (see the Receptor-mediated elimination subsection) and is recognized as a major process influencing the overall disposition of macromolecules.

One must carefully interpret the volumes of distribution of peptides and proteins reported in the literature. Most studies rely on a so-called noncompartmental analysis to estimate primary pharmacokinetic parameters. However, this method is only valid for linear systems, assuming that the site of drug elimination is in rapid equilibrium with the sampling site (plasma). The former condition is often assumed for compartmental models as well, including those with nonlinear mechanisms of elimination. Therefore, uptake processes and relatively slow or complex tissue catabolism may confound reported distribution volumes of select macromolecules estimated by these common methods.

Binding proteins

For some therapeutic proteins, specific and nonspecific protein interactions can modulate distribution and activity. Soluble receptors are the best-characterized specific binding proteins and α_2 macroglobulin, an acute phase protein, has been implicated in the binding of several cytokines. Binding and neutralizing antibodies are another class of binding protein that will be discussed separately in the section on Immunogenicity, Binding, and Neutralizing Antibodies.

Soluble cytokine receptors (SR) occur naturally in human serum and urine and play a role in determining the disposition and biological activities of cytokines in health and in pathological states. Additionally, bioengineered soluble receptors and their immunoglobulin derivatives have been investigated as specific cytokine-inhibiting therapeutic agents. However, the physiological role(s) of naturally occurring SR is controversial and not well understood.

As expected, the SR can inhibit cytokine bioactivity by competing with the receptor and, when these antagonist-like effects are observed, the dose-response curve of the cytokine effect as a function of SR dose usually decreases monotonically, and almost complete inhibition is observed at the highest SR doses. In animal models, soluble receptors for interleukin-4, interleukin-7, interleukin-6, and tumor necrosis factor-α have been shown to enhance rather than inhibit cytokine responses under certain conditions. When these agonist-like effects are observed, the dose-response curve of the cytokine effect as a function of SR dose is bell-shaped, with no inhibition of cytokine bioactivity at low SR doses, maximal cytokine bioactivity at intermediate SR doses, followed by increasing inhibition of cytokine activity at higher SR doses. As the SR effects of the cytokines biological response is dependent on experimental conditions and can be either agonist-like or antagonist-like, the physiological roles of SR have been difficult to assess. Cytokines generally have short half-lives consistent with their physiological roles in cell-cell communication and the apparent SR-mediated agonism of cytokine activity occurs because the SR stabilizes the cytokine in vivo either by reducing the rate of spontaneous activity decay or by increasing the half-life of cytokine. The formation of SR-cytokine complex reduces cytokine-free concentrations, but the increases in circulation time can offset the effect of reduced receptor occupancy and contribute to overall increases in exposure. The binding half-life of insulin-like growth factor-1 (IGF-1) in rats deficient in IGF-1 binding protein is 20–30 min; but in rats with normal levels of the binding protein, the half-life of IGF-1 increases 8–12-fold to 4 hours. In the plasma, nearly 40% of human growth hormone (GH) is also bound to binding proteins; the high-affinity component of the GH binding activity consists of the extracellular domain of the GH receptor. The metabolic clearance of the SR-bound GH fraction is 10-fold slower than free GH because the bound GH is not filtered by the kidney and the competitive inhibition of receptor binding reduces elimination via receptor- mediated pathways. Indirect evidence for the physiological role of SR binding is provided by the data from short-stature Mountain Ok people of Papua, New Guinea who have SR levels 50% that of controls of normal stature; the levels of GH, IGF-1, and low-affinity GH-binding protein levels are comparable in the two groups.

Immunogenicity, binding, and neutralizing antibodies

The bioactivity and distribution of therapeutically administered proteins can be modulated by their immunogenicity; humoral responses to therapeutic proteins can result in binding and neutralizing antibodies. Generally, chronic or intermittently administered proteins are more likely to be affected by these pathways than proteins administered for acute conditions. The underlying protein structure, aggregation state, and protein formulation can contribute to the risk of binding and neutralizing antibodies. Factors related to the dosing regimen such as dose, frequency, and route of administration are also important determinants. The role of disease-related and individual-specific variables to the development of antibodies is poorly understood. The time to development of antibody depends on the dosing regimen and immunogenicity of the preparation. For some proteins, the development of antibodies to endogenous proteins can cause serious adverse events (e.g., red cell aplastic anemia can occur with anti-erythropoeitin antibodies). The impact of antibodies on drug efficacy in clinical trials should be assessed during the period the antibodies are present.

As a case study, consider interferon-β, an endogenous cytokine, recombinant forms of which are used chronically in multiple sclerosis (MS). Two types of IFN-β exist: IFN-β-1a and IFN-β-1b. IFN-β-1a is glycosylated and has the same amino acid sequence as endogenous IFN-β. IFN-β-1b is not glycosylated, lacks the N-terminal methionine, and is engineered with cysteine replaced by serine. Two approved IFN-β-1a products exist that are dosed by the once-weekly, intramuscular, 30-μg and three-times-weekly, subcutaneous, 44-μg dosing regimens; the IFN-β-1b product is an every-other-day, subcutaneous, 250-μg dosing regimen. As with other protein drugs, some patients develop neutralizing antibodies (NAB) upon chronic administration of all IFN-β products. The proportion of patients developing NAB ranges from 25% for three-times-weekly, subcutaneous IFN-β-1a regimen to 2% for the once-weekly, IM IFN-β-1a regimen. In a clinical trial where the weekly IM dose in the once-weekly, IM IFN-β-1a regimen was increased from 30 μg to 60 μg, the percentage of patients developing NAB titers greater than 20 after 3 years of treatment increased from 2.2% to 5.8% and suggests that, for a given route of administration, the frequency of IFN-β-1a administration is probably the major factor influencing the immunogenicity of an IFN-β product and the increase in dosage has relatively less impact. Published data from large randomized clinical trials demonstrate that disease activity in NAB-positive patients became similar to placebo-treated patients. Interestingly, skin necrosis, an adverse effect that occurs with SC IFN-β administration, occurred only in the NAB-negative patients. Despite the evidence from large clinical trials, some controversy exists regarding the appropriate clinical decisions for treatment of NAB-positive MS patients, especially those with a clinically stable disease, because (1) many NAB-positive patients test negative over the course of treatment, (2) no accepted IFN-β treatment biomarkers exist that are MS-relevant and, (3) market and competitive factors occur because of the availability of multiple IFN-â products for MS.

Metabolism

The cytochrome P450 enzymes, expressed in the endoplasmic reticulum of the liver, kidney, and intestine, are the predominant metabolizing pathways for small- molecule drugs. After the phase I oxidation reactions, small molecules typically are further modified by phase II conjugation reactions mediated by glucoronosyl transferases that render them hydrophilic for renal elimination. However, as noted earlier, the metabolism of protein drugs does not involve these small-molecule pathways: Endogenous pathways involved in protein homeostasis mediate protein drug metabolism.

As indicated earlier, proteolysis is the predominant mechanism for protein drug metabolism, but diverse endogenous proteolytic pathways exist in humans. Further, the half-lives of protein *in vivo* are, not surprisingly, regulated by a variety of intracellular mechanisms. The half-life of intracellular proteins is regulated via the ubiquitin pathway, which targets proteins to degradation in a large multimeric protease complex referred to as the proteasome. Ubiquitin is a widely expressed globular protein with a protruding carboxyl-terminus that tags proteins for degradation. Ubiquitin-activating enzymes activate through a process that requires ATP, and the activated ubiquitin is then transferred to a lysine on the target protein by another enzyme, the ubiquitin ligase. Multiple ubiquitin chains can be ligated on a single target protein lysine by conjugating glycine-lysine bonds between successive ubiquitin chains. Some target proteins are also tagged by binding proteins referred to as "*recognin*" that bind sequence elements called "*degrons*" that specify half-life. Sufficiently ubquitinated proteins are recognized and degraded in the proteasome. Although the ubiquitin pathway is critical for cellular protein homeostasis, its involvement in the metabolism of exogenously administered proteins is probably minor.

Some circulating proteins, most notably albumin and immunoglobulin G (IgG), have anomalously long half-lives because they are protected from degradation by specific mechanisms after cellular uptake. The best characterized of these protein-stabilizing mechanisms is the neonatal Fc receptor or FcRn, which is present on a variety of cell types and tissues including the kidney, liver, and lung endothelial cells, hepatocytes, monocytes, and intestinal macrophases. It confers a long half-life to IgG (mean half-life in humans = 23 days) relative to other types of immunoglobulins (half-lives for IgA, IgD, IgE, and IgM are 6, 3, 2.5, and 5 days, respectively). Most proteins generally undergo degradation in lysosome after pinocytosis and receptor-mediated endocytosis from the cell surface. However, the constant Fc region of immunoglobulin G and antibody-based drugs are internalized by pinocytosis or, when they bind, the cell surface antibody- binding Fcγ receptors. However, upon internalization into the endosomes, immunoglobulin G is bound by FcRn and the complex, upon endocytosis, is protected from proteolysis and recycled to the cell surface instead of being processed for degradation in lysosomes. The FcRn receptor for IgG is often referred to as the Brambell receptor after the authors who postulated their existence to explain the relatively long half-life and the increased rates of IgG degradation at higher IgG concentration. Mice that are β_2 microglobulin-deficient do not express FcRn and have IgG half-lives that are 10–15-fold shorter than mice with intact FcRn. Overall, 3 major mechanisms for clearing protein drugs exist: (1) renal, (2) hepatic, and (3) receptor-modulated.

Excretion

The rate of elimination of proteins is strongly dependent on the size, structure, and, in the case of chronically administered protein drugs, the presence or absence of antidrug antibodies. Renal clearance is relatively uncommon for protein drugs with molecular weights greater than 50 kD. Specific primary structural features such as the presence of a humanized immunoglobulin constant (Fc) region can confer prolonged stability via endogenous recycling pathways. Likewise, glycosylation and the addition of polyethylene glycol moieties (a synthetic modification often referred to as PEGylation) can also prolong circulation times.

Protein drugs with molecular weights less than 20 kD are filtered out of circulation in the Bowman's capsule of glomerulus of the kidney and enter the luminal space of the nephron. Even under pathological conditions, urinary excretion of intact protein is unusual. The filtered protein drugs are reabsorbed from the lumen and released into the circulation either as intact drugs or degraded into peptides. The proximal tubule is the predominant site for reabsorption, which transfers proteins into apical vacuoles that fuse with lysosomes. Lysosomal proteases degrade proteins into amino acids that re-enter the circulation. Small peptides can also be directly degraded by proteases on the luminal side of the renal tubule and the resulting amino acids can be reabsorbed by transport mechanisms.

Hepatic metabolism is important to the clearance of therapeutic proteins with molecular weights greater than 20 kD, although renal clearance can contribute to proteins as large as 50 kD. The Kupfer cell and hepatocytes of the liver are involved in clearing protein drugs.

Pegylation

Pegylation refers to the covalent modification of proteins by polyethylene glycol (PEG) moieties. As PEG is a hydrophilic, degradation-resistant polymer, pegylation can increase the circulating half-life of proteins, reduce renal elimination, alter the distribution, and reduce the immunogenicity of proteins. The addition of PEG increases the molecular weight of the protein, which is instrumental in reducing renal filtration, and it provides a hydrophilic shield containing tightly associated water molecules that protects against proteolysis and some nonspecific interactions that mitigate therapeutic protein immunogenicity. However, pegylation can reduce receptor-binding affinity. When engineering pegylation during drug development, the effects of reduced receptor binding can be offset by the increased drug exposures; the improvements in circulating half-life and protein disposition effects and reduced immunogenicity benefit of this modification. The chemistry of PEG conjugation involves chemical activation of PEG followed by covalent attachment at the reactive amino groups of lysine or the N-terminal amino acid or the sulfhydryl groups of cysteine. As a rule of thumb, the molecular weight of the PEG moiety has to be comparable with that of the therapeutic protein for pegylation to be effective.

Pegylation chemistry is also capable of conjugating branched PEG polymers that can increase the mass of PEG added at a each site and can better protect the protein therapeutic from degradation and immune recognition. The pegylation approach is quite general and has also been used for liposomes: It prolongs the circulation times of liposomes by reducing the rapid elimination by the reticuloendothelial system.

Interferon-α-2b (IFN-α-2b, PEGINTRON), which is used for treating hepatitis, is a case study on the impact possible with the pegylation approach because considerable preclinical and clinical data are also available for the IFN-α-2b unmodified by pegylation (INTRON-A). As a result of pegylation, the molecular weight of IFN-α-2b is increased from 19 kilodaltons to approximately 31 kilodaltons and the half-life increases from 3–8 hours to 65 hours. Other pharmacokinetic variables altered include a decreased volume of distribution (from 31–73L to 8–12L) and decreased systemic clearance (from 6.6–29.2 L/hour to 0.06–0.1 L/hour). The pharmacodynamic effects of anti viral and antitumor activities of pegylated IFN-α-2b are 12–136-fold and 18-fold, respectively, greater than the unpegylated form. The net result of these pharmacokinetic and pharmacodynamic improvements is that the frequency of pegylated IFN-α-2b administration for treating chronic hepatitis C is once weekly compared with three times weekly for the unpegylated form.

Hyperglycosylation

Hyperglycosylation is the addition of sugar moieties to proteins and can be engineered using molecular biology techniques to specific locations on a protein. Many cellular proteins have N-linked or O-linked glycan modification that are added in posttranslational and cotranslational processes in the endoplasmic reticulum and in the Golgi apparatus. The N-linked glycosylations occur at amino groups of the asparagine in Asn-X-Ser/Thr sequences, although not all potential glycosylation sites may be modified and heterogeneity can occur within given protein molecules. The O-linked glycosylations occur at the hydroxyl groups of serine and threonine.

Receptor-mediated elimination

For some proteins, pharmacokinetic nonlinearities can occur because of receptor-mediated elimination. When therapeutic proteins bind their cognate cell-surface targets, the bound therapeutic protein can be internalized by receptor-mediated or fluid-phase endocytosis and traffic to the lysosomes where it may be degraded. The capacity-limited nature of these systems can manifest as saturable dose-dependent drug clearance and may be susceptible to further modulation through functional adaptation mechanisms such as receptor up-regulation or down-regulation. The saturable internalization of erythropoietin (EPO) in erythroid progenitor cells is a classic example. Chapel et al. have shown that the bone marrow, a major site for erythropoietic cells, represents a significant EPO elimination pathway. Busulfan or 5-fluoruracil-induced bone marrow ablation in sheep was associated with a decrease in EPO clearance, revealing the *in vivo*

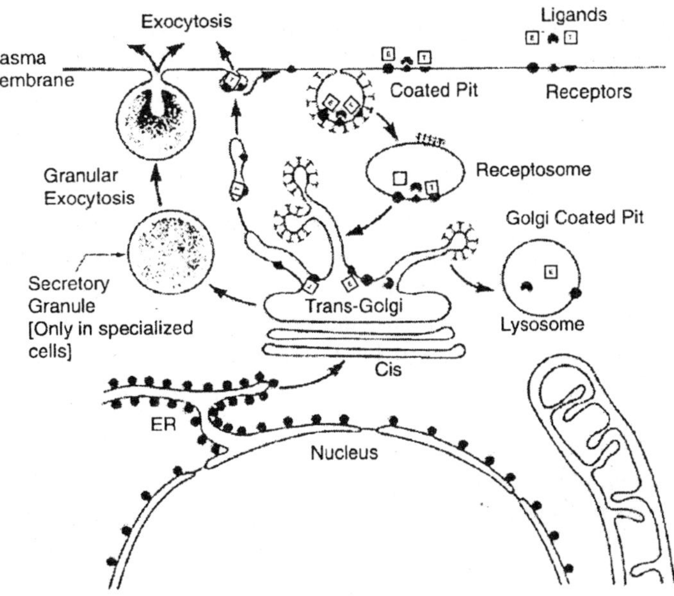

Fig. 6.2. Schematic for the pathway of receptor-mediated endocytosis.

significance of target-mediated uptake and elimination for this therapeutic protein. Complex target-mediated clearance mechanisms suggest that both pharmacokinetics and pharmacodynamics might have to be considered concurrently to understand the disposition of select macromolecules. Peptide and protein drugs that alter the expression of target cells may have the ability to modulate their pharmacokinetic properties. For example, thrombopoietin (TPO) is an endogenous hematopoietic growth factor that stimulates the proliferation and differentiation of megakaryocytes and thus the production of new platelets, which, in turn, would yield a net increase in the density of available TPO receptors (c-Mpl) and reconcile the reciprocal relationship between platelet count and circulating plasma TPO concentrations.

Pharmacokinetic Data Analysis

The primary objective of pharmacokinetic data analysis is to characterize quantitatively the drug disposition processes discussed above. Sufficient knowledge of the preclinical pharmacokinetics of macromolecules, which can only be obtained via mathematical formalisms, may be used to anticipate relevant pharmacokinetic properties in humans, thereby serving to guide dose selection in subsequent clinical trials. The two most commonly used methods for characterizing pharmacokinetic data are noncompartmental analysis and compartmental modeling. Basic assumptions and techniques are presented in this section and are placed within the context of biotechnology pharmaceuticals, which may provide guidance for selecting the most appropriate and desirable method for a given dataset. It is important to recognize that no method of data analysis can offset shortcomings in experimental designs and assays, and that careful consideration of such details is a sine qua non in pharmacokinetics.

Noncompartmental Analysis

Intravenous drug disposition

The estimation of primary pharmacokinetic parameters using noncompartmental analysis is based on statistical moment theory. The relationships defined by this theory are valid under the assumption that the system is linear and time-invariant. For simplicity, we further assume that drug is irreversibly removed only from a single accessible pool (e.g., plasma space). Regardless of the route of administration, the temporal profile of plasma drug concentrations, $C_p(t)$, can represent a statistical distribution curve. As such, the zeroth and first statistical moments (M_0 and M_1) are defined as:

$$M_0 = \int_0^\infty C_p(t)dt = AUC \quad \ldots(1)$$

$$M_1 = \int_0^\infty t \cdot C_p(t)dt = AUMC \quad \ldots(2)$$

where AUC and $AUMC$ are the so-called area under the plasma concentration-time curve and area under the first-moment curve. Several methods have been described for estimating the values of these moments, some of which will be presented in this section, and may be used to calculate relevant pharmacokinetic parameters.

Under linear conditions, the time-course of plasma drug concentrations following a single IV bolus dose can be characterized by a sum of exponentials:

$$C_p(t) = \sum C_i \cdot e^{-\lambda_i \cdot t} \quad \ldots(3)$$

where the coefficients (C_i) and exponentials (λ_i) may be obtained via curve- stripping, or more appropriately, from curve-fitting using nonlinear regression analysis. One advantage of fitting Equation (3) to pharmacokinetic data is the relative simplicity in calculating AUC and $AUMC$ values:

$$AUC = \sum C_i / \lambda_i \quad \ldots(4)$$

$$AUMC = \sum C_i / \lambda_i^2 \quad \ldots(5)$$

Primary pharmacokinetic parameters such as total systemic clearance (CL) and the volume of distribution at steady state (V_{ss}) can be defined as:

$$CL = D_{iv}/AUC \quad ...(6)$$

and

$$V_{ss} = \frac{D_{iv} \cdot AUMC}{AUC^2} CL \cdot MRT_{iv} \quad ...(7)$$

where D_{iv} represents the IV bolus dose and MRT_{iv}, or mean residence time, is the average time a drug molecule resides in the system before being irreversibly removed. Also, the central volume of distribution (V_c) can be calculated as:

$$V_c = D_{iv} \Big/ \sum C_i \quad ...(8)$$

Additional advantages to resolving AUC and $AUMC$ from curve-fitting the sums of exponentials are the stability of the estimates and that nonlinear regression procedures provide measures of error about the pharmacokinetic parameter estimates.

Peptide and protein drugs requiring an IV route of administration may also be given as a constant rate infusion. Pharmacokinetic data from experiments designed to achieve a steady-state plasma concentration (C_{ss}) allow for the direct calculation of drug clearance according to the equation:

$$CL = k_0/C_{ss} \quad ...(9)$$

where k_0 is the constant zero-order rate of drug infusion. The steady-state volume of distribution can be obtained from:

$$V_{ss} = \frac{k_0 \cdot T - CL \cdot AUC_0^T}{C_{ss}} \quad ...(10)$$

where T is the duration of the IV infusion. For short-term constant rate infusions, when plasma concentrations do not attain C_{ss}, Equation (6) is valid for calculating clearance by substituting $k_0 \cdot T$ for D_{iv}. Moment analysis also may be used to generate V_{ss} under these conditions from the equation:

$$V_{ss} = \frac{k_0 \cdot T \cdot AUMC}{AUC^2} - \frac{k_0 \cdot T^2}{2 \cdot AUC} \quad ...(11)$$

Extravascular drug disposition

In general, peptide and protein drugs exhibit poor systemic bioavailability following oral administration owing primarily to gastrointestinal enzymatic degradation. On the other hand, IV drug administration may not result in a desirable time-course of drug exposure and certainly lacks appeal for patients requiring chronic therapy. One of the most common routes of extravascular peptide and protein drug administration is subcutaneous injection, with additional routes, such as inhalation, intranasal, and transdermal delivery representing the targets of current investigation.

The time-course of plasma drug concentrations following extravascular administration is often irregular, and simple analytical solutions for calculating AUC and $AUMC$, such as Equations (4) and (5), are not readily available. For these cases, numerical integration methods may be used to evaluate the integrals in Equations (1) and (2), such that:

$$AUC = \int_0^{t^*} C_p(t)dt + \frac{C_p^*}{\lambda_z} \quad ...(12)$$

and

$$AUMC = \int_0^{t^*} t \cdot C_p(t)dt + \frac{t^* \cdot C_p^*}{\lambda_z} + \frac{C_p^*}{\lambda_z^2} \quad ...(13)$$

where C^*_p and t^* are the last observed plasma concentration and time values, respectively, λ_z is the terminal slope of the curve, and the quotients provide estimates of the area extrapolating from t^* to infinity. The trapezoidal and log-trapezoidal rules are the most common methods for numerically evaluating the integrals in Equations (12) and (13). The trapezoidal rule for calculating the area under a curve within an interval t_i and t_{i-1} is given as:

$$\int_{i-1}^{i} y \cdot dy = 0.5 \cdot [(y_i + y_{i-1})(t_i - t_{i-1})] \qquad \ldots(14)$$

where y is $C_p(t)$ for AUC and $t \cdot C_p(t)$ for $AUMC$. For the log-trapezoidal rule, the equation is:

$$\int_{i-1}^{i} y \cdot dy = \frac{1}{\ln\left(\dfrac{y_i}{y_{i-1}}\right)} . [(y_i + y_{i-1})(t_i - t_{i-1})] \qquad \ldots(15)$$

The cumulative sum of the interval areas thus provides an estimate of the *AUC* and *A UMC* from time zero to t^*. Yu and Tse have evaluated the performance of several numerical integration algorithms for calculating *AUC*. In practice, it is most common to employ the trapezoidal rule for ascending ($y_i > y_{i-1}$) and plateau ($y_i \approx y_{i-1}$) regions of the curve and the log-trapezoidal rule when measured values are decreasing ($y_i < y_{i-1}$). Such an approach is used for noncompartmental analysis in the computer program WinNonlin, a nonlinear regression analysis program specifically designed for pharmacokinetic and pharmacodynamic data analysis.

The noncompartmental analysis of pharmacokinetic data after extra vascular drug administration, when coupled with that of IV dosing, can yield additional relevant pharmacokinetic parameters, particularly regarding absorption processes. For example, the systemic availability (*F*), which represents the net fraction of the drug dose reaching the systemic circulation after extravascular administration, is defined as:

$$F = \frac{D_{iv} \cdot AUC_{ev}}{D_{ev} \cdot AUC_{iv}} \qquad \ldots(16)$$

where catabolism at the extravascular site of administration and other processes may result in incomplete drug absorption. Also, the mean absorption time (*MAT*), or the average time a drug molecule remains unabsorbed, can be calculated from the relationship:

$$MAT = MRT_{ev} - MRT_{iv} \qquad \ldots(17)$$

where the mean residence times derive from the ratios of *AUMC* and *AUC* [e.g., Equation (7)].

Overall, the relative simplicity of noncompartmental analysis, as compared with the methodological challenges of developing and validating structural mathematical models, forms the basis for it being the most common method for ascertaining the major pharmacokinetic properties of drugs. It is beyond the scope of this chapter to contrast the merits of these two methods, and the reader is referred to more complete treatments and the references therein. However, various pharmacokinetic processes of many peptide and protein pharmaceuticals are inherently nonlinear, which violate the fundamental assumptions of linearity and time-invariance in statistical moment analysis. For such compounds, the construction of mechanism-based mathematical models is required and essential for characterizing the *in vivo* pharmacokinetics of the drug. In any event, noncompartmental analysis represents a highly useful starting point for any pharmacokinetic data analysis. For simple linear systems, this technique may be sufficient for calculating primary pharmacokinetic parameters from preclinical experiments and anticipating dose-concentration relationships in humans. Additionally, moment analysis of plasma concentration-time profiles resulting from a suitable range of dose levels may be used initially to identify whether nonlinearities exist, such as disproportionate *AUC* values (relative to dose) indicating dose-dependent clearance or bioavailability, thus necessitating the implementation of more sophisticated methods of pharmacokinetic systems analysis.

Pharmacokinetic Models

Compartmental modeling involves the specification of a structural mathematical model (commonly using either explicit or ordinary differential equations) and system parameters are estimated from fitting the model to pharmacokinetic data via nonlinear regression analysis or population mixed effects modeling. The methodological issues involved in the development, application, and interpretation of pharmacokinetic models are beyond the scope of this chapter and are discussed in detail elsewhere. The most popular structural model applied to macromolecule pharmacokinetic data is the open two-compartment. This system is described, in general, by the following differential equations:

$$\frac{dA_p}{dt} = \frac{Input}{V_c} - \left(\frac{CL}{V_c} + \frac{CL_D}{V_c}\right) \cdot A_p + \frac{CL_D}{V_t} \cdot A_t \qquad ...(18)$$

$$\frac{dA_t}{dt} = \frac{CL_D}{V_c} \cdot A_p - \frac{CL_D}{V_t} \cdot A_t \qquad ...(19)$$

where A_i represents the amount of drug in the plasma ($i = p$) or tissue ($i = t$) compartments, *Input* represents a function describing the appearance of drug based on the route of drug administration, CL_D is the distributional clearance between compartments, and V_t is the volume of the second or tissue compartment. Plasma drug concentrations are thus specified as $C_p = A_p/V_c$.

The drug input function in Equation (18) will depend on the experimental design. For rapid IV injection, the input function is set equal to zero and the dose (D) is reflected in the initial condition for Equation (18) [$A_p(0) = D$]. A constant rate IV infusion also is easily handled by setting *Input* equal to the zero-order infusion rate (K_0) for time (t) less than or equal to the infusion time (T_{inf}), otherwise $Input = 0$. The remaining equations typically are used to describe extravascular drug administration. The simplest function assumes a linear first-order absorption process (k_a) from an extravascular site following a short time-lag (t_{lag}). If a time-lag is not observed, t_{lag} may be set to zero, resulting in a simple linear absorption model, as exemplified in a pharmacokinetic model for recombinant human growth hormone following SC dosing in monkeys. As mentioned in the previous section, IV pharmacokinetic data must be analyzed simultaneously with SC data to estimate drug bioavailability (F).

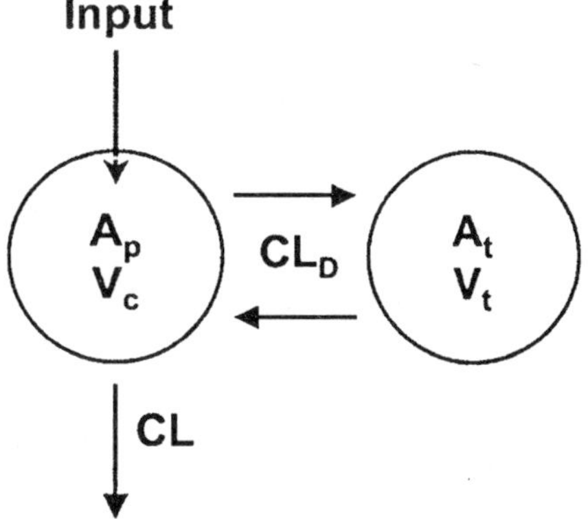

Fig. 6.3. Schematic of a two-compartment mammillary model commonly used to characterize macromolecule pharmacokinetics.

Owing to the complexities of drug absorption from extravascular sites, peptide and protein drugs may require an additional delay compartment comprising two consecutive first-order processes, which may be accompanied by an initial rapid input of a fraction of the dose as defined by Equations. Such a dual absorption model was used to describe the input of recombinant erythro poietin after SC administration in monkeys. Interestingly, the bioavailability was shown to be dose-dependent and ranged from 0.268 to 1.0, increasing with increased dose level. This property may be caused by saturation of catabolism at the site of drug administration; however, further research is needed to elucidate the specific processes involved in drug disposition following extravascular dosing. Many other complex functions are available, such as an inverse Gaussian model, which may be sub stituted into pharmacokinetic models to describe the absorption of macromolecules.

The clearance of several macromolecules may be characterized using simple linear first-order elimination as shown in Equation (18), but may depend on the animal species and range of dose levels being evaluated. In contrast, many peptide and protein drugs demonstrate saturable or capacity-limited clearance, and CL in Equation (18) may be defined with a concentration-dependent function, such as:

$$CL = \frac{V_{max} \cdot V_c}{K_m \cdot V_c + A_p} + CL_{ns} \quad \ldots(20)$$

where V_{max} and K_m are the traditional Michaelis–Menten parameters and CL_{ns} represents a linear nonsaturable clearance pathway. The nonlinear Michaelis–Menten function [quotient in Equation (20)] may be specified alone or in parallel with CL_{ns}. Thus, at high plasma drug concentrations (i.e., $C_p >> K_m$), the saturable clearance function approaches a limiting value (V_{max}), and at relatively low concentrations will represent a first-order elimination rate (V_{max}/K_m).

Receptor-mediated clearance is an example of target-mediated drug disposition (TMDD), where binding of a compound to a pharmacological target (e.g., enzyme, receptor, or other proteins) influences the pharmacokinetics of the drug. Such systems often exhibit a dose-dependent decrease in the apparent volume of distribution (approaching a limiting value). The general pharmacological expectations of TMDD and techniques for characterizing this phenomenon have been reviewed recently. A general pharmacokinetic model of TMDD has been described, and the operative equations defining the rate of change of plasma drug concentrations typically include:

$$\frac{dC_p}{dt} = -k_{on} \cdot R_f \cdot C_p + k_{off} \cdot RC \quad \ldots(21)$$

$$\frac{dRC}{dt} = k_{on} \cdot R_f \cdot C_p - (k_{off} + k_{int}) \cdot RC \quad \ldots(22)$$

where k_{on} and k_{off} are second- and first-order rates of association and dissociation, R_f and RC represent free and bound receptor (or pharmacological target) concentrations, and k_{int} is a first-order internalization rate constant of RC. Under certain conditions, the total receptor concentration (R_{tot}) may be assumed to be time-invariant, and thus $R_f = R_{tot} - RC$. Therefore, at high drug concentrations, $RC \rightarrow R_{tot}$ and effectively limits the distribution and elimination of drug from the central compartment. This approach has been used to characterize the complex nonlinear pharmacokinetics and pharmacodynamics of IFN-β 1a in monkeys. Alternatively, an additional equation may be introduced that describes the rate of change of R_f directly. Also, an equilibrium solution to the general TMDD model is available, where the drug-binding microconstants (k_{on} and k_{off}), which are often difficult to estimate from routine pharmacokinetic data, are replaced with an equilibrium dissociation constant ($K_D = k_{off}/k_{on}$).

Predicting Macromolecule Pharmacokinetics in Humans

One of the major goals of preclinical pharmacokinetics is to obtain relevant information on the *in vivo* disposition of drugs early in the drug development process and to apply such knowledge to anticipate probable pharmacokinetic properties in humans for initial dose selection in phase I clinical trials. Allometric scaling and physiologically based pharmacokinetic (PBPK) models are the most popular techniques for predicting pharmacokinetic properties of drugs in one species from data collected in one or more other species. Although these methods have been applied to small-molecular-weight compounds for decades with variable and often limited success, it is hypothesized that these techniques are more accurate for peptide and protein drugs owing to the relative species conservation of mechanisms that control the biodistribution and elimination of such compounds.

Allometric Scaling

Many physiological processes and organ sizes scale across species according to the well-known power-law relationship or allometric equation:

$$Y = a \cdot W^b \qquad \ldots(23)$$

where Y is a physiological parameter of interest, W represents body weight, and a and b are the allometric coefficient and exponent. The linearized form of Equation (23) is obtained by taking its logorithm:

$$\log Y = \log a + b \cdot \log W \qquad \ldots(24)$$

where log a and b represent the intercept and slope of the physiological data presented on a log-log plot. The units of a will depend on the units of Y and W, and its absolute value will depend on the specific property of interest. In contrast, b is a unitless parameter characterizing the rate of change of Y with respect to W. According to the power-law relationship, Y may increase more rapidly than W ($b > 1$), less rapidly than W ($0 < b < 1$), or be directly proportional ($b = 1$). For rates of metabolism and clearance processes, the allometric exponent tends to be around 0.75, whereas organ sizes or physiological volumes tend to be proportional to body weight. Physiological times or the duration of physiological events (e.g., heartbeat and breath duration, lifespan, or turnover times of endogenous substances or processes) scale across species with b values around 0.25. These inter-species relationships appear to manifest from the fractal nature of biological systems.

Retrospective analysis suggests that primary pharmacokinetic parameters of many small synthetic molecules scale across species according to allometric principles, primarily reflecting the physiological processes controlling such characteristics. However, the use of allometric scaling for prospective predictions of human pharmacokinetic parameters and dose selection of these compounds is controversial and is the topic of considerable debate. In addition, several correction factors and techniques have been suggested for improving the prediction of drug clearance in humans from preclinical values. Few studies have been conducted that specifically address the role of parameter uncertainty and species selection; however, those that have been reported suggest careful study designs and caution for prospective allometric scaling predictions. Research directed toward improving the understanding of interspecies pharmacokinetic relationships is likely to continue and necessary for resolving key methodological issues.

Notwithstanding concerns associated with prospective allometric scaling, primary pharmacokinetic parameters of select macromolecules appear to follow allometric relationships, possibly resulting from a conser vation of processes controlling peptide and protein disposition. Mahmood reviewed the prediction of total clearance of 15 therapeutic proteins from inter- species scaling, confirming the need for a suitable number of animals and that simple allometry may be used for most proteins. As an example, log-log plots of total systemic clearance and the volume of distribution at steady state

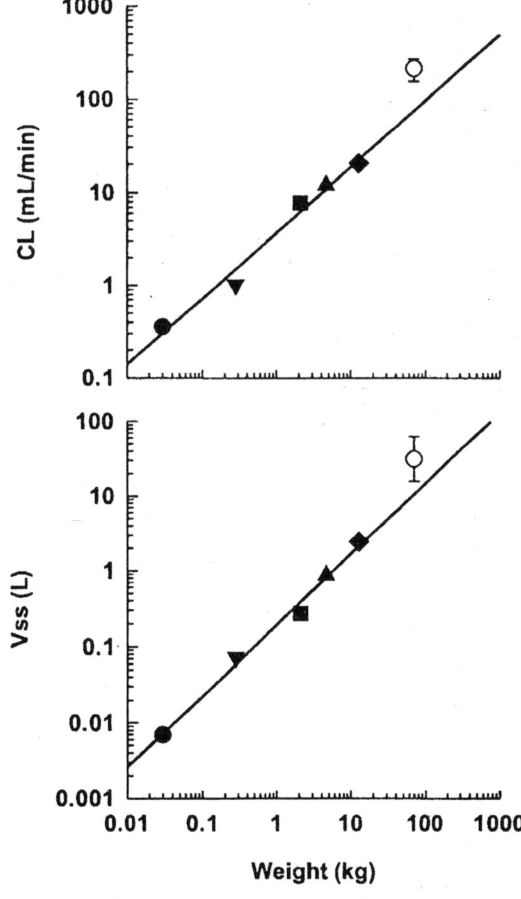

Fig. 6.4. Interspecies scaling of total systemic clearance and steady-state volume of distribution of interferon-α as a function of total body weight.

for interferon-α in mice, rats, rabbits, dogs, monkeys, and humans. The lines of regression were generated without considering human values and the relationships were as follows: $CL = 3.7W^{0.71}$ ($r^2 = 0.98$) and $V_{ss} = 0.2W^{0.94}$ ($r^2 = 0.99$). Typical values in man (open symbols) were slightly underestimated using these equations, and Lave et al. suggest that transformations of plasma concentration- time profiles make more use of preclinical data and may provide improved predictions of human pharmacokinetic parameters. Building on this concept, Cosson et al. described a method of fitting preclinical pharmacokinetic profiles and estimating allometric relationships simultaneously using a population mixed effects modeling technique. Such an approach has been applied to characterize the interspecies pharmacokinetic relationships of pegylated human erythropoietin. The final model was used to predict typical pharmacokinetic parameters in humans, as well as to simulate expected concentration-time profiles from IV and SC administration.

Despite successful applications of interspecies scaling to macromolecule pharmacokinetics, potential complicating factors exist, the most significant of which relate to saturable or dose-dependent pharmacokinetic processes. As discussed above, nonlinear behavior may manifest from several sources including receptor capacity and binding kinetics, macromolecule physico-chemical properties, and major mechanisms of peptide and protein transport and elimination. Thus, evidence of nonlinear pharmacokinetics in preclinical experiments would raise concerns as to the utility of allometric scaling for predicting such properties in humans. It remains to be determined whether a combination of *in vivo* preclinical data, compartmental modeling, and *in vitro* uptake studies might reliably anticipate macromolecule pharmacokinetics in humans under such nonlinear conditions.

Physiologically Based Pharmacokinetic Modeling

Classic pharmacokinetic modeling attempts to characterize drug disposition with systems comprised of a relatively small number of compartments. In contrast, PBPK models seek to mimic physiological pathways and processes controlling the time-course of plasma drug concentrations and represent the state-of-the-art in advanced pharmacokinetic systems analysis. As Dedrick has noted, "Physiologic modeling enables us to examine the joint effect of a number of complex inter-related processes and assess the relative significance of each". Basic concepts of PBPK modeling and applications to macromolecule pharmacokinetics are described in this section, and several reviews may be consulted for further details regarding the specification, implementation, and evaluation of PBPK models.

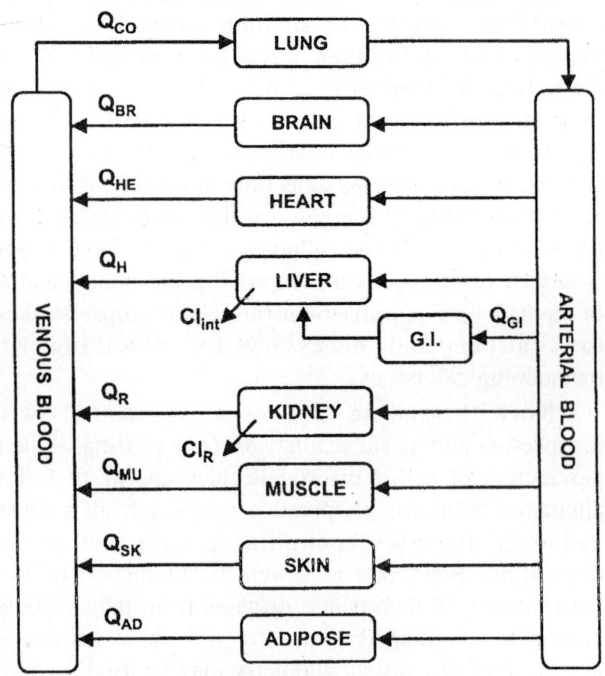

Fig. 6.5. Model structure of a hypothetical physiologically based pharmacokinetic model.

The compartments in PBPK models represent organs and tissues of interest and are arranged and connected according to anatomical and physiological relationships. Most PBPK models contain principal components, such as arterial and venous blood pools, liver, and kidney, along with additional tissues depending on its role in specific disposition processes (e.g., absorption, transport, and elimination), whether it represents a potential site of action (biophase) or is likely to account for a significant proportion of the administered dose. A series of mass-balance equations are specified that define the time-course of drug concentrations within each compartment. In the simplest case, it is assumed that mass transfer is blood-flow or perfusion-rate limited and compartments are well-stirred spaces. Under this assumption, the rate of change of drug concentration (C) in a noneliminating tissue (T) may be described by the following ordinary differential equation:

$$V_T \cdot dC_T/dt = Q_T \cdot (C_A - C_T/K_{pT}) \qquad \ldots(25)$$

where V and Q represent the volume and blood flow associated with a particular tissue, K_p is the tissue:plasma partition coefficient, and C_A is arterial drug concentration. Drug elimination (via excretion or metabolism) in speci fic organs often is described using a first-order approximation or a Michaelis–Menten function, separately or in parallel. Physiological parameters (e.g., V and Q) are frequently fixed to experimentally-measured values or literature-reported estimates; however, these terms have also been estimated during model fitting with a Maximum *a Posteriori* Bayesian method. Several *in vitro* and *in vivo* experimental methods have been described for determining drug-specific parameters. Again, most contemporary applications of PBPK modeling involve estimating such terms from fitting the model to pharmacokinetic data.

Sugiyama and Hanano constructed a simple "minimal" PBPK model, consisting of plasma, liver, and kidney compartments, to evaluate the role of receptor- mediated clearance in the overall disposition of epidermal growth factor (EGF) in rats. A remainder compartment was included to account for the rest of the body of the animal. The kinetics of the liver compartment incorporated receptor turnover processes (i.e., synthesis and degradation), binding of drug to free cell-surface receptors, and internalization of the drug-receptor complex (endocytosis and degradation). Computer simulations were conducted to evaluate this model, revealing that nonlinear kinetics of EGF may result from capacity limitation produced by either a saturation of free receptors or dose-dependent receptor downregulation.

The simple assumptions that constitute blood-flow-limited PBPK models often are inadequate for characterizing the pharmacokinetics of macro molecules. Instead, a membrane- or permeability-rate-limited model is more common, where it is assumed that mass transfer across the cell membrane is rate-limiting. For these models, organ compartments are subdivided into at least two well-stirred spaces representing vascular ($C_{T,V}$) and extravascular ($C_{T,EV}$) compartments. Such a system might be described by the following equations for a noneliminating tissue:

$$V_{T,V} dC_{T,V} / dt = Q_T \cdot (C_A - C_{T,V}) - F_{uB} \cdot PS_T \cdot (C_{T,V} - C_{T,EV} / K_{pT}) \qquad \ldots(26)$$

$$V_{T,EV} dC_{T,EV} / dt = f_{uB} \cdot PS_T \cdot (C_{T,V} - C_{T,EV} / K_{pT}) \qquad \ldots(27)$$

where f_{uB} is the free fraction in blood and PS_T is the permeability surface area product. Examples of membrane-limited models developed for protein molecules include β-endorphin, a 31 amino acid straight-chain polypeptide, and ISIS 1082, a 21-mer phosphorothioate oligonucleotide.

Monoclonal antibodies represent a diverse group of therapeutic proteins typically presenting with complex pharmacokinetic properties. For these compounds, more comprehensive, mechanism-based PBPK models have been described. Baxter et al. developed and evaluated a bifunctional antibody PBPK model in mice and scaled the model to predict its pharmacokinetics in humans. A membrane-limited model was used; however, additional equations were required to describe up to nine molecular species in each tissue (resulting from specific and nonspecific binding), and mass transport across the membrane included convective and diffusive components (so-called two-pore system). The latter model, by Friedrich et al., further incorporated lymphatic circulation and identified critical properties requiring optimization for this treatment modality to be successful.

Although the PBPK approach has existed for several decades, reports of its use in characterizing macromolecule pharmacokinetics have been relatively sparse. The technological requirements for PBPK modeling are often seen as formidable; however, advances in computer hardware and software are bringing this methodology within common reach. The significant potential for scaling preclinical models to anticipate human pharmacokinetics in various relevant tissues (including target sites) represents a strategic advantage of PBPK modeling in drug development. Furthermore, this systems approach provides a means of understanding the pharmacological implications of the complexities associated with the disposition of macromolecules. The pharmacokinetic properties of biotechnology pharmaceuticals are complex relative to small-molecule drugs, and preclinical studies are critical to the discovery and development of these therapeutic agents. Understanding the mechanisms and implications of *in vivo* disposition of macromolecules provides a means for investigating and designing novel drug candidates and delivery systems to optimize exposure-response relationships or therapeutic efficacy. Mathematical modeling of preclinical pharmacokinetic data is necessary for characterizing such properties, and techniques like allometric scaling and PBPK modeling may be used to anticipate human pharmacokinetics under certain conditions. The utility of these approaches may be further enhanced by coupling pharmacokinetic data with mechanism-based pharmacodynamic modeling of biomarkers and surrogates of drug effects.

7

CLINICAL PHARMACOKINETICS

The term "*pharmacokinetics*" refers to the time course of the passage of a drug and its metabolites through the body. It can be thought of as "what the body does to the drug" in contrast to pharmacodynamics, which can be thought of as "what the drug does to the body". The processes involved are absorption, distribution, metabolism and excretion. Together, these processes play an important role in determining the duration and magnitude of both the desired and undesired pharmacodynamic effects of drugs. It is not usually possible to measure the concentration of a drug at its sites of action. Plasma, which can be conveniently sampled, is generally used instead, but drug concentrations may be determined in other bodily fluids such as saliva and cerebrospinal fluid, as well as, of course, the excreta, urine and faeces. There is often a relationship between plasma concentration and response, although this may sometimes be complex. Therefore, estimation of plasma concentrations, and how they are altered by the many factors that can affect drug handling, may be used to make predictions about dosage in the otherwise healthy individual and in the presence of organ failure or concomitant medications.

A growing appreciation of the predictive value of pharmacokinetics, together with a change in the attitude of European and American regulatory authorities to the whole question of dosage, has led to increased importance of the clinical pharmacokinetics regulatory submission. It is no longer acceptable to register a dosage regimen based on a single empirically derived dose of proven efficacy and safety. Drug developers are now rightly required to demonstrate, wherever possible, that the optimum dose and frequency of dosing have been selected to give the greatest benefit for the least risk of adverse reactions. Regulatory authorities also require pharmacokinetic information to support clinical data in order to make recommendations on how dosage should be modified for particular patient populations. The clinical significance of altered pharmacokinetics, and hence the requirement for dosage adjustment, will, to some extent, depend on the therapeutic index of the drug. Thus, while a clinical pharmacokinetics package forms a mandatory part of every regulatory submission for a systemically administered drug, a more comprehensive package will be generally required for drugs of low therapeutic index. Although, like statistics, the details of pharmacokinetic analysis are best left to the experts, a pharmaceutical physician who is familiar with

- the study of the time course of a drug's passage through body fluids and tissues
- "what the body does to the drug"

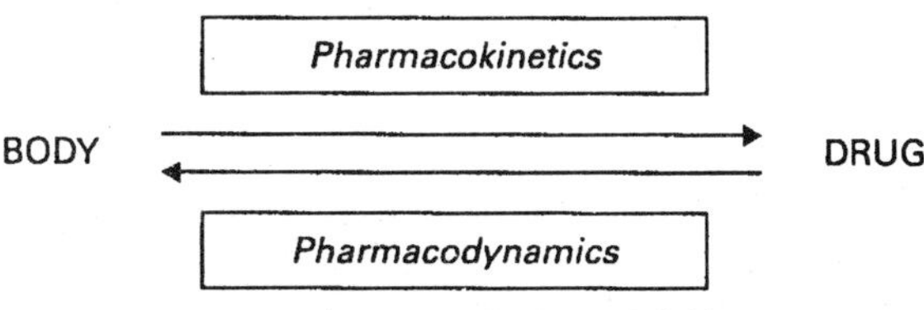

Fig. 7.1. Pharmacokinetics – definition.

the basic concepts of how pharmacokinetic information contributes to a dossier will be able to interact more effectively with company colleagues and regulatory authority staff. It is the aim of this chapter to provide such a preliminary grounding.

Basic Concepts

However, an understanding of the basic concepts is essential in order to appreciate how pharmacokinetic data can provide insight into the physiological processes that determine the time course of a drug in the body, and implications this has for the toxicity and therapeutic efficacy of drugs, particularly new active substances in development.

Overview of the Fate of Administered Drug

A drug can be administered directly into the vascular compartment or by an alternative route such as orally. It can usually be assumed that all of the dose administered by the intravenous route reaches the systemic circulation. After oral administration, only a proportion may reach the systemic circulation because of incomplete *absorption* or because absorbed drug may be metabolised in the mucosa of the gastrointestinal tract or liver, a process known as *first-pass metabolism*. Once in the systemic circulation, drug is transferred from one site in the body to another and back again; this is called *distribution*. Rates and extent of distribution to different tissues may depend on blood perfusion, diffusion and binding to plasma and tissue proteins. Also, once the drug is in the plasma, it can start to be removed, either by changing it to another molecule (*metabolism*) or by removal from the plasma into urine, bile or, more rarely, breath (*excretion*). Collectively, metabolism and excretion are known as *elimination*.

Plasma Concentration–Time Curve

The effects of the processes listed above on the time course of the plasma concentration with time is as follows. Initially, as absorption starts, the plasma drug concentration will rise. As soon as there is some drug in the plasma, distribution and elimination will start. Absorption will start to slow down as there is less drug to be absorbed. Eventually, the rate of drug going into the plasma from absorption will be equalled by the rate of drug leaving the plasma by distribution and elimination, so temporarily a plateau of maximum concentration is reached. Absorption continues to slow (as by now most of the drug has been absorbed) and the plasma concentration will continue to fall because of ongoing distribution and elimination. Often, elimination is slower than distribution, resulting in an initial fast fall, due mainly to distribution and then a slower fall due largely to elimination. Most physicians will be familiar with the basic shape of a plasma concentration–time curve following oral or intravenous administration, and are likely to be familiar with, or at least readily understand, the simple terms that relate to this shape. Such terms – maximum plasma concentration (C_{max}), time to maximum plasma concentration (T_{max}), area under the plasma concentration–time curve (AUC) and half-life ($t_{1/2}$) – are illustrated below.

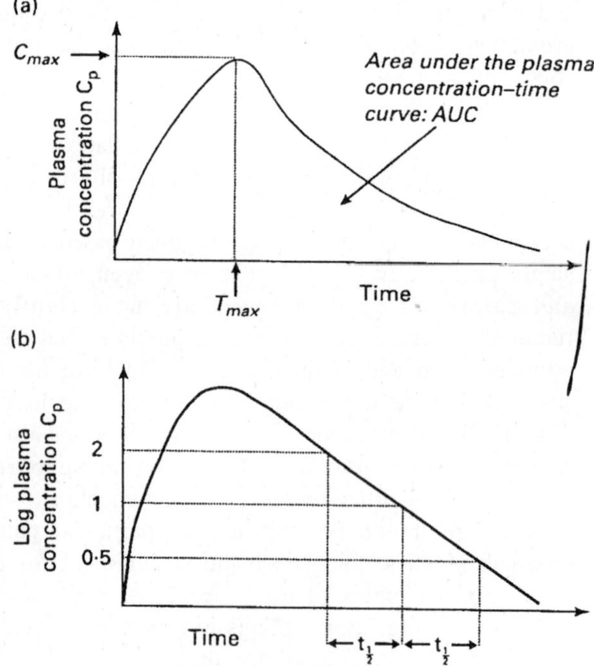

Fig. 7.2. Descriptive pharmacokinetic parameters.

Descriptive versus Conceptual Parameters

These simple descriptive terms can be used for any concentration–time profile, and do not require any conceptual understanding of how the drug is handled by the body. Although these descriptive terms are useful in designing a dosage regimen (as we shall see later), there is no way of understanding why two drugs dosed at the same nominal dose could have very differing values of C_{max} and half-life. To understand why the values are as they are, it is necessary to use a new set of parameters, which assist in the conceptual understanding of how the drug is handled by the body. These parameters are clearance (CL), bioavailability (F) and volume of distribution (V), and are discussed in turn below.

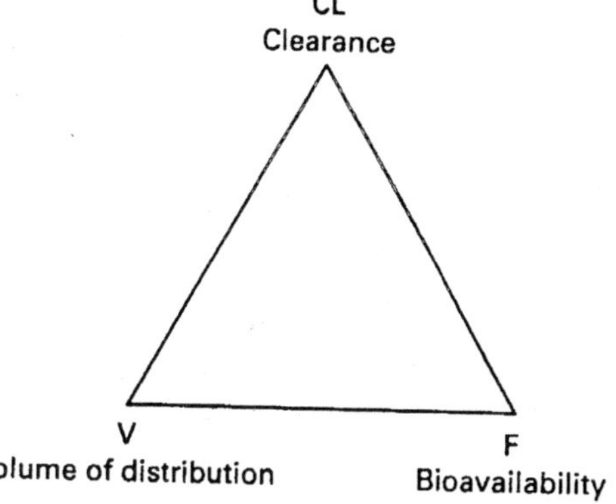

Fig. 7.3. The triad of primary pharmacokinetic parameters.

Clearance

Clearance is a measure of the body's ability to eliminate the drug substance from the plasma by either metabolism or excretion. The main organs undertaking the clearance function are therefore the liver and the kidneys, although other organs can take part as well (gut, lung, peripheral tissues, etc.). Clearance is an important parameter because it is the property of a drug that determines the maintenance dosing rate needed to maintain a desired plasma concentration.

When clearance is otherwise unspecified, the term "*clearance*" is used to mean "*total plasma clearance*", which is the sum of the individual organ clearances (hepatic clearance, renal clearance, etc.). Measuring or estimating individual organ clearances can be used to predict changes in drug handling under different physiological circumstances. Given that one of the definitions of clearance is "the volume of plasma completely cleared of drug in unit time", it can be readily seen that this is equal to the total plasma flow multiplied by the proportion of drug removed by the organ during the passage. This latter proportion defines the concept of "*extraction ratio*" of an organ. If there is a high (>70%) extraction ratio across an organ, increasing the blood flow is likely to increase clearance. Conversely, when the extraction ratio is low (<20%), changes in blood flow are unlikely to change clearance because the eliminating capacity is not limited by the amount of drug being supplied.

Clearance units and range for values

As indicated in the definition, clearance has units of flow, for example ml/min or l/h; it can also be corrected for body weight. For drugs that undergo negligible renal elimination and are very stable metabolically, clearance values can be <1 ml/min. The maximum values for organ clearance approach total organ plasma or blood flow. Hence, the maximum limit for hepatic clearance is about 1500 ml/min. Higher values for clearance would suggest that more than one organ is responsible for clearance or that the drug is metabolised in the plasma. For example, diamorphine has a systemic clearance of about 3000 ml/min because it is deacetylated in the plasma.

The kidney is a special case because, unlike with other organs, we can measure the amount of drug eliminated by that organ, in this case by measuring the amount of drug in urine. For all small molecules, the unbound drug in plasma is readily filtered at the glomerulus where the normal glomerular filtration rate (GFR) is about 120 ml/min. Hence, if the renal clearance of a drug is much higher than the GFR, we can conclude that active tubular secretion must exist as a renal excretion pathway. This is important because, unlike filtration, which is a passive process, competition for tubular secretion, and hence the potential for clinically relevant drug interactions, can occur. Conversely, if the renal clearance is substantially lower than the filtered free drug clearance, we can conclude that tubular reabsorption must be occurring. This raises the possibility of renal clearance being dependent on urinary flow rate or pH. In addition to metabolism, the liver is also able to secrete unchanged drug into the bile, sometimes against a high concentration gradient. This is also a form of hepatic clearance. An example of a drug that is almost exclusively eliminated by biliary secretion is the antimalarial drug atovaquone. Whether a drug is eliminated largely unchanged in urine or primarily metabolised is a function of its physicochemical properties and its suitability as a substrate for metabolising enzymes. As a broad generalisation, hydrophilic (water-loving) drugs will be eliminated in the urine and lipophilic (fat-loving) drugs will be primarily metabolised.

For most drugs, clearance values for an individual subject are independent of dose. This would mean that, for example, when you double the dose, the plasma concentration is doubled. However, for some drugs, clearance may change with dose. This usually occurs when a drug is eliminated primarily by metabolism (and this is a saturable process) and the mass dose of the drug is high. For example, alcohol is a drug that is consumed in gram doses where the rate of metabolism is saturated after a small intake. A more clinically relevant example is phenytoin, where metabolism is saturated within the therapeutic dosage range. Terms used to describe this include "*non-linear kinetics*" and this results in disproportionately high increases in plasma concentration when the dose is increased. Under such circumstances, clearance is concentration dependent.

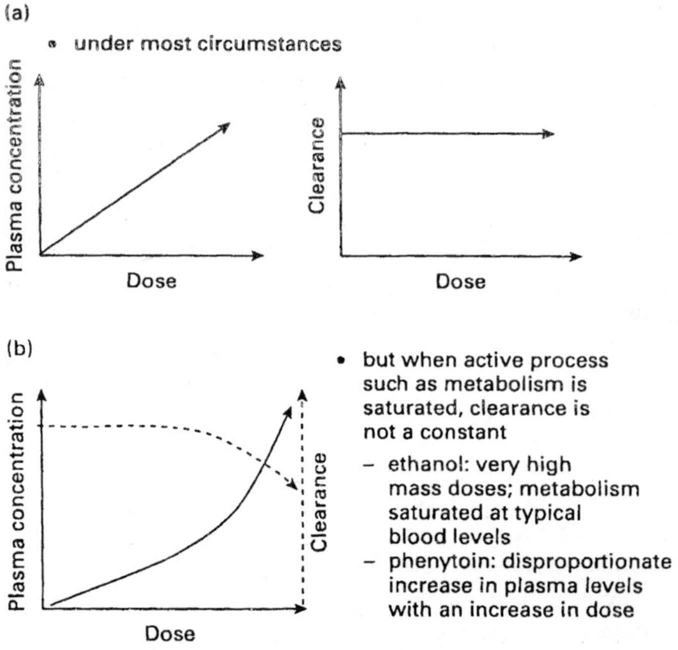

Fig. 7.4. (a) Clearance is a constant; (b) saturation of metabolism.

Bioavailability

Bioavailability is the other important conceptual pharmacokinetic parameter, in addition to clearance. Bioavailability is defined as "the proportion of an administered dose that reaches the systemic circulation". It has no units and is usually expressed as a percentage. Values range from 0 to 100%, and will be 100% or "complete" for an intravenously administered drug. After oral administration, only a proportion of the drug may reach the systemic circulation because of incomplete absorption or because absorbed drug may be metabolised in the gut wall or liver (first-pass metabolism). For orally administered drugs, bioavailability will be the product of the fraction of the dose absorbed into the body and the fraction of the dose that escapes gut and hepatic first-pass metabolism. For example, if a drug is 50% absorbed but the absorbed drug undergoes 75% first-pass metabolism, the bioavailability is $0{\cdot}5 \times 0{\cdot}25 = 12{\cdot}5\%$. As an approximation, first-pass extraction is equal to the hepatic extraction ratio. Examples of drugs with low bioavailability because of high first-pass metabolism include propranolol, verapamil and morphine.

As with clearance, the physicochemical properties of a drug can determine its absorption and hence contribute to bioavailability. Hydrophilic drugs may dissolve well in the gut lumen and hence cause few formulation problems, but cross cell membranes poorly and hence may be poorly absorbed, although there are some mechanisms of absorption of hydrophilic drugs between cells. In contrast, lipophilic drugs may dissolve poorly and hence cause formulation problems, but they may be well absorbed. These opposing constraints mean that very hydrophilic or very lipophilic drugs are often poorly bioavailable, and intermediate values are often sought by drug discovery to retain good bioavailability.

Volume of distribution

Volume of distribution is the third parameter to complete the triad of primary pharmacokinetic parameters. The key concepts are summarised in Box 5.4. Volume of distribution is defined as a proportionality constant relating the total amount of drug in the body to the plasma concentration. It is also sometimes described as the apparent "volume" into which the drug distributes if all the drug in the body is at the same concentration as in plasma. Overall, volume of distribution is a complicated concept and can be one of the most difficult to understand. It is also not a single parameter, as the volumes of distribution can vary depending on when it is calculated following the dose. For example, it can be readily understood that shortly after an intravenous bolus, the volume of distribution may be quite small because the drug is still largely in the plasma compartment. However, once steady state has been reached, the volume of distribution may be larger. In the terminal elimination phase, when tissues are loaded with drug and the plasma concentrations are being reduced by clearance, the volume can be even larger again.

It is a rare for the volume of distribution to represent a real volume. It can occur – the smallest possible distribution volumes will occur for drugs that are largely physically confined to the plasma compartment, for example large, highly protein-bound drugs, such as some intravenous contrast agents. However, there is no upper limit to volume of distribution and it can be very much larger than body volume. Under such circumstances one can conclude that the drug must be highly concentrated in at least one tissue. This may have important implications for therapeutic potential or for toxicity. For example, a lipophilic drug is likely to penetrate and be concentrated in the CNS, which may be desired or undesired.

The units of volume of distribution are those of volume and can be adjusted for body weight (l/kg). The two main uses of volume of distribution are in the calculation of loading doses for rapid onset of drug effect, and in understanding changes in half-life.

Calculation of primary parameters

It is important to understand that the primary parameters clearance and volume of distribution can only be routinely calculated following intravenous administration of drug. This is because it is necessary to know the amount of drug that has reached the systemic circulation for these calculations. This is not known for a non-intravenous dose, unless one makes an estimate of bioavailability, for example from urinary recovery of unchanged drug. Given the usefulness of knowing these primary parameters in being able to make physiological predictions about the drug, this is one reason why some regulatory authorities insist on having this information, which requires intravenous administration of the drug, even when there are no plans to administer the drug therapeutically intravenously. Calculation of bioavailability requires a comparison of the area under the plasma concentration–time curves following a non-intravenous and an intravenous dose, after correction for dose size. Without knowing the bioavailability, only "apparent" clearance and volume of distribution can be calculated and the ability to make predictions from these values is very limited.

Half-life

Physicians may be surprised to see that mention of half-life has been dealt with so late in this chapter, as it is likely to be the pharmacokinetic term most familiar to them. As mentioned earlier, half-life is not a primary pharmacokinetic parameter but is one of the descriptive terms. Although many physicians will readily accept that changes in clearance will alter half-life, what is not quite so obvious is that half-life is equally determined by volume of distribution and in fact there is an equation relating these three terms:

$$t_{1/2} = 0{\cdot}7\ V/CL \qquad \ldots(1)$$

Thus, if we are comparing half-life values between two groups of patients, or in an individual before and after a potentially interacting drug, we cannot automatically assume that a prolonging of the half-life is the result of a reduction in clearance. This may well be the case, but is also possible that there are differences in volume of distribution. Furthermore, if drug has a long half-life it cannot be assumed to have a low clearance. For example, digoxin has a half-life of over a day but this is the result of a large volume of distribution because the drug is concentrated in tissues. In fact, its clearance is relatively high, and this is why measures to increase clearance (such as haemodialysis) are ineffective in removing a significant amount of drug from the body in cases of overdose, unless additional measures are taken to reduce volume of distribution, for example digoxin antibodies.

The plasma elimination half-life can be determined from a semilogarithmic plot of the plasma concentration–time plot as the time taken for the plasma concentration to fall by 50%. The elimination half-life of some drugs is very short (seconds or minutes) whereas for others it may be very long (weeks). Clearly, half-life is related to clearance but, perhaps less obviously, it depends on the volume of distribution. To appreciate this, consider two drugs A and B that have the same clearance, i.e. they will be eliminated from plasma at the same rate if present in the same concentrations. However, if B has twice the volume distribution of A, plasma concentrations of B after the same dose will be half those of A. Since systemic clearance is equivalent to the volume of plasma (per unit time) from which drug is removed, it will take twice as long for the same amount of drug B to be removed from the body, because the concentration is lower. Thus, half-life may be prolonged by reduced clearance, by an increased volume of distribution or by a combination of the two mechanisms.

Half-life determines the time it will take to achieve steady state and is useful for determining a dosing regimen. However, it does not give any clue to the processes involved in handling of the drug, so that knowledge of the half-life alone cannot be used to make predictions about factors which are likely to affect the rate of elimination.

Predictions from Pharmacokinetic Parameters

Earlier I stressed the utility of being able to make predictions from knowledge of the primary pharmacokinetic parameters, and some examples have been given. A further example is as follows. Imagine we have undertaken a "first-in-man" study where the drug has been given intravenously. Negligible amounts of unchanged drug were recovered in the urine, and the total plasma clearance was calculated to be 750 ml/min. From *in vitro* data it is likely that the drug is metabolised. It is reasonable to assume that the total plasma clearance is likely to be largely due to hepatic clearance and hence we have a hepatic extraction ratio of about 50% (750/1500 ml/min). Already we can assume that the drug will have oral bioavailability no higher than 50% (because first-pass metabolism is likely to be about 50%) and that changes in hepatic blood flow and/or metabolising capacity will affect steady-state plasma concentrations. This is without having yet given an oral dose of the drug.

Use of Pharmacokinetic Information to Design Dosage Regimens

An understanding of the pharmacokinetic properties of a drug is one of the major sources of information used in designing a dosing regimen.

1. The volume of distribution can be used to determine the size of the dose required to reach a desired target plasma concentration with the first dose.

2. Clearance will determine the maintenance dosing rate to maintain an average plasma concentration.
3. The half-life will determine how the maintenance dosing rate should be divided in time to keep fluctuations in plasma concentration within acceptable limits.

However, there are other major factors in determining the dosing regimen, such as the nature of the concentration–response relationship for both efficacy and toxicity (therapeutic window) and commercial/ compliance factors. There are additional reasons why caution should be applied in assuming an efficacy–time profile from a given plasma concentration–time profile.

Furthermore, it should not be assumed that a constant plasma concentration is desirable. For example, aminoglycoside antibiotics are safer and more effective for systemic gram-negative infection when given once daily rather than three times daily for the same total daily dose, despite a plasma half-life of less than two hours. Secondly, although traditionally pharmaceutical companies have tried to have the "one dose for all" approach for dose selection, this may be increasingly hard to maintain with the increasing amount of genetic and related information on an individual's capacity to handle and respond to a drug.

Bioavailability and Bioequivalence

Bioavailability and bioequivalence are related terms but they can be confused. Bioavailability as defined above is also known as *absolute bioavailability* and is simply the fraction of the administered dose that reaches the systemic circulation; it is therefore defined only in terms of the *extent* of drug absorption. However, in the CPMP guideline for the investigation of bioavailability and bioequivalence, bioavailability is defined as the "the rate and extent to which the active substance of therapeutic moiety is absorbed from a pharmaceutical form and becomes available at the site of action". The reason that bioavailability has been defined in this way is because *rate*, as well as extent, is important when comparing bioavailability of two pharmaceutical forms of an active substance to determine whether they are bioequivalent. Bioequivalence and comparative bioavailability are discussed below but the absolute bioavailability will be described first.

Bioavailability

It would seem that when developing a drug that is intended purely for oral administration there would be no need to administer the drug intravenously. However, as mentioned above, the primary pharmacokinetic parameters cannot be determined without giving the drug intravenously. As drug regulators find these parameters helpful, they like to see this information. Currently the European regulators make this mandatory but it is only advised by the FDA.

It can be assumed that the bioavailability of an intravenous dose is 100% and a calculation of oral bioavailability can therefore be obtained by comparison of the AUCs after oral and intravenous administration, after correction for the exact dose:

$$F = \frac{AUC_{oral}}{AUC_{iv}} \times \frac{Dose_{iv}}{Dose_{oral}} \quad \text{...(2)}$$

The AUCs can be obtained by administration of intravenous and oral formulations in a crossover study. It is important to use the exact dose rather than nominal doses: the oral and intravenous formulations should be assayed, and the syringes or giving sets used for the intravenous administration carefully weighed before and after dosing. The size of the intravenous dose should be reduced compared with the oral dose in proportion to the expected bioavailability so that the AUCs will be similar. This avoids assumptions about linear kinetics and maximises safety, since high plasma concentrations by the intravenous route are avoided. Similarly, it is appropriate to infuse the intravenous drug over a period comparable with the time to maximum concentration (T_{max}) after oral administration in order to avoid transient high peaks.

There may not be any intention to develop an intravenous formulation for therapeutic use but it will usually be a necessary to produce one for the purposes of the study. For prodrugs (i.e. where the main pharmacological activity comes from a metabolite), the appropriate intravenous comparator is the active metabolite. There are, however, some drugs that cannot be administered by the intravenous route, either because it would not be safe or because it is not technically feasible to develop a suitable formulation. If there is a very high recovery of unchanged drug in urine, it may be possible to obtain a reasonable estimate of absolute bioavailability from oral administration. However, metabolites in urine cannot be assumed to derive from drug that was bioavailable since they may have been formed in the gut by the action of intestinal bacteria, for example, and subsequently absorbed and excreted in urine. An alternative to intravenous administration is a reference oral solution; if this is not feasible, an oral suspension of standardised fine particles size may be the best option. Clearly these do not enable calculation of absolute bioavailability but might indicate whether the test formulation has less than optimal bioavailability. For a drug that exhibits high intra-individual as well as interindividual variability of clearance, or which has time-dependent kinetics, it may be useful to give the intravenous and oral formulations simultaneously. Drug administered by one route will need to be labelled with either a radioactive or stable isotope so drugs administered by the two routes can be distinguished.

Bioequivalence

Two medicinal products containing the same active ingredients are bioequivalent if they produce the same clinical effect. However, assessment of clinical response would require a clinical trial for every new formulation, which is simply not feasible or justifiable. It is reasonable to assume that the effects of drug molecules, once they have reached the systemic circulation, should be independent of the formulation from which they came. Therefore, two products can be regarded as bioequivalent if they produce the same plasma concentration–time profiles. It should be recognised that pharmacokinetic bioequivalence may not be a perfect surrogate for therapeutic equivalence since adverse reactions may differ because of biological effects of excipients. Furthermore, equivalent plasma concentrations may not imply indistinguishable clinical effects in the case of topical agents acting locally on the skin, lung, eye or within the gut lumen.

In contrast to the measurement of absolute bioavailability, for which only the extent of absorption is important, establishment of bioequivalence requires demonstration that the rates of absorption are also indistinguishable. This can be clinically important; for example, a capsule formulation of phenytoin produced higher and earlier peak plasma concentrations, which were associated with a higher incidence of adverse reactions although the extent of absorption was similar to the standard formulation. Fortunately, a comparison of plasma AUCs is universally accepted as a valid means of comparing the extent of absorption, although there is little agreement as to the best measure of the rate. Since peak concentration (C_{max}) is obviously of great importance for many drugs, it is generally taken as the second important kinetic parameter for tests of comparative bioavailability or bioequivalence. Nevertheless, as mentioned earlier, as C_{max} occurs at the time after drug administration (T_{max}) when the rate of entry of drug into the plasma equals the rate of its removal, therefore T_{max} is determined by the rate of distribution and elimination as well as the rate of absorption. T_{max} is also dependent on discrete sample times, in contrast to a continuous variable like concentration, and it therefore has less statistical power to reflect a real change in absorption rate. Another approach to the problem of absorption rate is the calculation of *mean residence time*, a measure of the average time a drug molecule resides in the body.

Testing of bioequivalence is an area where drug regulatory authorities have produced extremely detailed and specific guidelines, not only on the design and conduct of the study but also on statistical analysis, sample analysis and drug sample retention. One reason for this is that manufacturers of generic medicines can obtain registration of a generic version of a drug of proven clinical safety and efficacy on the basis of a single bioequivalence study, without the need to perform clinical trials. Commercial pressures are clearly great and there have been a number of examples of misconduct, and a scandal involving gross fraud. The result is that the guidelines are extremely strict, and for products of high therapeutic index and excellent safety records they seem excessive. However, there is little room for flexibility, and adherence to the guidelines is strongly recommended. It has been frustrating being required to undertake bioequivalence studies for minor changes in formulation which are unlikely to affect bioavailability. Recently, there have been regulatory moves to propose a classification of drug bioavailability which stratifies the need for a human study, depending on the physicochemical characteristics of the compound and its bioavailability. This may reduce the need for bioequivalence studies in the future.

Although the two-period crossover design has certain intrinsic weaknesses, intra-individual variation is usually smaller than variation between subjects, and bioequivalence can usually be established using a smaller number of subjects in a crossover study. The order in which subjects receive single doses of the different formulations must be randomised and an adequate interval allowed between doses to ensure washout. The number of subjects will depend on the variability of the kinetics of the compound. A power calculation should be performed using historical data, if possible. In practice, the minimum number of volunteers needed is 12 and the maximum usually about 24 but is occasionally more. The number and times of blood samples is a critical: a sufficient number of samples is required around the T_{max} to permit T_{max} and C_{max} to be identified with adequate accuracy. Sampling should continue for at least 3–4 half- lives and later samples should be spaced so that no more than about 15% (or ideally 10%) of the AUC has to be determined by extrapolation or interpolation between points. Model-fitted data are usually not acceptable; Cmax should be obtained directly from the observed concentration data and AUC calculated by the trapezoidal method with extrapolation of the terminal slope to infinity using linear regression.

If pharmacokinetics are dependent on dose or time, or a slow-release formulation is being studied, it is necessary to examine bioequivalence at steady state. For controlled-release formulations which are intended to produce relatively flat concentration–time profiles, an index of fluctuation is required, for example $(C_{max} - C_{min})/C_{avg}$. A study at steady state may also be needed if the assay is not sensitive enough to quantify plasma concentrations of drug up to four half-lives after a single dose. Sometimes it is not technically feasible to assay a drug in plasma and it may then the justifiable to compare bioavailability by the total amount of drug excreted in urine, or pharmacodynamic data may be used, but these cases are exceptions.

In general, regulatory authorities expect proof of bioequivalence of every marketed formulation relative to the one that was used to establish pivotal safety and efficacy data. However, because differences between formulations may sometimes be very small, there are some situations when it is not necessary to demonstrate bioequivalence *in vivo*. Different strengths of the same formulation do not usually need to be studied, for example tablets of 100 mg and 200 mg, where the lower dose tablet is a direct scale down of the larger, with the same proportions of excipients. However, if kinetics are dependent on dose, it may be necessary to compare them. If two formulations differ with respect to either types or proportions of excipients or the way in which they were manufactured, an *in vivo* comparison would generally be required. In other cases, such as an additional film coat, addition of a colouring agent for brand identity, a change a shape of tablet or a minor change in a common excipient, the guidelines are far from clear as to whether a bioequivalence study is required.

In all this, it should be remembered that the role of regulatory authorities is to protect the public. For entirely justifiable reasons, they will apply very strict criteria to products with a low therapeutic index, non-linear kinetics or unfavourable physical properties. Digoxin, phenyotin and primidone provide notable examples of drugs where bioinequivalence issues have led to clinical problems.

Table 7.1. Factors to be considered when deciding whether a new formulation requires a study to establish bioequivalence

Factors to be considered	*Suggests study is required*
Difference from reference	Substantial
Bioavailability	Low
Therapeutic index	Low
Kinetics	Non-linear
Dispersal/dissolution properties	Poor
Relationship to another drug	Other drug has known poor bioavailability or bioequivalence problems
Likely attitude of a strict regulatory authority in a commercially important territory	Likely to require a study
Importance of drug to your portfolio	Commercially important drug

Drug Interactions

Selection of Studies

It is reasonable that data should be required to demonstrate whether the response of patients to a new active substance is likely to change or be changed by concomitant medication. However, there is clearly a huge number of potential drug combinations and some rational selection is required. To assist with the selection of drug combinations for which data are required, the following seven questions should be asked.

What are the ADME characteristics of the drug?

For example, a drug that is mainly excreted in the urine, with a renal clearance much greater than GFR, is likely to be actively secreted by the renal tubule. If the drug is an organic acid, probenecid is likely to reduce its elimination; if it is basic, its renal clearance may be reduced by cimetidine. For drugs that are metabolised, there are a number of enzyme inhibitors and inducers which may potentially affect the same pathway. Selection of a drug interactions study at the level of hepatic metabolism is becoming much more rational with the identification of a variety of isozymes of hepatic cytochrome P450 and the association of specific drug metabolising processors with each isozyme.

Does the drug belong to a class of compounds known to interact with many other drugs?

For example, drugs containing an imidazole ring, such as cimetidine and many antifungal agents, inhibit many reactions mediated by cytochrome P450. Therefore, a new compound of this chemical class is likely to behave similarly, and evaluation of its potential interactions will be required.

What is the therapeutic index of the drug?

If the drug has a low therapeutic index, interactions are much more likely to have clinical consequences, so a variety of kinetic studies will be needed.

Is the drug likely to be co-prescribed with a drug of narrow therapeutic index?

For example, a drug for angina, cardiac failure or an antiarrhythmic agent is likely to be co-prescribed with warfarin. If there is any evidence of enzyme induction or inhibition, a clinical study with warfarin may be required.

What are the chances of the drug being co-prescribed with a wide range of medicines?

A drug that is to be given to young adults in single doses (for example for migraine) is far less likely to cause many clinically significant interactions than one that is intended for long-term administration, particularly in an elderly population who often receive several concomitant medications.

Pharmacodynamics

Although this chapter concentrates on clinical pharmacokinetics, it would be wrong to omit mention of pharmacodynamic interactions in a section on drug interactions. It is difficult to generalise, but drugs with marked pharmacological effects, particularly on the cardiovascular system and CNS are potentially subject to clinically important pharmacodynamic interactions.

Does the drug share a common mechanism of absorption or disposition with another likely co-prescribed drug?

Two drugs that are intended to be coadministered might compete for active absorption or a common route of elimination.

Study Design

There are several factors to take into account in the design of drug interaction studies. Single-dose studies have been criticised but may be useful to exclude major effects. If an interaction is detected with single doses, it may be necessary to conduct a study at steady state, mimicking the dosage used in clinical practice to determine the true clinical consequences of interaction. Whenever possible, interaction studies should not only be pharmacokinetic but should also include pharmacodynamic measurements in order to assess the likely clinical effect of an observed pharmacokinetic interaction. Furthermore, if possible the design should go some way to explaining the mechanism of interaction. For example, measurement of a metabolite in plasma or urine may help to distinguish changes in elimination from changes in absorption as the reason for the change in AUC of the parent drug.

There are certain special cases which can seem difficult. For example, chronic full dosing of warfarin to volunteers has safety concerns, and the concentrations following a single standard dose can be regarded as subtherapeutic. To address this, a design using a single large dose of warfarin has been shown to be reliable in detecting or excluding clinically significant interactions with warfarin.

Enzyme Induction and Inhibition

Drugs that cause induction or inhibition of enzymes may affect the metabolism of concomitantly administered drugs, as well as of hormones and other endogenous substances. For this reason, such properties are considered undesirable and sometimes they might constitute sufficient reason to discontinue drug development. At the very least, studies will be required to assess the magnitude of effect of likely interactions. Metabolic and toxicity studies in animals will usually provide the basis for suspicion, and studies in human liver slices, cultured hepatocytes and microsomal preparations can be extremely valuable in establishing metabolic pathways and the likelihood of enzyme induction or inhibition in man. There have been some important developments in this field in recent years and it is now possible to identify:

- which cytochrome P450(s) is/are responsible for the metabolism of the test compound
- which cytochrome P450(s) is/are inhibited by relevant multiples of the therapeutic concentrations of the test compound.

These data will help predict other drugs which may affect the handling of the test drug and alternatively, concomitant medication for which the handling, and hence clinical response, may be altered by administration of the test drug. There is an increasingly extensive library of known inhibitors, inducers and substrates for each isozyme. This information can be used to predict which groups of drugs are unlikely to interact with the test drug, which can be justification for not performing unnecessary studies. Unfortunately, extrapolation from the *in vitro* data is not perfect and hence *in vivo* data may be required with a likely concomitant medication of narrow therapeutic index.

Once the *in vitro* screen has been performed, it is an increasingly common practice to use well-validated markers of each individual cytochrome P450 in order to make generalisations about the presence or lack of interactions of a certain group of compounds. Several reference probe compounds can even be given simultaneously using the "cocktail" approach so that, for example, the presence of absence of an effect of the test compound on several cytochrome P450s can be studied conveniently in a single human study. This can be a powerful tool and can be very cost-effective.

One potentially serious consequence of enzyme induction relates to the oral contraceptive pill (OCP), which may be rendered ineffective by induction of its metabolism. The effect of a period of drug administration on circulating concentrations of the appropriate oestrogen and progestogens over the course of menstrual cycles may be examined in women taking the OCP, with additional non-hormonal precautions taken to avoid unwanted pregnancy. Another approach is to investigate whether the drug causes *autoinduction* - whether its own clearance is increased by a period of drug administration compared with that after a single dose. This has implications for starting and maintenance dosage of the drug, as well as potentially for other drugs.

Environmental factors which may affect drug handling include changes in the diet (barbecued meat causes enzyme induction; grapefruit juice can inhibit cytochrome P450 3A4), smoking (induction), and alcohol (acutely causes inhibition; chronically causes induction) and these must be avoided for a period before the study and until its completion. The duration of dosing with the test drug also needs some consideration. While enzyme inhibition may occur after a single dose, it may take 7–10 days for enzyme induction to be fully develop as the new protein synthesis occurs.

Protein Binding

Although at one time, displacement from plasma protein binding sites was thought to be an important cause of clinically significant drug interactions, it is now recognised that it is only likely to produce a temporary increase in drug effect. Thus, a pure displacement interaction is only likely to be clinically significant for a drug with a narrow therapeutic index, a long half-life and small volume distribution, which is best exemplified by warfarin. For clinically significant drug interactions that have been attributed to displacement of plasma protein binding, alternative mechanisms, such as inhibition of metabolism, have been found to be responsible, for example, warfarin–phenylbutazone and tolbutamide– sulphonamide interactions. If the drug is highly protein bound, screening *in vitro* for protein binding displacement may help guide a search for suitable probe drugs to assess the clinical effect. However, displacement *in vitro* does not necessarily mean a clinically significant interaction *in vivo*. I have reviewed this subject and the implications for drug development elsewhere.

ELDERLY

The elderly, who for the purposes of drug regulation are generally defined as over 64 years of age, are a disproportionately large group of consumers of medicines. In the developed world, the proportion of the elderly in the population is increasing and will continue to do so for at least the next quarter of a century. Many drugs in development, such as those for ischaemic and degenerative diseases, are targeted almost exclusively at the elderly. It therefore becomes much more than a "box-checking exercise" to evaluate both the dynamics and kinetics of new active substances in this population.

Age-related differences in pharmacokinetics between the elderly and young are primarily due to:

1. diminished renal function
2. altered proportions of body fat and water

3. reduced cardiac output
4. some degree of altered hepatic metabolism
5. disease
6. general debility
7. concomitant medication.

For a drug that is to be developed for a disease that occurs mainly in the elderly, it is often advisable to evaluate tolerability and pharmacokinetics in healthy elderly volunteers before clinical trials in the patient population. Dosage may need to be reduced and particular care taken when the kidney is the major organ of elimination, which should be established in the healthy young before administration to the elderly. It should be remembered that the GFR in the healthy elderly with normal plasma creatinine and urea is generally much lower than that in the young. One reason why "healthy elderly" studies have attracted heavy criticism is that the carefully selected well-preserved subjects with normal ECGs, laboratory results and physical examinations do not really resemble the frail heterogeneous elderly population that they are meant to represent. This might result in a poor appreciation of the range of pharmacokinetic alterations in the elderly patient group. It has been suggested in an FDA guideline that the "population approach" can be adopted to obtain information about pharmacokinetics in the elderly. Although this approach has a certain appeal, it also has serious drawbacks.

Renal Impairment

As the kidney is one of the major organs of drug elimination, renal impairment is likely to affect the kinetics of many drugs. Although a wide range of processes (filtration, tubular secretion, and active and passive tubular reabsorption) underlie renal drug handling, the overall renal clearance of drugs generally declines in parallel with GFR or creatinine clearance ("the *intact nephron hypothesis*"). However, the extent to which this affects total clearance depends on the proportion of renal clearance to total clearance. Pharmacokinetic studies in patients with renal impairment might therefore seem to be redundant for drugs that are cleared predominantly by non-renal processes, but experience has shown that studies may still be needed. For example, if a highly metabolised compound has a renally cleared metabolite with pharmacological activity, metabolite accumulation will occur if standard doses are given. Clinically significant effects resulting from an accumulation of an active metabolite from a highly metabolised drug include:

1. seizures produced by the accumulation of norpethidine after administration of pethidine
2. toxicity from thiocyanate accumulation following administration of nitroprusside
3. rash and allergy from accumulation of oxipurinol following administration of allopurinol
4. narcosis due to morphine 6-glucuronide after administration of morphine.

Even when the major metabolite is inactive, clinically important pharmacokinetic changes may occur in patients with renal failure. The non-steroidal anti-inflammatory drugs that derive from propionic acid (for example, ibuprofen, naproxen, ketoprofen, indoprofen and benoxaprofen) are metabolised to ester glucuronides in the liver. These are inactive and are normally rapidly eliminated by the kidney. However, when renal function is impaired, elimination of the glucuronide is delayed and plasma esterases convert the metabolite back into the parent compound, producing accumulation of the parent drug ("the *futile cycle*"). In the light of these examples, it is reasonable that if the drug is to be prescribed to patients with renal impairment, an appropriate study should be performed, even for drugs which are highly metabolised. A single-dose study is usually conducted before patients with chronic renal failure are included in clinical trials. The dose employed can be similar to that used for studies in subjects with normal renal function since Cmax is unlikely to be increased greatly. The study of pharmacokinetics and tolerability at steady state may then be necessary, for which a lower dosage should be used if clearance was shown to be reduced in the initial study. When it is expected that renal disease will have only a modest effect on drug handling, it may be sufficient to compare the pharmacokinetics in a group of patients with advanced renal disease with those in healthy controls. However, when the kidney is the main organ of elimination, it would usually be necessary to examine the changes in kinetics in several groups of patients graded with respect to renal function. The effect of dialysis in patients with end-stage renal disease should also be investigated.

Liver Disease

As with renal impairment, a study in patients with liver disease is required to avoid a contraindication in this patient population. Unlike renal disease, there is no single clinical variable that can be used to predict reliably the extent of change of hepatic drug clearance of a given compound. However, the most widely used is the Child–Pugh classification, which is based on several clinical and laboratory variables and has been useful in producing dosing information. In general, drug handling is more likely to be affected in advanced decompensated cirrhosis than when the disease is well compensated. Reactions mediated by mixed function oxidases (Phase 1) are thought to be affected earlier in the disease and to a greater extent than are large capacity conjugation (Phase 2) reactions. Alcohol further complicates the metabolic picture since it has a significant enzyme- inducing effect when taken chronically but when present in high concentrations it may acutely inhibit oxidative capacity.

In addition to changes in clearance, drug distribution may be altered in liver disease by the resulting low plasma protein concentrations and ascites. Intrahepatic and extrahepatic cholestasis are also likely to affect biliary transport of more drugs and studies in patients with these conditions may need to be considered for some drugs. Pharmacodynamic changes that are not related directly to alterations in pharmacokinetics also occur in liver disease, for example increased sensitivity to anticoagulants.

When designing a pharmacokinetic study in patients with liver disease, it is important to keep the target population for the disease indication in mind. Patients with severe liver disease are ill, and may not be likely to take medications for relatively minor illnesses. This is in contrast to patients with advanced renal failure, who may be otherwise relatively well. Given that the hepatic drug handling for a highly metabolised drug may be disturbed by advanced liver disease in a highly unpredictable manner (unlike in renal disease), it may be prudent to limit a study with the test drug to patients with relatively mild and compensated cirrhosis rather than decompensated cirrhosis, where marked changes and perhaps adverse clinical consequences could be expected. This restricted approach might be appropriate for a non-life-threatening indication (for example, migraine) but for the treatment of Gram-negative sepsis it would be essential to study the kinetics and tolerability in advanced liver disease.

Disposition, Rates and Routes of Elimination of Radiolabelled Drug

In the development of most new active substances, it is desirable to investigate the disposition of the compound and its metabolite(s) and their rates and routes of elimination. This is generally carried out with radiolabelled compound, usually ^{14}C. In the UK, approval of the Administration of Radioactive Substances Advisory Committee is required for administration of radiolabelled compound to man. The purpose of the submission is to demonstrate that the dose of absorbed radiation is minimised by administration of the lowest dose that is consistent with meeting the objectives of the study. In general, the estimated absorbed radiation dose should be less than 500 μ Sv, but higher amounts are permissible if they can be justified. The estimate is based on tissue distribution of radioactivity in animals and the pharmacokinetics in animals and man. The ARSAC application is in three parts, pertaining to:

- the applicant
- the radionuclide
- the staff and facilities where the work will be done.

In addition to ARSAC approval, the protocol must also be approved by ethics committees in the normal manner for studies in man. The study should be conducted in between four and eight consenting subjects, in facilities where any spills of radiolabelled materials can be contained and monitored. Normally, subjects will be required to provide blood samples and to collect all excreta for a period determined by the known or estimated half-lives of the parent compound and metabolite. With co-operative subjects, recoveries of radioactivity should be close to 100%. Samples will be assayed for radioactivity and by cold chromatographic methods, and every attempt should be made to identify major metabolites which may be revealed by radiochromatographic profiling.

The study should provide unique information on the plasma-concentration profiles of parent drug and metabolite. The rates and extended excretion in urine, faeces and if appropriate, expired air can be defined. Given the increasing public concern over radioactivity, it is becoming increasingly difficult to recruit adequate numbers of subjects to such studies. A new approach to undertaking these studies has recently become available. In conventional studies, drug-related material is detected by measuring the disintegration of ^{14}C. Accelerator mass spectrometry, in contrast, can count individual atoms of ^{14}C and this can enable measurements of 14C concentrations even when the dose is reduced by a thousand-fold or more compared with conventional studies. Such low doses may not require ARSAC approval or specific measures for dispensing of study drugs.

Pharmacokinetic–Pharmacodynamic Modelling

As mentioned earlier in this chapter, there is usually a relationship between drug concentration and the effect. Sometimes this relationship is not obvious. For example, the effect–time curve may be delayed in relation to the plasma concentration–time curve if diffusion of the drug to its receptor site is slow. In this situation, a plot of simultaneous plasma concentration and effect points may not show a clear pattern. However, if the individual points are joined by a drawn sequentially from the first time point through all other points in time order, it will be seen that at early time points a high plasma concentration is associated with little effect but at later time points a low concentration is associated with greater effects. This time-dependent effect on the relationship between plasma concentration and drug effect is referred to as *hysteresis*. If concentrations are plotted on the abscissa and effect on the ordinate, the situation described above would produce anticlockwise hysteresis.

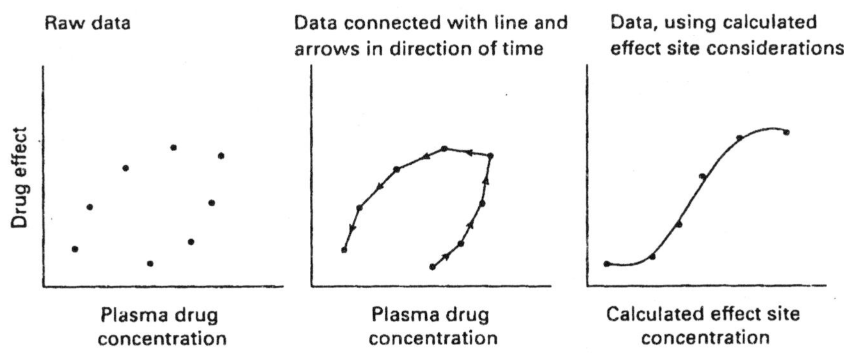

Fig. 7.5. The relationship between pharmacodynamic effects and plasma drug concentrations showing anticlockwise hysteresis and the derived concentration-effect relationship at the effect site.

Another situation in which the plasma concentration–effect relationship may be confounded by time is one where there is very rapid development of tolerance to the drug, even within a single dosing cycle. In this case, for a given plasma concentration, drug effect will be lower as concentrations are falling than when they are rising and will produce clockwise hysteresis; this has been demonstrated for nicotine. Several methods have been developed to try to elucidate the underlying concentration–effect relationship in the presence of hysteresis. Sheiner's initial approach involved postulating a hypothetical effect compartment and derivation of a rate constant for the transfer of drug between the plasma and effect compartments. The resulting correction for time delay would result in collapse of the hysteresis loop and display the underlying concentration–effect relationship. Recently this has been refined and modified using a non-parametric method to reduce the area contained within the loop, without the need to estimate a first-order rate constant. Once the hysteresis loop has been collapsed by either method, the relationship between plasma concentration and effect is apparent and can be fitted to various models; this may be linear, sigmoidal or hyperbolic. Such information can then be used to model effect–time profiles for a variety of dosing regimens and support the choice of a dosing regimen.

Population Kinetics

The usual way to examine the effect of a clinical variable (such as age, disease, concomitant medication, etc.) on the pharmacokinetics of a drug is to perform a small controlled study in which the experimental and control groups are homogeneous and closely matched and differ only in the variable of interest. This classic scientific method is well accepted by the scientific and regulatory communities and enables examination of a variable in a small group of subjects before including patients with that variable in a large clinical trial. However, there are some deficiencies with this approach. Perhaps the most important is that the small sample may not be truly representative of the population intended on the elderly. Similarly, small samples may miss the significance of genetic polymorphisms that determine drug metabolism in the population at large. It must also be appreciated that pharmacokinetic studies are usually distinct from clinical trials and it may be difficult to correlate altered pharmacokinetics with adverse reactions or other changes in clinical response.

Table 7.2. Advantages and disadvantages of detailed pharmacokinetic studies in small groups of specific patients – the traditional approach

Advantages	*Disadvantages*
Well accepted	Not usually useful for "screening"
Causation between factor and altered pharmacokinetics to be established, for example in interaction studies	Relationship between altered pharmacokinetics and clinical response cannot be examined directly
Early results from specific studies enable expansion of patient population in Phase III studies; not usually difficult to perform	Study sample may not represent the population Small sample may fail to elicit extremes of altered kinetics

An alternative approach, which is now been frequently recommended by the FDA, is population kinetics. In order to appreciate the difference in approach, it is necessary to describe how pharmacokinetic analysis is traditionally performed. In a typical conventional pharmacokinetic study, a large number of samples is taken from each subject and pharmacokinetic parameters are calculated for each individual data set, with estimation of errors associated with these calculations. Average values of each parameter can then be calculated for the group and between-subject variability determined, but the data subjected to analysis is derived from individuals. By contrast, in the population approach, the raw data set that is analysed consists of concentration–time points taken from a large number (up to hundreds to thousands) of patients. Only a few data points (perhaps 1–4) are obtained from each patient. The unit of analysis then becomes the population rather than the individual. In the illustration, all the data from all patients are plotted together, there is clearly an underlying shape, and we could simply derive a line of best fit to these data points to describe the mean pharmacokinetics of the whole population, but the variability will be very large and the parameters are of limited predictive power. Since the variability is partly attributable to the different characteristics of the individual patients within the population, clinical data relating to demographics, laboratory safety data, concomitant medication and diseases, efficacy, and adverse experiences can be used to explore their effect on the variability of pharmacokinetic parameter estimates. The importance of some of these factors can thereby be determined.

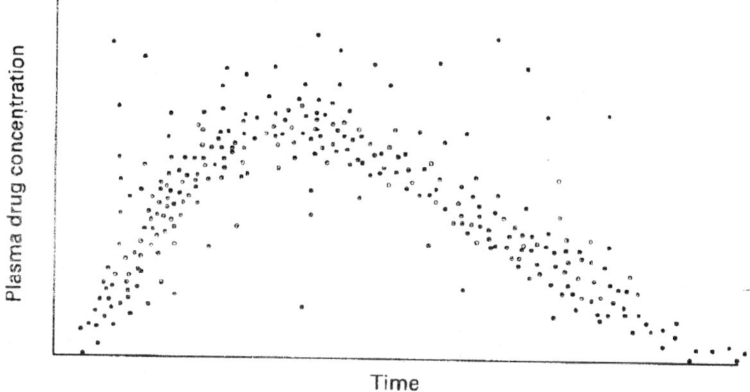

Fig. 7.6. The population approach: plasma drug concentration-time data obtained from a large population of patients.

In practice, one starts with a simple model, for example clearance being a fixed value (the mean) plus a random error. Adding a factor related to body weight, it may be possible to reduce the error term and hence account for some of the variability. In this way, a model can be built in a stepwise manner, with inclusion of clinical variables that appear to be associated with pharmacokinetic variability and excluding those which do not, until as much variability as possible has been accounted for statistically. One of the most widely used computer programs to perform this type of analysis is NONMEM (non-linear mixed effect modelling). It can be used to examine the contribution towards the variability of pharmacokinetic parameter of both continuous variables (like age and weight) and categorical variables (such as sex, race, the presence or absence of drugs, smoking, etc.).

In this way, a predictive model is developed for pharmacokinetic parameters of individuals within the population. Compared with the traditional approach, there is some important additional information that can be obtained from this technique. Firstly, the factors contributing to pharmacokinetic variability in the target population can be identified and quantitated. Secondly, the effects of many variables can be screened, in fact as many variables as are collected on the case report form. This may enable identification of important drug interactions, or of other patient factors affecting pharmacokinetics that may not have been suspected. Thirdly, as efficacy and tolerability data have been collected in the same patients, this analysis might help to establish a range for therapeutic concentrations.

Despite these attractions, there are disadvantages in using the population approach. The extra resource required to collect, transport and assay large number of samples (may be thousands) is considerable. An extremely demanding aspect is that for a meaningful analysis to be performed, exact sampling times must be recorded in relation to the previous dose and several preceding doses over 2–3 half-lives. The population pharmacokinetic technique may work relatively well where a pharmacokinetic model is relatively simple, but when the model is complex the number of parameters to be estimated many be so large that meaningful correlations may be difficult to find because of the errors involved. The demonstration of a statistical association does not necessarily imply causation. If an unlikely clinical variable is associated with altered pharmacokinetics, it might be necessary to perform a specific study to confirm or refute this. The approach is not appropriate to detect for the first-time clinical variables that are likely to have a major effect on pharmacokinetics. For example, for a renally cleared drug which is likely to require a reduced dose in patients with renal failure, it is necessary, for safety reasons, to perform a careful traditional pharmacokinetic study to determine the appropriate dosing regimen before these patients can be included in the main Phase III trials. The FDA has suggested that the population method is a suitable method with which to explore the changes in pharmacokinetics in the elderly, but because age is often associated with altered pharmacokinetics, it is often necessary, again for safety reasons, to explore this before including elderly patients in the main efficacy studies using a standard dose. The results of a population pharmacokinetic analysis are not usually available until several months after the end of the main Phase III trials programme. This is likely to be around the time of the regulatory submission, and it is very late to find out about important clinical variables that affect handling of the drug. Current programs such as NONMEM are not user-friendly; few people have adequate expertise to obtain reliable results and, at present, there is no validation standard for this and similar programs.

With the development of new programs, combined with feedback from regulators and greater experience in the industry, it is likely that population analysis will be used increasingly in the future. The main utility of population analysis (including population dynamics) to be as follows.

1. It can be used to confirm the effects of concomitant medication and other clinical variables predicted from classical studies.
2. It can be used to rule out other factors unlikely to be important.
3. It is particularly suitable for studying kinetics in children.
4. The therapeutic concentration range can be defined, particularly if therapeutic drug monitoring is likely to be useful because of a narrow therapeutic index and/or a clear concentration–effect relationship.
5. It is suitable for studying populations in which there is an unusually large number of potentially important variables, for example immunosuppressed patients who are receiving many concomitant medications.

Table 7.3. Advantages and disadvantages of the population approach

Advantages	*Disadvantages*
Can be used for screening for the effect of a large number of variables	Can demonstrate correlation but not causation
Possible to establish relationship between concentration, clinical response and adverse reactions	Logistically difficult with large number of plasma samples, exact sample times and dosing history required
Limited sampling per patient makes the technique particularly useful for children	Technically difficult; complex software; lack of validation standards; few experienced operators
Enables prediction of the kinetics of an individual from demographic data	Data not usually available until after the end of the Phase III clinical programme

At present we believe that a judicious mix of the traditional approach combined with population analysis of selected drugs is appropriate.

Ideal Drug from the Point of View of Pharmacokinetics

There are many examples of drugs which are successful in the marketplace but which have less than optimal pharmacokinetics. However, when a compound which has desirable pharmacokinetic characteristics is selected for clinical development, this can lead to a smoother clinical development programme, fewer regulatory concerns, a more straightforward data-sheet, and, ultimately, better clinical utility. In today's competitive marketplace such characteristics may be key determinants of commercial success.

Role of Pharmacokinetic Properties in Determining a Dosage Regimen

Determining the optimal dosing regimen for a new drug can be very difficult. However, considerable commercial superiority can be obtained by one drug over another by thoughtful selection of the dosing regimen, even if the two drugs have comparable pharmacokinetic and pharmacodynamic properties. Because pharmacokinetic properties of the drug determine the time course of plasma concentration, it is obvious that this information will have some role in determining a dosing regimen. However, there are many other important types of information which are also relevant in determining a dosing regimen, and excessive reliance on pharmacokinetic properties alone can result in a suboptimal dosing regimen. To summarise, pharmacokinetics describes the absorption, distribution, metabolism and excretion of a drug by the body. Plasma concentration profiles, and in particular half-life, are important factors to consider in designing a dosage regimen. Calculation of primary pharmacokinetic parameters such as clearance and volume of distribution can provide insight into the physiological processes affecting plasma concentrations and enable some predictions to be made about the effects of age, disease and concomitant medication of these concentrations. The clinical pharmacokinetic regulatory package can therefore be assembled in a rational manner, providing sound support for the clinical trials regulatory submission.

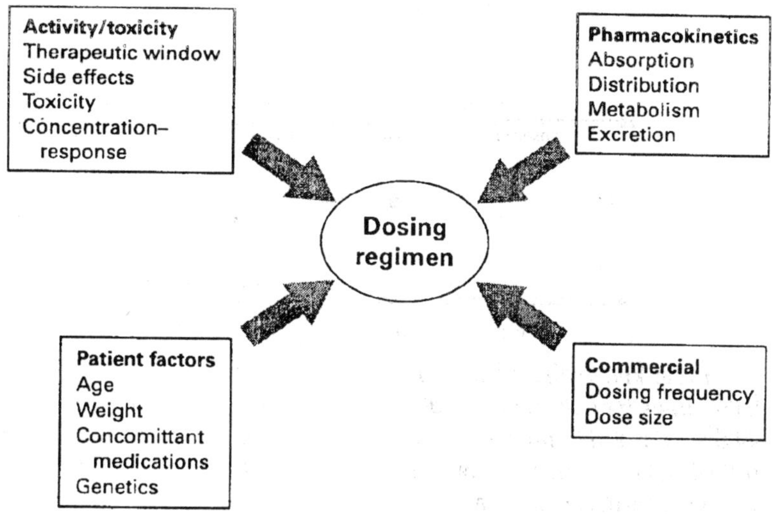

Fig. 7.7. Factors affecting a dosage regimen.

Clinical Pharmacodynamics

Therapeutics relates drug administration to physiological effects, both beneficial and toxic, in patient populations. The important intervening steps or processes, which occur following drug dosing that lead to therapeutic effects in the body, are described below. This scheme illustrates the dose-effect relationship. The discipline of pharmacokinetics provides an understanding of drug absorption, disposition, and elimination, as these relate to the physiological effects of drugs. Pharmacodynamics relates the measured response, either efficacious, toxic, or both, to the drug's pharmacokinetics. Pharmacokinetics has become increasingly important, as it has proven to be a very useful tool in understanding not only drug dosage in relation to achievable drug concentrations in plasma, but also the influence of disease states on the behavior of a drug in the body. A very powerful interpretative instrument becomes available when the disciplines of pharmacokinetics and pharmacodynamics are combined. Clinical pharmacokinetics specifically deals with optimizing drug dosage in individual patients. By using plasma concentration measurements, and clinical pharmacokinetic principles, doses can be adjusted to achieve maximal therapeutic utility, with minimum toxic risks for individual patients.

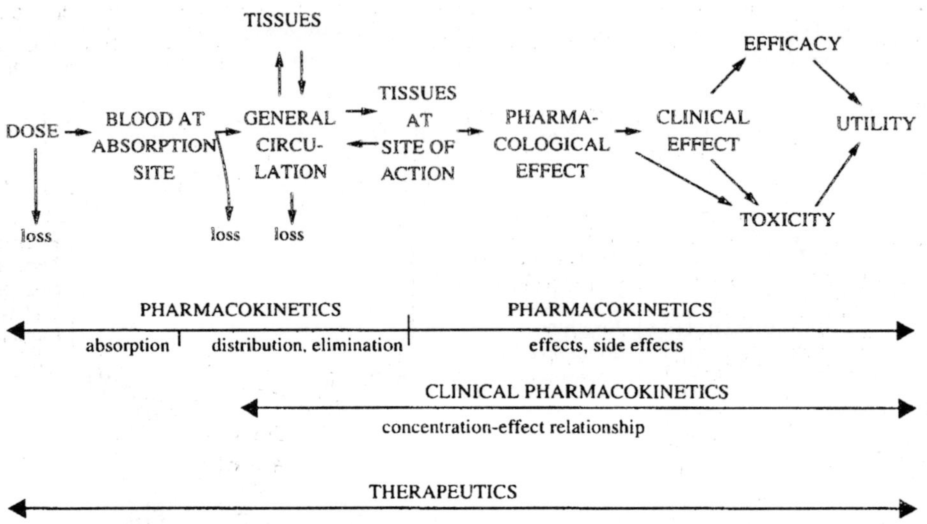

Fig. 7.8. Schematic representation of the dose-effect relationship for a drug.

Basic knowledge of pharmacokinetic principles is important not only for the clinician to understand basic drug–patient interrelationships, but also for the drug industry to facilitate the design of relevant studies for drug discovery candidates. The gain from designing proper pharmacokinetic studies can probably be counted not only in better therapy for the patient but also in long-term economic savings for the pharmaceutical industry.

In this article the basic principles of pharmacokinetics and pharmacodynamics will be addressed, and examples of how these principles can be used to increase the understanding of drug therapy and drug dosage formulation are given.

Pharmacodynamic Considerations

The fundamental hypothesis in clinical pharmcokinetics asserts that a relationship exists between a drug concentration in some measurable biologic fluid and observed drug effects. Many drugs, for example, antiarrhythmics, anticonvulsants such as phenytoin, and diuretics such as furosemide, show an apparent direct relationship; that is with every change in plasma drug concentration, there is an immediate and corresponding change in effect. For other drugs the relationship is more complicated; the drug level of warfarin for instance, triggers a cascade of events leading to prolonged clotting time. Here, the mean steady-state level rather than the time course of concentrations can be most closely correlated to the therapeutic effect. In some instances, the effect itself is difficult to quantify, and demonstrating any relationship is difficult. When unbound concentrations are maintained at a particular steady-state concentration across a population, then an observed difference in response between individuals must be due to pharmacodynamic receptor-level variability across the population. However, most traditional relationships of drug effects have been developed relative to drug dose rather than steady-state unbound concentrations. When comparing the dose given to the effect, the variability in drug absorption, first-past metabolism, protein binding, and clearance must also be included, thereby giving a significantly more variable and complicated relationship.

The full model for the concentration (C) and effect (E) relationship is the Hill equation, also called the extended E_{max} model:

$$E = \frac{E_{\max} C^s}{EC_{50}^s + C^s} \qquad \ldots(3)$$

where E_{max} is the maximal effect, EC_{50} is the concentration giving 50% of maximal effect, and s is the slope factor. The Hill equation can be simplified to different extents, for example, if $s = 1$.

Between 20 and 80% of the maximal response, the relationship is logarithmic:

$$E = m \log C + e \qquad \ldots(4)$$

where m is the slope and e is the intercept. This equation has the limitations of not being able to predict effects outside this range of responses (i.e., <20% and >80%).

Below 20% of maximal response, the relationship is linear:

$$E = m\,C + e \qquad \ldots(5)$$

This relationship has been used for up to 50% of maximal response; however, it then is a coarse approximation, depending upon the value of s (the lower the value of s, the better the approximation).

The Hill equation should be used only when a reasonable estimation of E_{max} is possible and when data are gathered over the whole effect range. If data are available only from the lower part of the curve, the linear equation might just as well be used. The difference between the Hill equation and the linear or log-linear equation is that only the Hill equation gives a mechanistic–physiologic understanding of the effect. The other equations are merely descriptive.

Sheiner and associates have developed the relationship where the pharmacodynamic model [Eq. (3)] is integrated together with the pharmacokinetic model. This makes possible describing both the steady-state concentration–effect relationship (i.e., EC_{20}, EC_{50}, EC_{90}, etc.) and the time lag between the measured rapidly changing plasma concentration and the corresponding steady-state effect at that concentration level. This time-lag parameter is described by the equilibration half-time. Using both these parameters, that is, the expected effect and the time required to obtain the effect, allows investigators to model the effect–concentration relationship when patients are not at steady state.

The relationship between the measured effect and steady-state plasma concentration sometimes yields bell-shaped (e.g., nortriptyline) or U-shaped (e.g., clonidine) curves. Several unusual concentration–effect curves, including the U-shaped curve describing the blood pressure lowering effect of clonidine, have been explained by Paalzow and associates as being a result of multiple receptor responses. The drug then acts on several different receptors that can have opposite effects and that are triggered at different concentrations.

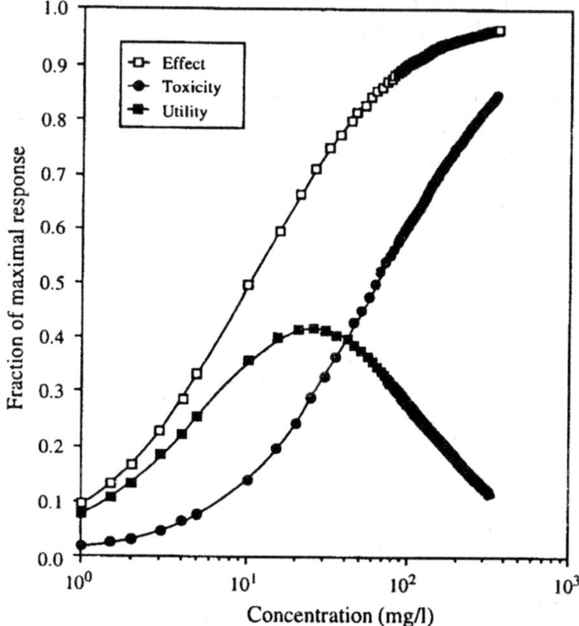

Fig. 7.9. Utility curve and concentration-effect/toxicity relationships for a theoretical drug.

Tolerance to the drug effect, that is, a decrease in the effect with time, also obscures the dose-response relationship. Pharmacokinetic and/ or pharmacodynamic causes for tolerance development are possible. Pharmacokinetic tolerance, for example, can be caused by induction of metabolic enzymes, thereby causing a decrease in drug concentrations. Pharmacodynamic tolerance can be characterized mainly in two different ways: the receptors down-regulate in response to the drug, giving a smaller response with time, or other physiologic mechanisms counteract the drug effect. The blood pressure lowering effect of hydralazine that is diminished by a compensatory increase in heart rate, and the diuretic effect of furosemide that is decreased as a result of the drug's volume and salt-depleting actions are two examples.

Depending upon the steepness of the concentration–effect relationship [the size of s in Eq. (3)], an increase in concentration will result in different changes in effect. An all-or-none relationship is obtained when the curve is very steep ($s > 6$). Theophylline shows a shallow relationship with plasma concentration for its antiasthmatic effect; a big increase in concentration results in a small increase in effect. However, as the side effects of theophylline show a much steeper relationship with plasma concentration, it is critical not to increase theophylline concentrations above 20 mg/L. With a lower limit for antiasthmatic effect of 10 mg/L, theophylline exhibits a narrow range of concentrations where therapy is beneficial.

Another measure of utility is in terms of the ratio between the concentration level causing an undesirable side effect to the concentration level giving the desired therapeutic effect (therapeutic index). For theophylline this ratio is 2, for digoxin it is 1.6, and for furosemide it is 40. The higher the therapeutic index, the less critical are dosing recommendations with respect to the risk of serious side effects.

Clearance

Clearance is the measure of the ability of the body to eliminate a drug, and as such is one of the most important pharmacokinetic parameters, as it gives a well-defined, physiologically relevant measurement of how drugs are eliminated by the organism as a whole, or by a particular organ. Clearance relates drug concentration to the elimination rate from the body, or at steady state the average concentration C_{ss} to the dosing rate because at steady state the input rate into the body will equal the output rate:

$$\text{Elimination rate} = \text{CL}\ C \qquad \ldots(6)$$

$$\text{Dosing rate} = \text{CL}\ C_{ss} \qquad \ldots(7)$$

The clearance concept has been used in defining the pharmacokinetics of drugs since the mid-1970s. The clearance concept is based in physiology, where it is used as a measure of renal function (creatinine clearance). Creatinine is formed from muscle breakdown at a constant rate, and thus a constant creatinine concentration in plasma results. The magnitude of this concentration is dependent on the elimination rate of creatinine and the size of the muscle pool (formation rate). By measuring the plasma concentration and the renal excretion of creatinine, renal clearance can be estimated and thereby kidney function indicated, as creatinine is mainly filtered into the urine

$$\text{CL}_{\text{creatinine}} = \frac{\text{Urine volume} \times \text{Urine concentration}}{\text{Plasma concentration}} \qquad \ldots(8)$$

Drugs are not only eliminated via the kidneys but also eliminated in the bile by the liver and metabolized in the liver and elsewhere, which makes direct measurement of the elimination rate of a drug difficult. Indeed, other routes of elimination could include loss in expired air, saliva, sweat, partition into tissue stores, efflux from the blood into the gut lumen, and gut metabolism as well as other sites of metabolism such as the lung. The total clearance, CL, can be defined as

$$CL = \frac{Dose_{iv}}{AUC} \qquad \ldots(9)$$

where $\text{Dose}_{\text{i.v.}}$ is the intravenous dose, and AUC is the resulting area under the plasma concentration time curve. Total clearance can also be measured during continuous drug therapy as dosing rate divided by C_{ss} according to Eq. (7).

Clearance is referenced to plasma (plasma clearance, CL_p), blood (blood clearance, CL_b) or plasma water (unbound clearance, CL_u), depending upon where the concentration is measured. Total clearance can be divided into the contributions of each of the eliminating organs, the most important being renal clearance, CL_R, and hepatic clearance, CL_H.

$$CL = CL_R + CL_H + CL_{gut} + CL_{other} \quad \text{...(10)}$$

Renal clearance can be separately determined by measuring the excretion rate of unchanged drug into the urine, as for creatinine. The difference between total clearance and renal clearance is usually called *non-renal clearance*, meaning the clearance that is not accounted for by excretion of unchanged drug into urine, be it metabolism in the liver or elimination by any other organ.

Clearance is measured in units of volume per time (ml/min or L/h) and thus is defined using the same units as blood or plasma flow. By definition, clearance gives the volume of plasma (blood) from which a drug is completely removed per unit time. For some drugs the liver or kidneys have the ability to clear drug from all the blood flowing through the organ; for example, *p*-aminohippuric acid (PAH) has a renal plasma clearance of 600–700 ml/min, which equals renal plasma flow. Because PAH does not partition into red blood cells, PAH renal blood clearance will equal renal blood flow (see imipramine in the next paragraph for calculations according to Eq. (11), $C_{RBC}/C_p = 0$). So, when the eliminating organ has a high capacity to eliminate a drug, the blood clearance equals the blood flow to that organ. As the organ cannot eliminate drug any faster than the rate at which drug is presented to the organ, blood flow becomes the limiting value for clearance. Thus, hepatic blood clearance cannot exceed 1.5 L/min, and renal blood clearance cannot exceed 1.2–1.3 L/min.

Some drugs show a higher plasma clearance than the corresponding plasma flow through the eliminating organ. Imipramine has a plasma clearance of 1050 ml/min, thus exceeding the rate of plasma flow to the liver, where it is predominantly eliminated. Looking at whole blood, the concentration of imipramine in blood is higher than its concentration in plasma because of a considerable partitioning into red blood cells ($C_{RBC}/C_p = 2.7$). Thus, the amount of drug delivered to the liver by the blood is much higher than that assumed from measuring its plasma concentration alone. The relationship between plasma and blood clearance at steady state is given by

$$\frac{CL_p}{CL_b} = \frac{C_b}{C_p} = 1 + H\left(\frac{C_{RBC}}{C_p} - 1\right) \quad \text{...(11)}$$

Imipramine blood clearance can be calculated by substituting the red blood cell to plasma concentration ratio and the average value for hematocrit (H = 0.45) into Eq. (12). The resulting blood clearance is calculated to be 595 ml/min, a value within the physiologic range of liver blood flow The higher plasma versus blood clearance for imipramine also indicates that the drug present in the red blood cells is readily available for the metabolizing enzymes by being in rapid equilibrium with the drug present in plasma water. Thus, the plasma clearance may assume values that are not "physiologic." However, if the concentration in blood is used to define clearance, the maximal clearance possible is equal to the sum of blood flow to the various organs of elimination. If a drug shows a higher blood clearance than the combined blood flow, a probable cause is extrahepatic or extrarenal elimination, such as the metabolism of nitroglycerin in blood and tissues. The *rate of elimination* of a compound by an organ is the difference between the rate of presentation to the organ and the rate of exit from the organ. *Rate of presentation*

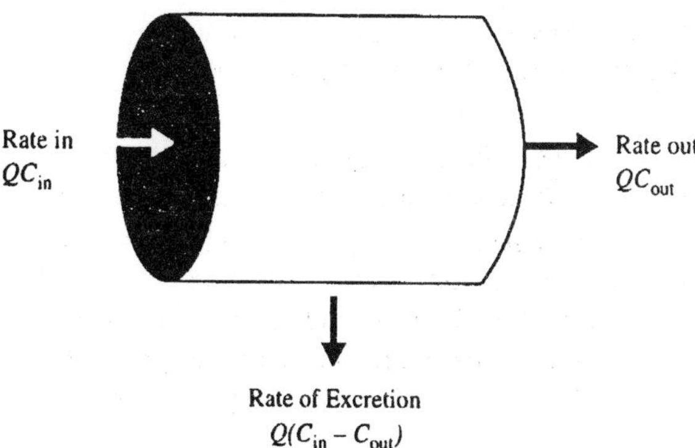

Fig. 7.10. Extraction of drug in an organ of elimination.

equals the organ blood flow multiplied by the entering concentration (QC_{in}), and the rate of exit equals the blood flow multiplied by the exiting drug concentration (QC_{out}).

$$\text{Rate of elimination} = QC_{in} - QC_{out} \qquad ...(12)$$

By relating the rate of elimination to the entering concentration [Eq. (4)], an expression for organ clearance of drug can be obtained

$$CL_{organ} = \frac{Q(C_{in} - C_{out})}{C_{in}} = Q\,ER \qquad ...(13)$$

in terms of blood flow and ER, the extraction ratio, which equals $(C_{in} - C_{out})/C_{in}$. A high organ clearance signifies that the organ has a high capacity to extract drug from the blood.

For a compound for which the organ has a high extraction capacity, the exiting concentration is very low relative to the entering concentration, and ER approaches unity. For an organ with a low extraction capacity, the exiting concentration is not very different from the entering concentration, and ER approaches zero. Extraction ratio can thus be expressed as the fraction of the organ blood flow that is cleared by the organ ($ER = CL_{organ}/Q_{organ}$). Several models relating the hepatic clearance to physiologic parameters have been suggested, including the well-stirred and the parallel tube models, the distributed model, and the dispersion model. The well-stirred model is the most easily understood and most commonly employed model, and the following discussion will be based on this approach.

The well-stirred model assumes that the unbound drug concentration leaving the organ, for example the liver, is equal to the unbound concentration within the organ, thus assuming an instant "mixing" at the entrance of drug into the organ. The intrinsic ability to metabolize or otherwise clear unbound drug and the protein binding (unbound fraction, f_u) together with the blood flow through the liver (Q_H) all contribute to the resulting hepatic clearance, which may be mathematically expressed as

$$CL_H = Q_H \frac{f_u CL_{u,\text{int}}}{Q_H + f_u CL_{u,\text{int}}} \qquad ...(14)$$

Thus, an example of a high-extraction drug is when the capacity of the liver to metabolize a drug is large compared to the rate at which drug enters the liver ($f_u\ CL_{u,int}\ Q_H$), clearance approximates liver blood flow

$$CL \cong Q_H \qquad ...(15)$$

An example of low-extraction drug is when the capacity of the liver to metabolize a drug is small relative to the rate of presentation ($f_u\ CL_{u,int} \ll Q_H$), because of a low intrinsic ability to metabolize or because of diffusion problems to the enzyme site. Under these conditions, hepatic clearance approximates

$$CL \cong f_u\ CL_{u;int} \qquad ...(16)$$

Between these extremes, hepatic clearance is dependent on all three factors: Unbound fraction of drug, intrinsic clearance, and hepatic blood flow. The unbound clearance, CL_u, equals CL/f_u.

A reasonable assumption is that the active secretion mechanism in the kidney can also be described by the well-stirred model. However, the kidneys have several mechanisms that may determine renal clearance of a drug, including passive filtration and reabsorption. The renal clearance is the sum of filtration and secretion minus reabsorption. It can be described as

$$CL_R = CL_{filtration} + CL_{secretion} - CL_{reabsorption} \qquad ...(17)$$

or,

$$CL_R = (CL_{filtration} + CL_{secretion}) \times (1 - \text{fraction reabsorbed}) \qquad ...(18)$$

Filtration in the kidneys is determined by the glomerular filtration rate, GFR (120 ml/min in a healthy young person), and by the fraction of the drug that is dissolved in plasma water, that is, the unbound fraction, f_u. Thus,

$$CL_{filtration} = f_u \text{ GFR} \qquad \ldots(19)$$

Suppositions regarding the mechanisms by which a drug is renally eliminated can be made by comparing the filtration clearance with the measured renal clearance. Drug is always passively filtered to some extent, depending of the value of f_u. If $CL_R > CL_{filtration}$, the drug is also secreted and may be reabsorbed but to a smaller extent than it is secreted. If $CL_R < CL_{filtration}$, however, this is an indication of reabsorption but does not exclude secretion. If $CL_R = CL_{filtration}$, the drug can still be both secreted and reabsorbed, but to the same extent. Conclusive evidence on whether a drug is reabsorbed cannot be made solely on the basis of clearance values.

Intestinal metabolism or clearance

Recently, it has been recognized that small intestinal metabolism and active efflux of orally absorbed drugs, are major determinants of oral drug bioavailability. Many elements, including patient specific ones, determine the extent of oral drug delivery. The observed oral bioavailability (F_{oral}) of any particular drug is dependent upon the following processes: delivery to the intestine (gastric emptying, pH, presence of food), absorption from the lumen of the intestine (dissolution, lipophilicity, particle size, active uptake), intestinal metabolism (phase I/phase II), active extrusion (drug efflux pumps), and then first pass hepatic metabolism.

The enzymes of the cytochrome P 4503A family are the predominant phase I drug metabolizing enzymes in man. The major isoform of the CYP3A family is CYP3A4, the predominant form found in adult human liver and small intestine. Members of the 3A4 family are estimated to be responsible for the metabolism of more than one half of all drugs that are substrates for the P450 system of metabolic enzymes in man. The levels of CYP3A4 found in human liver and small intestine is highly variable, with 10–100 fold variations observed in liver and as much as 30-fold variation in the small intestine, respectively. Levels of CYP3A4 in the small intestine are generally 10–50% of the levels found in the human liver, and these levels as well as the activity of the enzyme decrease longitudinally along the small intestine. The enzymes of the CYP3A4 subfamily comprise approximately 30% of all hepatic cytochromes and at least 70% of all intestinal cytochromes responsible for drug metabolism.

Previously, drug absorption from the gut was assumed to occur by passive processes, and little attention was paid to the activity of counter transport systems. It has now been recognized that P-glycoprotein (P-gp), an ATP-dependent efflux transporter, is expressed at high levels on the apical surface of the columnar epithelial cells in the jejunum of the small intestine. P-gp represents the best studied member of the ATP binding cassette (ABC) family of transporters, and is the product of the multidrug resistance gene MDR1 in man. P-gp is expressed in a wide variety of tissues including the adrenal glands, the bladder, the cells of the blood-brain barrier, kidney, liver, lungs, pancreas, rectum, spleen, and most importantly for the purpose of oral bioavailability, in the esophagus, stomach, jejunum, and colon. In an apparent contrast to the situation noted above for CYP3A, levels of P-gp increase longitudinally along the intestine, with the lowest levels found in the stomach and the highest levels found in the colon.

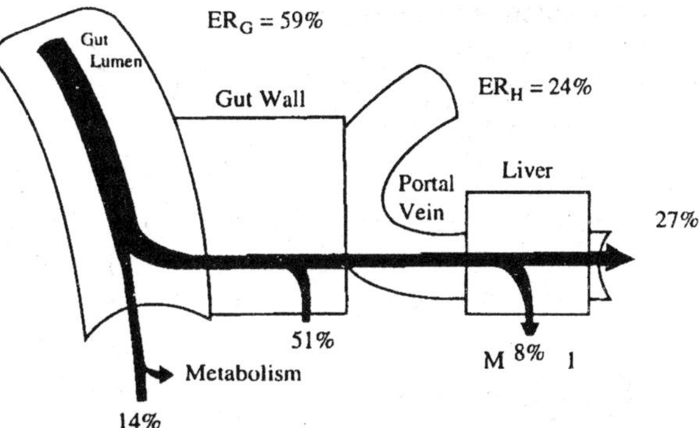

Fig. 7.11. This cartoon depects the various processes leading to an oral bioavailability of 27%, following an oral dose of the Sandimmune formulation of cyclosporine.

The co-importance of CYP3A and P-gp for the oral bioavailability of drugs is suggested by their shared locations within the enterocytes of the small bowel, as well as a significant overlap in their substrate specificities. Intracellularly, P-gp is found traversing the plasma membrane of enterocytes while CYP3A is found within the cytoplasm on the endoplasmic reticulum. Although gene expression of these two proteins does not appear to be coordinately regulated, their proximal spatial relationship suggests that P-gp may act to regulate exposure of drug (substrates) to metabolism by CYP3A. Repeated absorption and extrusion processes would then, result in repeated exposure of drug to CYP3A, resulting in enhanced overall metabolism, and correspondingly lower oral bioavailability. This spatial juxta-position, coupled with the large number of overlaps between CYP3A and P-gp substrates, suggests a strong complementary role for these proteins in the pharmacokinetics of drug absorption.

Oral bioavailability (F_{oral}) is equal to the product of the fraction of dose absorbed (F_{abs}), the fraction of the absorbed dose which passes into the hepatic portal blood flow unmetabolized (F_G), and the hepatic first-pass availability (F_H), as seen in Eq. (20).

$$F_{oral} = F_{abs}\, F_G\, F_H \qquad \ldots(20)$$

Gut and hepatic availability may be defined as one minus the extraction ratio (ER) at each site.

$$F_{oral} = F_{abs}\,(1 - ER_G)(1 - ER_H) \qquad \ldots(21)$$

The hepatic extraction ratio (ER_H) can be determined after intravenous dosing from the ratio of hepatic clearance (CL_H) to hepatic blood flow (Q_H).

$$ER_H = \frac{CL_H}{Q_H} = \frac{f_u CL_{u,\text{int}}}{Q_H + f_u CL_{u,\text{int}}} \qquad \ldots(22)$$

$$F_H = \frac{Q_H}{Q_H + f_u CL_{u,\text{int}}} \qquad \ldots(23)$$

The ability to estimate the gut extraction ratio requires further experimental manipulations and assumptions, such as evaluating the effects of an enzyme inducer, e.g., rifampin, on oral and i.v. drug dosing as first utilized by Wu et al. for cyclosporine, or measurement of portal concentrations as first utilized by Thummel and coworkers for midazolam.

It is apparent that the greatest impact on oral bioavailability, that would result from the concerted activity of intestinal CYP3A and P-gp, will be observed in drugs that are characterized by low to intermediate hepatic first-pass extraction. High hepatic extraction will probably obscure the gut effects. The inhibition or induction of intestinal CYP3A directly translates into changes in the oral bioavailability of drugs. Inhibition and induction of P-gp in contrast, manifests as a change in the rate of absorption, T_{max}, which can also affect the extent of oral availability, since the T_{max} changes reflects the access of the drug to the intestinal enzymes.

Many commonly prescribed drugs are joint substrates for CYP3A and P-gp, which as has been discussed, both reside in the human intestine, associates within the enterocytes. It is therefore very likely that changes in bioavailability for a number of drugs could result from intestinal metabolism and/or efflux counter transport of absorbed drug back into the intestinal lumen. Selective inhibition of one or both of these processes could theoretically increase bioavailability, while decreasing the variability inherent in absorption. An approach using specific modifiers of intestinal metabolic and counter transport activity could conceivably transform the therapeutic efficacy of many drugs now in use.

Distribution

The systemic circulation transports drug molecules from the site of administration to all tissues and organs in the body. Depending upon the physicochemical properties of the drug (lipophilicity, degree of ionization), the drug partitions into different tissues to different extents. The rate at which distribution takes place into a tissue is dependent on both the drug partition coefficient (concentration in tissue/concentration in blood at equilibrium) and the blood flow to that tissue. The higher the perfusion rate (blood flow per unit volume of tissue), the more rapid is equilibrium achieved between blood and tissue. The higher the partitioning into the tissue, the longer reaching equilibrium takes, as more drug has to be transported to the tissue. Within the blood, drug is dissolved in the plasma water (unbound concentration, C_u). Drug can also be bound to plasma proteins and concentrated in the red blood cells. It is the unbound drug molecules that diffuse across the membranes into the tissues. At equilibrium, the unbound concentration of drug is thought to be the same throughout the whole body.

Volume of Distribution

To measure drug concentrations, a blood sample is centrifuged and the plasma concentration analyzed. The relationship between the amount of drug in the body and the concentration (C) is called volume of distribution:

$$V = \text{amount in body}/C \qquad \ldots(24)$$

Depending on the fluid being measured, blood (C_b), plasma (C_p) or plasma water (C_u), different values for the volume term can be obtained as the concentrations in these fluids differ.

The volume of distribution is a proportionality constant. It can be smaller or larger than the true physiologic fluid spaces of the body, depending upon whether the affinity of the drug is highest in plasma constituents or in other tissues. For a normal 70-kg man, the plasma volume is 3 liters, blood volume is about 5.5 liters, extracellular fluid outside plasma is 12 liters, and total body water is approximately 42 liters.

To determine the volume of distribution of a drug, an i.v. dose is necessary. The volume of distribution can be calculated from the plasma concentration versus time data by means of non-compartmental methods as described by Benet and Galeazzi for a bolus i.v. dose

$$V_{ss} = \frac{Dose_{i.v.} AUMC}{AUC^2} \qquad \ldots(25)$$

Here V_{ss} represents the volume in which a drug would appear to be distributed during steady state, AUC is the area under the plasma concentration time curve, and AUMC is the area under the first moment of the plasma concentration time curve, that is, the area under the curve of the product of time, t, and plasma concentration, over the time span zero to infinity. The volume of distribution at steady state can also be determined by compartmental methods, that is, by using the coefficients and exponents of a multiexponential fit to the data.

An alternative measure of volume of distribution is V_{area}. This parameter is dependent on the terminal half-life or, expressed differently, the terminal rate constant λ_z, where λ_z, is equal to $0.693/t_{1/2}$

$$V_{area} = \frac{Dose_{i.v.}}{\lambda_z AUC} = \frac{CL}{\lambda_z} \qquad \ldots(26)$$

as $Dose_{i.v.}/AUC = CL$, according to Eq. (7). Although V_{area} is a convenient and easily calculated parameter, the value of V_{area} can show differences when the half- lives differ, for example, between different patient populations, without a true difference in the distribution space. Contrary to V_{area}, V_{ss} is theoretically independent of changes in elimination. Thus, to determine whether a particular disease state is influencing the clearance process and/or the distribution of the drug, the V_{ss} volume term should preferentially be used. The pharmacokinetic parameters for cefamandole in six normal volunteers and in three uremic patients are compared. As cefamandole is almost exclusively eliminated via the kidneys, uremia results in a dramatic decrease in clearance (24-fold). The terminal half-life increases, but only by a factor of 11, resulting in more than a twofold difference in V_{area} between the two groups [Eq. (26)]. Based on these data, conclusions could be made that a decreased renal function not only influences the ability to excrete cefamandole but also results in a decrease in the distribution of the drug in the body. However, when comparing Vss the conclusion is that no significant difference exists in the distribution of cefamandole between the two patient populations.

Half-Life

Half-life is the "oldest" and best known of all pharmacokinetic parameters. It is a measure of the time required for the amount of drug in the body to decline to half of its value. Half-life is a useful measurement to determine the time to reach steady state for chronic dosing, or the time for the amount or concentration of drug to decline, for example, after an intoxication. To reach 90% of steady state or to eliminate 90% of the drug from the body takes 3.3 half-lives because 50% of the steady-state level is reached in one half-life, 75% in two, 87.5% in three, and 93.75% in four half-lives. The corresponding values hold for elimination of drug from the body. Half-life can be readily determined from a plot of log plasma concentration versus time and was for many years considered to be the most important characteristic of a drug. Early studies examining drug disposition in disease states were compromised, by a reliance on half-life as a sole measure of disposition changes. It is now appreciated that half-life is a secondary, derived parameter that relates to and depends on the primary parameters of clearance (CL) and volume of distribution (V) according to the following relationship in Eq. (27):

$$t_{1/2} \approx \frac{0.693V}{CL} \qquad \ldots(27)$$

Thus, to look at half-life only as a measure of, for instance, the effect of liver disease on drug pharmacokinetics is not sufficient, as a change in half-life can be caused by either a change in clearance or a change in volume of distribution. Furthermore, half-life may be unchanged in a particular disease state due to parallel changes in both V and CL. Clearance and volume of distribution are two separate and independent characteristics of a drug. They are closely correlated with physiologic mechanisms in the organism (thereby the term primary parameters). Clearance defines the body's ability to remove the drug, that is, by metabolism or by renal or biliary excretion. Volume of distribution is a measure of the physical interrelationship between the drug and body constituents, such as binding to plasma proteins or partition into muscle, tissue, or fat.

Protein Binding

At steady state, the distribution of any drug in the body is dependant upon its binding to plasma proteins, blood cells and tissue receptors. Only unbound drug is capable of entering and exiting from plasma and tissue compartments. Therefore, an apparent volume of distribution can be expressed as follows,

$$V = V_p + V_{TW}\frac{f_u}{f_{u,T}} \qquad \ldots(28)$$

where V_p represents the volume of plasma, V_{TW} is the volume of tissue fluid (non-plasma), f_u represents the fraction unbound in plasma, and $f_{u,T}$ is the fraction unbound in tissue. Human plasma contains over 60 proteins. Albumin is the major component of this protein family responsible for the binding of most drugs in plasma. Acidic drugs bind primarily to albumin, the major drug-binding protein in plasma. Some acidic drugs bind with very high affinity, for example, furosemide, which is 98–99% bound and warfarin, which is 99.5% bound. Basic drugs bind to albumin with lower affinity but are more avidly bound to proteins like α_1-acid glycoprotein and various plasma lipoproteins. These proteins have lower concentrations in plasma relative to albumin. Binding is therefore more easily saturable, as is the case with some drugs such as prednisolone and disopyramide, yielding fluctuations in the free fraction of drugs falling within the therapeutic plasma concentration range. Because the binding of drugs to plasma proteins and tissue binding sites is largely non-selective, many drugs with similar chemical properties can compete with each other for access to binding sites. The concern over the potential for adverse drug events based on competitive displacement from plasma protein binding sites has been overstated however. Indomethacin has been shown to markedly decrease warfarin binding to human serum albumin, in vitro. However, this in vitro drug interaction has not been confirmed by in vivo studies. Steady- state unbound drug concentrations in vivo are largely independent of factors which alter protein binding, unless a drug is very highly protein bound, for example, greater than 90%. A dynamic equilibrium exits between tissue and plasma stores of any drug. Binding at these sites is reversible and changes so rapidly that equilibrium is re-established within milliseconds. Therefore, changes in the free fraction of drugs brought about by competition with higher avidity ligands or saturable kinetics are quickly compensated for by movement of drug from tissue stores into plasma, precluding the need for adjustment of dosage regimens.

Variation in plasma protein concentrations can occur secondary to decreased albumin concentrations associated with hepatic cirrhosis, and nephrotic syndrome. Increased (α_1-acid glycoprotein concentrations are associated with the stress response to disease states such as myocardial infarction, inflammatory disease, and postsurgically. A more relevant problem resulting from competition between drugs for plasma protein binding is the misinterpretation of the measured concentrations of drugs in plasma, as most assays are not able to differentiate between bound and unbound drug. Concentration-dependent binding of a drug to a plasma protein is expected when the total drug concentration approaches the protein concentration. For albumin this concentration is 0.6 mM, and for α_1-acid glycoprotein in healthy individuals it is 0.015 mM, assuming that one drug molecule binds per protein molecule. For a drug with a molecular weight of 250, this corresponds to concentrations in plasma of 150 mg/L and 4 mg/L, for saturation of albumin and α_1-acid glycoprotein, respectively.

Influence of Protein-Binding Changes on Volume of Distribution

As is obvious from the relationship shown by Eq. (28), a drug which is characterized by a high degree of binding to plasma proteins (i.e., a low f_u) will exhibit a small volume of distribution. Decreases in albumin concentration, for example, may result in a decline in the fraction of drug bound to plasma proteins. The increased amount of unbound drug is then free to distribute to other tissues. Unlike binding to plasma proteins however, binding to tissue receptors cannot be measured directly. This parameter is generally assumed to be constant. Again, from Eq. (28), this would appear to result in a volume of distribution increase. However, these changes are only important for drugs exhibiting a high degree of binding in plasma (>90%) and an even higher degree of binding in the tissues, that is, drugs with a high volume of distribution. Changes in protein binding will not significantly affect volume of distribution for low V drugs. Note that changes in volume of distribution do not influence the steady-state relationship between dosing rate and average concentration [Eq. (7)].

Influence of Protein-Binding Changes on Clearance

If we examine Eqs. (14)–(15), we can see that for drugs with a low extraction ratio (i.e., chlordiazepoxide), Q_{organ} is much greater than f_u, CL_{int}; clearance is then approximated by $f_u\ CL_{int}$. However in the case of a high extraction ratio drug (i.e. lidocaine), $f_u\ CL_{int}$ is much greater than Q_{organ}, and clearance approaches organ blood flow. Therefore, clearance of high extraction ratio drugs is perfusion rate limited, and not influenced by protein binding. Clearance of low extraction ratio drugs, in contrast to Eq. (14), is dependent upon both the fraction unbound and the intrinsic clearance (CL_{int}) of the metabolizing organ, for example, the liver.

Concept of Exposure

Most pharmacokinetic theory has concentrated on explaining changes in clearance and bioavailability in terms of the parameters of intrinsic clearance, blood flow and fraction unbound [Eqs. (14) and

(23)]. Yet the response of a patient to a dose or dosage regimen of a drug is dependent on the patient exposure to the drug, which is best characterized by AUC. Thus, it will be useful to consider the importance of individual parameters such as CL_{int}, Q and f_u in terms of exposure concepts. Consider first an intravenous dose of a drug where from Eq. (9).

$$AUC = \frac{Dose_{i.v.}}{CL} \quad \ldots(29)$$

and for a drug excreted exclusively by the liver substitution of Eq. (14) into Eq. (9) yields

$$AUC = \frac{Dose_{i.v.}(Q_H + f_u CL_{u,\text{int}})}{Q_H f_u CL_{u,\text{int}}} \quad \ldots(30)$$

For a high extraction ratio compound ($f_u\ CL_{u,int} \gg Q_H$), exposure will be inversely dependent upon hepatic blood flow

$$AUC \cong \frac{Dose_{i.v.}}{Q_H} \quad \ldots(31)$$

while for a low extraction ratio compound ($Q_H \gg f_u\ CL_{int}$), exposure will be inversely related to fraction unbound and intrinsic hepatic clearance.

$$AUC \cong \frac{Dose_{i.v.}}{f_u CL_{u,\text{int}}} \quad \ldots(32)$$

However, for an orally administered compound exposure will also be a function of oral bioavailability

$$AUC = \frac{F_{oral} Dose_{oral}}{CL} \quad \ldots(33)$$

Substituting, Eq. (20) for F_{oral}, Eq. (21) for $F_{H.}$ and Eq. (14) for CL into Eq. (32) above, and simplifying yields the following expression of exposure following an oral dose of a drug where elimination is via the liver.

$$AUC = \frac{F_{abs} F_G Dose_{oral}}{f_u CL_{u,\text{int}}} \quad \ldots(34)$$

Note that for oral dosing, exposure is inversely related to fraction unbound and intrinsic clearance for all drugs independent of whether they are low or high extraction ratio compounds.

Comparing Eqs. (31) and (34) for a low extraction ratio drug where elimination is primarily hepatic, it is obvious that similar oral and i.v. doses will yield similar AUC values, unless the product of F_{abs} F_G is low. A drug with $F_{abs}\ F_G \approx 1$, such as acetaminophen yields similar exposure following both oral and intravenous dosing, and also the variability of exposure will be similar for both routes, since the factors controlling variability, $f_u\ CL_{u,int}$, are the same in each case. Cyclosporine is an example of a low extraction ratio drug eliminated systemically by hepatic metabolism where exposure is markedly less following oral dosing vs. i.v., since $F_{abs}\ F_G$ is so low, in this case due to marked first pass gut metabolism. For this drug we would expect variability in exposure to the oral drug to be greater than i.v., due to the addition of the $F_{abs}\ F_G$ differences.

Propranolol is a good example of a high extraction ratio drug where systemic elimination is almost completely hepatic. Although there is some gut metabolism for propranolol following oral dosing, it is not extensive ($F_G \gg F_H$). The predicted differences in exposure following i.v. (10 mg) and oral (80 mg) dosing for this high extraction ratio drug. Note in comparing Eqs. (30) and (33) that exposure is less for the oral dose since $f_u\ CL_{u,\text{int}} > Q_H$. In addition, it is obvious that the variability following oral dosing is much greater than that following i.v. dosing. That is, hepatic blood flow from subject to

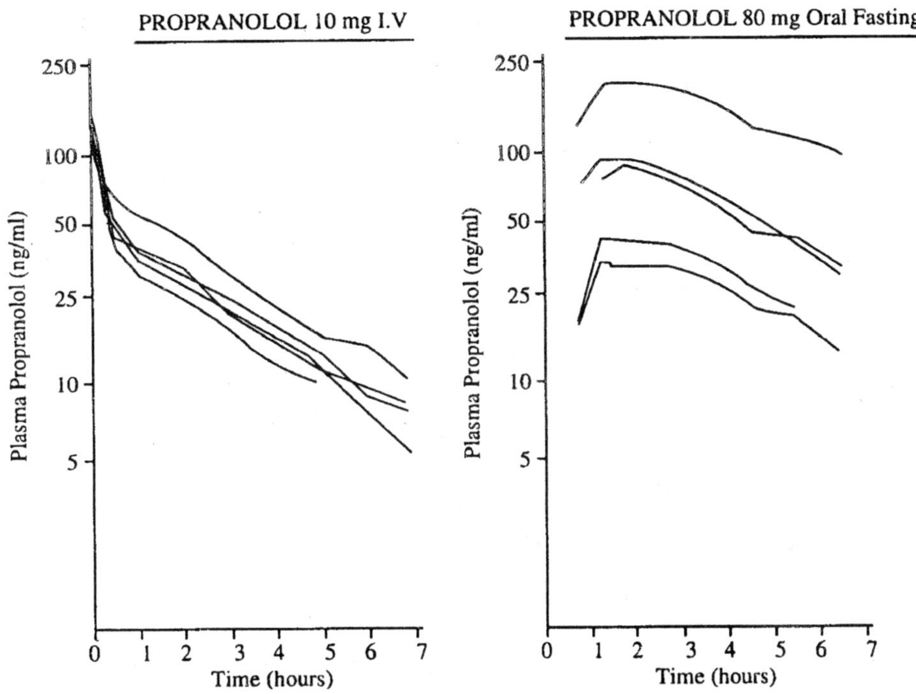

Fig. 7.12. Plasma propranolol leaves in 5 subjects after i.v. administration of 10 mg and oral administration of 80 mg of fasting subject.

subject shows much less variability than the intrinsic clearance of the hepatic enzymes. Returning to pharmacodynamic considerations, it is generally believed that drug responses, both efficacious and toxic, are related to exposure of the patient to unbound concentrations of the drug. For intermittent (not continuous infusion) dosing of drugs, Eq. (3) can be written as

$$E = \frac{E_{\max} AUC_u^s}{AUC_{u,50}^s + AUC_u^s} \quad \text{...(35)}$$

where $AUC_{u,50}$ is the unbound AUC that yields 50% of the maximal effect over a dosing interval. That is, the effect achieved over a dosing interval for a given dose of the drug is a function of the exposure to unbound concentrations of the drug. Unbound drug exposure is related to total exposure by f_u, fraction unbound.

$$AUC_u = AUC\, fu \quad \text{...(36)}$$

Note that unbound drug exposure will be independent of f_u for orally administered drugs that are predominantly eliminated by hepatic mechanisms. When AUC from Eq. (33) is substituted into Eq. (35) then

$$AUC_u = \frac{F_{abs} F_G Dose_{oral}}{CL_{u,\text{int}}} \quad \text{...(37)}$$

Similarly for intravenous dosing of low extraction ratio drugs, AUC_u is independent of f_u. Substituting, Eq. (31) into Eq. (35) yields

$$AUC_u \cong \frac{Dose_{i.v.}}{CL_{u,\text{int}}} \quad \text{...(38)}$$

For high extraction drugs predominantly eliminated by the liver, f_u does affect AUC_u

$$AUC_u \cong \frac{f_u Dose_{i.v}}{Q_H} \qquad ...(39)$$

For drugs where hepatic elimination is negligible, then $F_H = 1$ and following oral or intravenous dosing we may predict AUC_u as follows

$$AUC_u = \frac{f_u F_{abs} F_G Dose}{CL} \qquad ...(40)$$

CL and for a drug eliminated by renal processes

$$CL = \frac{Q_k f_u CL_{u,\text{int}}}{Q_K + f_u CL_{u,\text{int}}} \qquad ...(41)$$

where Q_K is blood flow to the kidney. Substituting Eq. (40) into Eq. (39), then

$$AUC_u = \frac{F_{abs} F_G Dose(Q_K + f_u CL_{u,\text{int}})}{Q_K CL_{u,\text{int}}} \qquad ...(42)$$

For a low extraction ratio drug in the kidney ($Q_k \gg f_u\ CL_{u,int}$), Eq. (43) becomes

$$AUC_u = \frac{F_{abs} F_G Dose}{CL_{u,\text{int}}} \qquad ...(43)$$

wheras for a high extraction ratio drug in the kidney ($f_u\ CL_{u,int} \gg Q_k$), Eq. (43) becomes

$$AUC_u = \frac{F_{abs} F_G Dose\ f_u}{Q_K} \qquad ...(44)$$

Note from the equations above that f_u becomes a determinant of AUC_u, and its thereby effect, only for a high extraction ratio drug given intravenously when the liver is the major route of elimination [Eq. (38)], and for a high extraction ratio drug given orally or intravenously when the kidney is the major route of administration [Eq. (43)]. Since most drug dosings do not fall into these very limited categories, it now becomes clear why changes in protein binding as a function of disease state or drug interactions are generally of irrelevant consequences.

Non-Linear Pharmacokinetics

Most drugs fortunately show linear pharmacokinetics within the therapeutic plasma concentration range (that is, with a doubling of the dose, the plasma concentration is also doubled), making possible the prediction of the impact of changes in drug dosing on the pharmacokinetic outcome.

Non-linear pharmacokinetics are caused mainly by saturation of the metabolizing enzymes during drug elimination or during the first passage of drug through the liver, and also by saturable protein binding as previously discussed. This leads to less predictable results in drug therapy and to the risk of a higher incidence of side effects.

Non-Linear Elimination/Clearance

All metabolic processes are saturable at a certain concentration of the substrate/drug. Thus, rate of elimination of the drug by metabolism as described by Eq. (7) can also be described by a Michaelis-Menten equation:

$$\text{Rate of metabolism} = \frac{V_m C}{K_m + C} \qquad ...(45)$$

From these equations metabolic clearance can be described as

$$CL = \frac{V_m}{K_m + C} \qquad \ldots(46)$$

where V_m is maximal velocity and K_m is the Michaelis-Menten constant. When kinetics are linear, $C \ll K_m$, and clearance equals V_m/K_m, but as the concentration approaches or exceeds K_m, clearance becomes dependent on the concentration, resulting in saturable metabolism. At steady state, when input rate (R_{in}) equals elimination rate, the steady-state concentration can be described by replacing rate of metabolism in Eq. (44) by R_{in} and rearranging

$$C_{ss} = \frac{K_m R_{in}}{V_m - R_{in}} \qquad \ldots(47)$$

Drugs that show saturable metabolism within the therapeutic range include phenytoin and salicylate. Because of the serious side effects encountered with phenytoin, and because of the genetic variability in metabolic capacity with respect to individual V_m and K_m values, phenytoin therapy is closely monitored using plasma concentration analysis. Phenytoin has a therapeutic concentration range of 10–20 mg/L, which is above K_m for most individuals. A small change of the dose in this region leads to a big change in plasma concentrations. An orbit graph of the relationship between V_m, K_m, and the average steady-state concentration of phenytoin based on Eq. (46) is shown.

The mean values of K_m and V_m within the population are 4 mg/L and 7mg/kg/day, respectively. The variation within the population is also depicted, where 50% of the population has K_m and V_m values within the innermost circle, 75% within the second circle, and so on. With the help of this graph, the suitable dosing rate of phenytoin for an individual patient can be determined. With two plasma concentrations at two different dosing rates of phenytoin in one patient, his/her individual V_m and K_m values can be obtained to further optimize the dosing schedule.

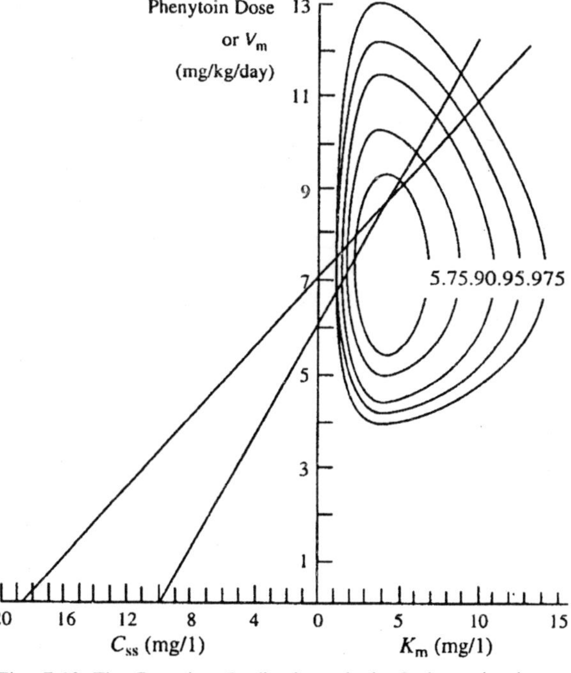

Fig. 7.13. The Bayesian feedback method of phenytoin dosage prediction.

Saturable first-pass effect

Because of very high drug concentrations entering the gut and the liver during the absorption of a drug after oral administration, the liver may often be exposed to drug concentrations that are much higher than after i.v. administration or much higher than the concentrations encountered during the elimination phase after oral administration. These initial hepatic portal vein concentrations after oral administration may exceed K_m even if the plasma concentrations measured in a peripheral venous sample do not exceed K_m. The higher the dose, the more of the drug escapes first-pass metabolism, which gives higher bioavailability with increasing dose. Virtually all PABA is eliminated into the urine as metabolite and unchanged drug within 24 h. However, the percent of the dose that has been metabolized to acetyl-PABA is dependent on dose size and rate of administration, with a clear decrease of the fraction of metabolite formed with increasing dose after oral administration. Also, the fraction of the dose that is metabolized increases dramatically with prolonged oral and i.v. administration. This may also have an impact on slow-release formulations, which for drugs exhibiting a saturable first-pass effect never yield portal vein concentrations as high as comparable immediate-release tablets, thus resulting in lower bioavailability for the slow-release formulation.

Steady-State Considerations in Design of Dosage Regimens

Most drug therapy is designed for chronic drug administration, such as for treatment of hypertension or diabetes. At steady state, the rate of input equals the rate of elimination [Eqs. (7) and (8)]:

$$\frac{F\,Dose}{\tau} = CL\ C_{ss,avg} \qquad \ldots(48)$$

where F is bioavailability, τ is the dosing interval, and $C_{ss,avg}$ is the average concentration during steady state. Note $C_{ss,avg}$ is another measure of exposure as discussed previously, since during the dosing interval $C_{ss,avg}$ is equivalent to AUC/τ. Multiplying both sides of Eq. (47) by τ and dividing by CL yields Eq. (33). From Eq. (47) dosing rate can be calculated knowing F and CL, or if $C_{ss,avg}$ is measured, CL/F can be estimated in a patient.Plasma drug concentration measurements as an aid in giving appropriate drug treatment may be useful when

1. The therapeutic index of the drug is low (e.g., theophylline, digoxin).
2. No pharmacodynamic measurements (e.g., blood pressure, minor side effects such as dry mouth during anticholinergic drug therapy) can be used as end points for therapy.
3. The drug shows non-linear kinetics within the therapeutic range (e.g., phenytoin).
4. The patient is "uncommon" (e.g., newborns, small children, pregnant women, or patients with decreased kidney function).

For the average steady-state concentration, the frequency of drug administration is not important as long as the dosing rate is the same. Thus, 1020 mg of theophylline can be given every 24 h or 340 mg every 8 h and still have the same average plasma concentration as when a constant infusion of 43.2 mg/h is given. However, the fluctuations around the mean value are influenced by the dosing interval. For drugs with a small therapeutic index, the fluctuations between maximum and minimum concentrations during a dosing interval must be kept within the therapeutic range, thus favoring shorter dosing intervals.

Maximum ($C_{ss,max}$) and minimum ($C_{ss,min}$) concentrations during a dosing interval tau (τ) can be estimated using the following equations, assuming rapid absorption compared to elimination, and a one- compartment model for the elimination, where lambda (λ) is the rate constant for drug elimination:

$$C_{ss,\max} = \frac{F\,Dose\,/\,V}{(1-e^{-\lambda\tau})} \qquad \ldots(49)$$

In Eq. (48) $(F\text{Dose})/V$ describes what is added to the concentration from the new dose. Thus, ($C_{ss,min}$) may be calculated as ($C_{ss,max}$) multiplied by the fraction remaining in the body at the end of the dosing interval:

$$C_{ss;min} = C_{ss;max}\,e^{-\lambda t} \qquad \ldots(50)$$

The difference between maximum and minimum concentrations at steady state is (FDose/V), and thus the amount that is eliminated during the dosing interval equals the available dose.

The factors that determine the average concentration at steady state are bioavailability and clearance. The maximum concentration is determined by the volume of distribution, the smaller the volume, the higher the concentration. The dosing interval compared to the half-life is most important in defining the fluctuations. A very convenient dosing interval is equal to the half-life of the drug. This results in a decline during the dosing interval to a minimum concentration that is 50% of the maximal concentration. However, administration of a drug every half-life might sometimes be difficult to achieve because of too short or too long half-lives compared to our 24-h cycle. A practical minimum dosing interval is 6 h, and the maximum is 24 h. For drugs with short half- lives, slow-release preparations might give smoother plasma concentration curves and decrease the number of dosings required. Compliance ultimately determines the therapeutic outcome; therefore, adjusting drug dosings to the daily routine of an individual, as much as possible, is important.

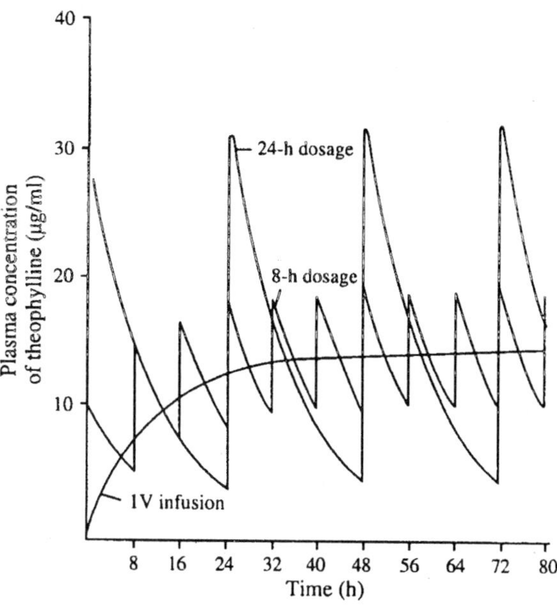

Fig. 7.14. Relationship between frequency of dosing and maximum and minimum plasma concentrations when a steady-state theophylline plasma level of 15 μg/ml is desired.

Loading Dose

A loading dose is given to attain the effective target concentration rapidly. It can be given as one dose or, more commonly, be divided into several doses over a relatively short period of time, such as one per day. The size of the loading dose depends on the target concentration and the volume of distribution and bioavailability of the drug. The loading dose should give the same amount of drug as will be present in the body during steady state

$$\text{Loading dose} = C_{ss}V/F \quad \text{...(51)}$$

A loading dose is used when the need for drug therapy is too urgent to wait 3–4 drug half-lives to reach the desired drug concentration in the body. The advantage is a more rapid attainment of steady state. The disadvantage is a higher risk of side effects if the drug concentrations become too high or if the individual is more sensitive to the drug than the average patient. However, in some instances, such as in dosing antiarrhythmics following an acute myocardial infarction, the only choice is to give a loading dose.

Individualizing Dosage Regimens: Individual Variations and Disease States

When starting a patient on a particular drug therapy, the clinician is dependent on general dosing information, such as from the PDR (Physicians Desk Reference) or other literature or experience, including an evaluation of the physical status of the patient. At that time the clinician cannot know exactly how this specific patient will react to the drug, pharmacokinetically or pharmacodynamically. For optimal therapy, the progress of therapy should be followed with measurements of relevant effect parameters, by titrating the dose to avoid certain known side effects, or by using therapeutic drug monitoring (drug plasma concentration measurements).

The need for individualized dosage recommendations has received increased attention in recent years parallel to the increased knowledge of what can cause interindividual variability in pharmacokinetic handling of drugs and in pharmacodynamic response. These causes include the influences of genetic variations, age, and disease states. Disease states influence the pharmacokinetics of drugs mainly by impairing drug transport and/or elimination, such as in heart failure or kidney or liver disease.

Kidney function and age show a close correlation. Glomerular filtration rate (GFR) is 100–125 ml/min/ 70 kg at 20–30 years of age, and then declines approximately 1ml/min per year as the patient ages. Decreased kidney function as a result of disease is usually detected by measuring serum creatinine levels and calculating the creatinine clearance as a measure of GFR, even though using creatinine as a marker for decreased kidney function has received increased criticism due to overestimation of GFR at medium–low kidney function. A GFR between 20 and 50 ml/min indicates moderate renal failure, and values < 10 ml/min indicate severe renal failure. If a major portion of the dose of a drug is eliminated unchanged via the kidneys, or if active or toxic metabolites are renally eliminated, corrections for kidney function may be necessary in dosing recommendations.

The influence of age on metabolic clearance is less clear than its influence on renal function. Metabolic clearance is more variable between individuals because of the genetic control and the influence of environmental factors on the metabolic capacity. The term metabolism also encompasses many different enzyme reactions that might be influenced to different extents by age, liver disease, or genetic variables. Unlike renal disease, in which creatinine clearance provides a reasonable estimate of kidney function, not one good indicator exists for the degree of liver function impairment with respect to drug metabolizing capacity.

Liver disease includes many diverse conditions. A distinction can be made between acute and chronic liver disease with respect to changes in clearance. Acute states do not generally seem to influence metabolic clearance of most drugs, but chronic states, such as cirrhosis, seem to decrease metabolic function to a greater degree. Also in cirrhosis, a portion of the blood flow may be shunted past the small capillaries within the liver or bypass the liver, causing even less exposure of the drug to the metabolizing enzymes and thereby greatly increasing the bioavailability of high-extraction-ratio drugs. Different drugs show different behavior with respect to the influence of liver disease on pharmacokinetics. Oxidative pathways seem to be more highly affected by liver disease than conjugation reactions such as glucuronidation. This is evident in the benzodiazepine group, where in cirrhosis patients oxazepam and lorazepam are preferred over diazepam and chlordiazepoxide due to the smaller changes in clearance for the former drugs, which are predominantly glucuronidated.

Cardiac failure may influence drug disposition by decreasing the cardiac output and increasing the peripheral resistance, thereby redistributing the blood flow from peripheral organs and tissues, such as kidneys and muscles, in favor of central organs, such as brain and heart. This might cause a slower than normal distribution of drug throughout the body and higher initial concentrations in the central organs that could cause an increased risk of side effects. Because of a lower blood flow to the gastrointestinal tract, heart failure might cause a slower rate of absorption of drugs. However, this seldom results in a lower bioavailability. A decreased and redistributed blood flow in liver and kidneys could yield a slower elimination of highly extracted drugs.

Pharmacogenetics

The 20th century yielded an enormous expansion in the chemical arsenal available to medical professionals, for the treatment of disease. The worldwide use of these drugs, particularly over the past several decades, has revealed substantial interindividual differences in the response to drugs. These differences, confirmed and explained by pharmacokinetic analysis, appear in individual patients as variations not only in expected therapeutic responses, but often in the frequency and nature of associated adverse events. Any particular drug or drug dose may be therapeutic in some patients, but ineffective in other individuals. Along the same lines, some individuals may experience drug related adverse effects from standard therapy, while others are unaffected.

Recognition of these interindividual differences in drug response is an essential first step in optimizing drug therapy. A great deal of evidence has accumulated over the past several decades indicating that a substantial portion of the observed variability in response to drugs is genetically determined, although age, nutrition, health, and environmental factors play important roles. Pharmacogenetics is primarily concerned with the genetic basis underlying this interindividual drug response, and focuses on genetic differences among individuals, and on the different patterns of drug response among geographically and ethnically distinct populations. The goal of pharmacogenetics is to make truly individualized drug therapy, one could say personalized medicine, possible, and with a reasonably predictive outcome.

The basic unit of inheritance is the gene, a specific DNA sequence of base pairs which codes for a particular protein. The genotype, is the configuration of genes in an individual, while the phenotype, is the outward physical expression of those genes. The mode of inheritance of any individual trait can be either monogenic or polygenic, depending on whether it is derived from a single gene at a single locus (position), or by multiple loci on the chromosomes respectively. An allele is one, two or more different forms of the same gene, containing specific inheritable differences, occupying corresponding positions on paired chromosomes. Genetic polymorphism, refers to monogenic traits existing in the population in at least two phenotypes, each of which exits at a frequency of at least 1%. An individual possessing a pair of identical alleles for a given trait is said to be homozygous for that trait. Individuals who are heterozygous for a given trait, possess a combination of dominant and recessive alleles for that trait.

The cytochrome P450 (CYP) monooxygenase system of enzymes is responsible for the primary portion of xenobiotic (foreign substance) metabolism in man. This large family of genes is composed of numerous subtypes, among which CYP2D6, CYP3A4/3A5, CYP1A2, CYP2E1, CYP2C9 and CYP2C19 play especially important roles in genetically determined responses to a wide spectrum of drugs. Examples to date of inherited variability in pharmacokinetics have been almost entirely restricted to drug metabolism. Renal clearance for any drug tends to be very similar for age and weight matched patients in good health. Similarly, the role of genetics in determining the absorption and distribution of drugs is poorly defined.

A number of examples of genetic polymorphisms in drug metabolism have now been identified, involving oxidation, S-methylation, and acetylation. These polymorphisms were initially identified by adverse drug reactions occurring in distinct groups, termed "*poor metabolizers*," following normal therapeutic doses of the initial, archetypic drugs.

Patients who are homozygous for the CYP2D6 "slow" alleles exhibit a poor metabolizer phenotype, with impaired metabolism and excretion of many drugs, such as metoprolol, nortriptyline and propafone. These "poor metabolizers" are more likely to experience adverse reactions to standard doses of these drugs. The frequency of this recessive trait ranges from 1–2% in Asians, approximately 5% in African Americans to 6–10% in Caucasian populations. More than 40 drugs now in clinical practice, particularly in the areas of cardiovascular disease and psychiatric disorders exhibit the same polymorphic pattern of metabolism by CYP2D6. Along similar lines, patients who are homozygous for the recessive allele of CYP2C19 are highly sensitive to omeprazole, diazepam, propranolol, mephenytoin, amitriptyline and other drugs metabolized by this isoform. The "*poor metabolizer*" phenotype of CYP2C19 comprises approximately 2–5% of Caucasians and 3–23% of Asians. Another polymorphically expressed enzyme of the P450 superfamily is CYP2C9. This enzyme is responsible for the metabolism of a range of therapeutically important drugs such as phenytoin, tolbutamide and warfarin. It has been estimated, that approximately 5% of Caucasians posses the genetic variant of CYP2C9 associated with a fivefold decline in metabolic activity. Drugs such as phenytoin and warfarin, for example, have narrow therapeutic indices, and individual genetically based variations in metabolism could have important clinical significance.

Individuals also vary widely in their elimination kinetics of isoniazid, procainamide, and other substrates of N-acetyltransferase (NAT2). Peripheral neuropathy associated with the use of isoniazid, an antituberculosis drug, first surfaced more than 40 years ago. It is now known that the "slow acetylator" phenotype represents approximately 40–50% of Caucasians, and results in decreased clearance of drug with increased potential for associated toxicities.

Genetic heterogeneity appears then, to be an important source of the observed variability in drug response. This strongly implies that information pertaining to interethnic and interindividual genetic differences can play an important role in drug discovery and development. New genetic tools for the rapid, inexpensive determination of patient genotypes could have important therapeutic implications. The need for a new, individualized approach to drug therapy is now, more obvious than ever. Every year approximately 3 billion prescriptions are issued in the United States, of which 2 million result in an adverse reaction, with as many as 1 million resulting in hospitalization. Some 100,000 patients die each year as a result of drug induced adverse reactions. Early or preventive therapy, guided by individual genetic information, could significantly improve clinical outcomes, while reducing the incidence of drug associated adverse events.

Use of Pharmacokinetic Information in Drug Formulation

Depending on the use of a drug, different parameters are important in designing a dosage form. For intermittent drug use, such as aspirin for headache, the ideal dosage form should give a rapid rate of absorption to yield quick relief of the pain. This objective has led to the formulation of buffered or soluble forms of acetylsalicylic acid, for which the absorption rate is limited mainly by the drug's ability to cross the GI membranes. With a different indication, such as aspirin used chronically for rheumatoid arthritis, low exposure to the stomach is desired; for this purpose, enteric-coated tablets and granules of the drug have been formulated.

For a drug intended to be used chronically, the clearance of the drug from the body, together with the extent of availability, determines the dose size for a given therapeutic drug level [Eq. (45)]. If clearance and volume of distribution of the specific drug result in a short half-life and keeping drug concentrations above a certain level is important, for example, during antiarrhythmic treatment, the dosing interval is crucial, leading to the demand for a controlled-release dosage form.

However, pharmacokinetic properties of a drug may pose limitations as to the possibility of attaining an ideal therapy. The choice of digoxin over digitoxin is mainly determined by the shorter half-life and in the minds of some clinicians a safer and more predictable drug therapy with digoxin. Oxazepam is an example of a drug with a slower than wanted rate of absorption, which decreases its use as a help in starting to sleep. This slow absorption rate is a characteristic of the drug itself and cannot be increased by drug-product formulation. Thus, dosage form development is limited by the basic pharmacokinetic properties of the drug.

The oral bioavailability of a high-extraction-ratio drug can never be improved by dosage form development if the reason for low availability is high first-pass metabolism. The ability to give an oral dosing regimen of a high-extraction-ratio drug is dependent on the ratio between therapeutic concentrations of the drug and toxic concentrations of the metabolites formed during the first pass and on how critical for successful therapy staying within the therapeutic range of drug concentrations is. Both lidocaine and propranolol have a high extraction in the liver with low bioavailability as a result (35 and 36%, respectively). However, propranolol is given orally and lidocaine is not.

Therapeutic concentrations of lidocaine are 1.5–6 mg/L, and side effects start to appear at concentrations of 6–10 mg/L. For lidocaine falling below the therapeutic concentration range is just as serious as going too high in concentration, as both situations may cause arrhythmias. With a half-life of only 1.8 h, oral doses would have to be given very often, which is not practical. Also, the variability in the first-pass effect between individuals, but the therapeutic index is much higher, and plasma concentrations falling below the "*therapeutic concentration*" are not as critical for the patient; therefore, larger fluctuations in plasma concentrations can be allowed during a dosing interval without loss of an acceptable therapeutic outcome.

The pharmacokinetic profile of a drug can in this way be used as a basis for dosage form development, together with the specific requirements of the particular drug concerning maximal and/or minimal concentrations desired, effectiveness versus toxicity, the desired rate of attaining an effect, and the convenience of drug administration for the individual. Thus, the knowledge of basic pharmacokinetic features, such as rate of absorption, degree of absorption, degree of renal elimination versus metabolism, whether the drug is a high or a low extraction drug, and the like, and knowledge of the pharmacokinetic–pharmacodynamic relationship are tools in optimizing drug product development to the needs of the patient

8

PHARMACOKINETICS IN ELDERLY

Clinical response to medication in an individual patient is the net result of the interaction of a number of complex processes. These processes can be categorized into two broad areas: those affecting pharmacokinetics or the relationship between the administered dose and the concentrations of the drug in the systemic circulation, and those affecting pharmacodynamics or the relationship between concentrations of the drug in the systemic circulation and the observed pharmacologic response. Absorption, distribution, metabolism, and excretion of a drug determine its pharmacokinetics. Drug–receptor interactions, concentrations of the drug at the receptor, and homeostatic compensatory mechanisms determine a drug's pharmacodynamics. Pharmacokinetics and pharmacodynamics are affected by a number of patient-specific factors including age, sex, ethnicity, genetics, disease processes, and prior and present drug exposure. This chapter focuses on the effects of advanced age on pharmacokinetics.

In clinical decision-making for the elderly patient it is important to recognize that the elderly may also experience an unexpected clinical response to a medication owing to the impact of factors other than their age, such as concurrent diseases and coadministered medications. Despite the fact that much less is known about pharmacodynamic changes in the elderly than changes in pharmacokinetics, the potential for altered pharmacodynamics must also be considered.

DEFINITION OF "ELDERLY"

"*Elderly*" has generally been defined as age 65 yr or older, although many other chronological definitions have been applied. Some researchers have enrolled patients as young as 50 yr old as "elderly" whereas others have studied only those patients in their 80s or older as "elderly." Although a chronological age is most often used to define elderly, it is important to recognize that the elderly are a heterogeneous group, with individuals aging at varying rates. Interindividual variation is much larger in the elderly than in the young. The aging process has been described as a condition of "*incipient disease*" with a variety of deteriorative changes taking place. When decline occurs more obviously in one organ system than another, a disease is diagnosed.

It is therefore difficult to distinguish between normal age-related changes and pathological states. Biological or physiological definitions of elderly have proved difficult to formulate, so chronological definitions of elderly remain the standard. The Food and Drug Administration's "Guideline for Industry Studies in Support of Special Populations: Geriatrics" arbitrarily defines the geriatric population as comprising patients aged 65 yr or older, although the inclusion of older patients is encouraged to the extent possible.

Elderly Patient

Although many older adults age successfully and lead healthy, productive lives well into their later years, the elderly as a group are more likely to suffer from chronic diseases and take more medications than their younger counterparts. The aging process itself is associated with changes in physiology that may alter drug pharmacokinetics and pharmacodynamics. When applying general knowledge of pharmacokinetic alterations in the elderly to the care of an individual patient in the clinical setting, it is necessary to consider the patient's overall condition, "*physiologic age*," disease states, and concurrent medications.

The elderly are especially vulnerable to adverse reactions to medications. The incidence of adverse drug reactions is two to three times that found in younger adults but may be underestimated because of lack of detection and underreporting. Many adverse reactions are preventable. Examples of preventable adverse effects include consequences of known drug–drug interactions or prescribing an inappropriate dosage for the elderly. The increased incidence of adverse reactions in the elderly results from altered pharmacokinetics, altered pharmacodynamics, increased opportunity for drug interactions, and inappropriate prescribing. While the changes in pharmacokinetics and pharmacodynamics are well recognized, age-related differences in dosing often are not noted in compendia such as the *Physician's Desk Reference* (*PDR*) that are used by prescribers. One recent study found many examples of evidence-based recommendations for dose alterations in the elderly that were reported in the literature but were not noted in the product labeling included in the *PDR*. This could explain, in part, the significant increase in adverse events in the elderly. Knowledge of basic pharmacokinetic differences in the elderly associated with age-related changes in physiology can be used to choose appropriate dosing regimens for the elderly and avoid preventable adverse drug reactions.

Pharmacokinetic Studies in the Elderly

Almost all of the information known about age-related changes in humans, including pharmacokinetics, has been obtained from cross-sectional studies. In these studies, the variable under investigation is measured in groups of subjects of different ages at a single point in time. Age differences are then inferred from a comparison of the mean values for each group or from a regression of the variable on age. The cross-sectional approach assumes that average differences between age groups reflect the change that occurs in an individual with the passage of time, which may or may not be valid.

When studying chronological changes in a particular variable, there are three primary time-related factors that must be considered: the effects of age, the effects of an environmental change or historical event at a specified period in time (period effects), and the effects of being part of the group or cohort of individuals born at a particular time (birth cohort). Cross-sectional studies often confound age effects with birth cohort effects. Findings in a group of individuals aged 65 today may differ from those in a group of 65-yr-olds studied 25 yr from now. These groups would be the same age but from different birth cohorts with different group experiences. Cross-sectional studies can also suffer from selective mortality effects, because the oldest study cohorts include only those individuals who survived to reach old age, and these individuals may be unique regarding the variable of interest.

Another approach to studying age-related changes is longitudinal studies. In these studies repeated measurements of a variable are made on the same individual at various points in time. This approach measures individual rates of aging for the specified variable, rather than differences between age groups as in cross-sectional studies. Although the results of longitudinal studies may be a more reliable approach to studying age-related changes, longitudinal studies tend to confound age effects with the effects of an environmental change or historical event at a specified period in time (period effects). These studies are also very difficult to conduct, taking many years to complete. For this reason, pharmacokinetic studies are virtually always cross-sectional in design.

Two general cross-sectional approaches are used to study pharmacokinetics in the elderly. The first is a formal pharmacokinetic study conducted either in healthy geriatric subjects or in elderly patient volunteers with the disease the drug is intended to treat. A relatively small group of subjects is studied using intensive blood sampling in each individual. In this approach, very healthy elderly people are selected for participation in an attempt to ensure that advanced age, and not disease, is the primary factor under investigation. Often these studies include only relatively young geriatric subjects that can meet the stringent inclusion criteria, limiting the generalizability of the results to the very old or frail patient. Results of these studies must be considered along with pharmacokinetic studies in other populations, such as patients with renal impairment, when making therapy decisions for individual patients.

The second cross-sectional approach is the pharmacokinetic screening or population pharmacokinetic study. These studies are typically conducted in conjunction with the main Phase III (or Phase II) clinical trials program. Under steady-state conditions, a small number of samples for drug level determinations are collected and analyzed. When appropriately designed, the influence of demographic and disease factors on pharmacokinetics can be examined in this type of study. Although the data analysis is more difficult, the advantage to this approach is that age and other factors, as well as their interactions, can be evaluated.

General Pharmacokinetic Changes Associated with Aging

Normal aging is associated with changes in human physiology, and many of these changes contribute to altered pharmacokinetics in the elderly. These changes are even more evident in frail or very old patients. Drug absorption and bioavailability, distribution, metabolism, and renal excretion may be altered in geriatric patients. If these changes are not considered when dosing elderly patients, preventable medication-related problems may result.

Absorption and Bioavailability

The bioavailability of a drug is defined as the fraction of drug reaching the systemic circulation after drug administration. Age-related changes in bioavailability depend on the route of drug administration, age-associated changes in the gastrointestinal tract and other organs of drug absorption, and age-associated changes in metabolism during the first pass through the liver or intestine. Despite changes in physiology with age, oral absorption and bioavailability of most drugs appear to remain unchanged in the elderly owing in part to the large functional reserve capacity of the gastrointestinal tract.

Gastric pH, gastrointestinal blood flow, active transport processes, and gastrointestinal motility have been reported to be altered in the elderly to a variable extent. Atrophic changes in the gastric mucosa may result in decreased acid secretion. The resulting increase in gastric pH could affect the ionization and solubility of some drugs. Decreased perfusion of the gastrointestinal tract and diminished active membrane transport processes could result in decreased rate or extent of drug absorption. These effects may be offset, however, by longer gastrointestinal transit times, with decreased gastrointestinal motility resulting in increased contact time for drug absorption. Most drug absorption in the gastrointestinal tract occurs by passive diffusion, and the majority of studies indicate that there are no clinically significant changes in the rate or extent of drug absorption from the gastrointestinal tract.

Intragastric metabolism and hepatic first-pass metabolism may be reduced in the elderly, resulting in increased drug bioavailability. Studies with levodopa, for example, have shown that the elderly experience a threefold increase in availability of levodopa related to a reduction in gastric wall content of dopa decarboxylase. Intestinal metabolism of verapamil, however, was well preserved in the elderly. Drugs that undergo a high rate of first-pass metabolism, such as propranolol, demonstrate increased bioavailability owing to decreased first-pass extraction.

Absorption and bioavailability for nonoral routes of administration (intramuscular, rectal, buccal, transdermal) and sustained release dosage forms have not been as well studied in the elderly. The rate of intramuscular absorption of antibiotics may be reduced in the elderly, but there are insufficient data to draw conclusions regarding the potential for age- related changes in drug absorption and bioavailability by these routes.

Distribution

Age-related changes in body composition and plasma protein binding may affect drug distribution in the elderly. The elderly tend to have decreased lean body mass, increased body fat, and decreased total body water. Interestingly, elderly individuals with high levels of physical activity are not different from those with low activity levels with respect to fat-free mass and fat mass. Lipid-soluble drugs may show an increased volume of distribution and water-soluble drugs may show a decreased volume of distribution in elderly patients related to these changes in body composition. For example, the elderly have an approx 20% lower volume of distribution for ethanol, which distributes in body water, than young individuals. Changes in body composition resulting in changes in volume of distribution may necessitate changes in loading doses of some drugs for the elderly.

Age-related changes in protein binding do not generally result in clinically significant changes in drug therapy for elderly patients. Generally, plasma protein binding of drugs remains unchanged or is decreased in the elderly. Serum albumin concentrations may be decreased in the elderly by 15–20%, but this is often related to renal dysfunction, hepatic disease, or frailty.

Hepatic Metabolism

Hepatic metabolism is one of the major routes of drug clearance in humans. The rate and extent of hepatic drug biotransformation depend on hepatic blood flow and hepatic enzyme content, affinity, and activity rate. Hepatic inactivation of drugs and environmental toxins occurs through phase I oxidative pathways (oxidation, deamination, or hydroxylation) or phase II conjugative pathways (acetylation, glucuronidation, or sulfation). Not all pathways of hepatic drug metabolism are equally efficient. Hepatic biotransformation results in a metabolite, which may be pharmacologically active or inactive, and may be eliminated from the body or further metabolized before elimination.

Interest in potential age-associated changes in drug metabolism is significant because of the need to reduce the risk of adverse drug reactions and drug interactions in the elderly. A number of age-related changes in physiology that may impact hepatic drug metabolism in elderly patients have been reported, but the effect of age on hepatic metabolism remains controversial. Much of the literature in this area has been conflicting. Early studies attributed observed changes in drug clearance in the elderly to changes in hepatic enzyme activity, and more recently to decreased liver size and hepatic blood flow. In vitro tests of enzyme have been inconsistent with results of in vivo studies. Despite these controversies, several generally accepted principles of the affect of aging on hepatic drug metabolism have emerged.

Hepatic blood flow has been shown to decline by approx 40% with age, in parallel with a decline in cardiac output. For drugs with a high hepatic extraction ratio, where clearance depends primarily on the rate of drug presentation to the liver through hepatic blood flow, aging is associated with decreased drug clearance. Phase I oxidative metabolism of some drugs appears to decline with aging, despite the fact that in vitro hepatic enzyme activity does not appear to be altered by age. Reduction in hepatic oxygen diffusion resulting from age-related changes in hepatocyte volume and surface membrane permeability and conformation is one proposed explanation for reduced oxidative drug metabolism observed with aging. Hepatic enzymes can be inhibited and induced by drugs and other compounds. Changes in hepatic enzyme induction with aging remain controversial. Phase II conjugative metabolic pathways appear to be unchanged with aging.

When prescribing for the elderly patient, age-related changes in drug metabolism should be considered. From a pharmacokinetic point of view, drugs that are metabolized exclusively by phase II conjugative mechanisms are preferred in the elderly. For oxidatively metabolized drugs with a high extraction ratio (high clearance drugs), dosages should generally be reduced owing to decreased hepatic blood flow. Dosages for drugs with a low extraction ratio (low clearance drugs) should be reduced as well. After initial dosing, doses can be adjusted based on patient response and tolerability. The potential for significant drug interactions, particularly resulting from hepatic enzyme inhibition in elderly patients on multiple medications, must be carefully considered.

Renal Excretion

Altered renal elimination of drugs is the most clinically important pharmacokinetic difference between elderly and young patients. Renal clearance depends, in part, on renal blood flow, which delivers drugs and metabolites to the kidneys for elimination. Elimination from the kidneys then occurs through glomerular filtration, tubular secretion, and tubular reabsorption. With aging, renal blood flow declines as cardiac output declines, resulting in decreased glomerular filtration rate as measured by creatinine clearance in the elderly. Although there is considerable interindividual variability, declining creatinine clearance with age (about 10% per decade after age 20) is consistently reported in the literature. Changes in the kidneys that occur with aging include a decrease in kidney weight, a thickening of the intrarenal vascular intima, sclerogenous changes of the glomeruli, and fibrosis and infiltration of chronic inflammatory cells in the stroma. Altered tubular function may also be present in advanced age.

The most important aspect of renal function to monitor clinically is the glomerular filtration rate (GFR). Most decisions about drug dosing for renally excreted drugs can be made based on the estimated GFR. Clinically, creatinine clearance is used to estimate GFR. Serum creatinine alone is not a good indicator of renal function in the elderly population because muscle mass, and therefore creatinine production, declines with age. A normal serum creatinine can result when both creatinine formation and elimination are reduced. Several algorithms have been proposed to estimate creatinine clearance. One frequently used method was developed by Cockcroft and Gault, where creatinine clearance (CL_{cr}) is calculated based on the patient's age, weight, and serum creatinine concentration:

$$CL_{cr} = \frac{(140 - \text{age in yr}) \times \text{weight (kg)}}{72 \times \text{serum creatine (mg / 100 mL)}} \quad \ldots(1)$$

For women, the result is multiplied by 0.85. This formula is less accurate for estimates in the very high or low range and when renal function is changing rapidly. For frail elderly patients with chronic muscle atrophy, an alternative formula has been proposed that takes into account serum albumin levels as well.

For men:

$$CL_{cr} = \frac{\{[19 \times \text{serum albumin (g / dL)}] + 32\} \times \text{body weight (kg)}}{100 \times \text{serum creatine (mg / dL)}} \quad \ldots(2)$$

For women:

$$CL_{cr} = \frac{\{[13 \times \text{serum albumin (g / dL)}] + 29\} \times \text{body weight (kg)}}{100 \times \text{serum creatine (mg / dL)}} \quad \ldots(3)$$

This approach provides more accurate and less biased estimates of CL_{cr} than the Cockcroft and Gault method in elderly patients with renal insufficiency or serum albumin levels < 2.8 g/dL.

Effects of Age on the Pharmacokinetics of Chemotherapeutics

Old age is playing an increasing role in the treatment of cancer, as the prevalence of cancer in elderly patients is high and increasing: 60% of all cancers occur in patients aged 65 yr and above, and the elderly constitute a growing portion of the overall population, with 20% of the population expected to be > 65 yr by the year 2030.

This will lead to an increased use of anticancer agents by elderly patients. In addition to the physiological effects that aging may have on the pharmacokinetic characteristics of these agents, it has to be noted that the likelihood of polypharmacy due to noncancer, age-related chronic illnesses may lead to an increased incidence of drug–drug interactions. Quite a few of these interactions are pharmacokinetically based, for example, inhibition of hepatic metabolism (cytochrome P450-dependent, CYP) by concurrent medications.

Examples

Previous articles have reviewed the primary literature describing the effects of aging on the pharmacokinetic properties of chemotherapeutic agents. Most of these clinical studies were small, cross-sectional trials and assess plasma concentrations of the drug of interest, and in some cases, their active metabolites. A large portion of these studies reports changes in systemic exposure (e.g., peak plasma concentration, area under the curve, and terminal half-life) rather than more meaningful pharmacokinetic parameters such as volume of distribution, specific organ clearances, and oral bioavailability, if appropriate. Therefore, as pointed out earlier, it is sometimes difficult to assess whether physiological aging, concurrent medications or other confounding covariates are responsible for the observed age differences in systemic exposure. In addition, it is sometimes very difficult to interpret the results mechanistically, that is, what pharmacokinetic process is affected by age-related changes.

Based on these general properties, individual drugs whose pharmacokinetics are known to be affected by age, the likely mechanism of that age effect, and the need for dose modification in the elderly. Note that f_e indicates the fraction of the total dose renally eliminated unchanged. The major reason for dose modification in the elderly is the age-related impairment in renal excretory function. Therefore, the dose modifications based on renal function for selected anticancer agents. Overall, it is apparent that age-related renal impairment is the major cause of dose modifications in the elderly, and the (estimated) creatinine clearance serves as a good predictor for a patient-individualized dosing regimen. Apparent age-related effects on hepatic metabolism/biliary excretion have been observed, but usually do not lead to dose adjustments. Age-related effects on absorption are rare since most agents are given intravenously, while age effects on drug distribution are difficult to observe and are unlikely to result in dose modifications. This overall conclusion may change in the future when cancer treatment will involve chemoprevention and disease modification, with the agents given orally and less likely to be renally eliminated. Furthermore, owing to polypharmacy the likelihood of clinically significant drug–drug interactions at the level of drug absorption, first-pass, and systemic metabolism will increase.

9

PHARMACODYNAMIC

Pharmaceutical industry is faced with more challenges than ever in recent years. The drug industry continues to consolidate and become more competitive. Highly publicized lawsuits have heightened sensitivities with respect to the balance between acceptable efficacy and safety. The U.S. Food and Drug Administration (FDA) reports that about 22% of the drugs had labeling changes after approval, most of which were safety-motivated and net dosage decreases. In addition, the industry has been struggling to increase productivity despite the advancement of basic research. In light of all these issues and the ever-increasing cost of drug development ($800 million/yr), the pharmaceutical industry is increasingly focusing on ways to streamline the drug development process through more efficiently designed clinical trials. Pharmacokinetic/pharmacodynamic (PK/PD) modeling and simulation, which generally have not been in wide use in drug development in the past, are useful and important tools that can improve the efficiency of the drug development process, from preclinical stage to the postmarketing phase and beyond.

The aim of this chapter is to provide a general perspective on PK/PD modeling and simulation and their applications in the drug development process. It is intended as an introductory reading for those who may not be intimately familiar with the concept and benefits of PK/PD modeling and simulations rather than providing intricate technical details. With the background information provided by this chapter, readers are encouraged to move on to more advanced technical references currently available for continued learning.

GENERAL PERSPECTIVE ON PK/PD MODELING AND SIMULATION

Basic Concept of PK/PD

Pharmacokinetics describes the time course of drug concentration in one or more biological specimen, normally plasma, serum, or whole blood, which reflects several processes including absorption, distribution, metabolism, and elimination. The overall kinetic process often can be characterized using various mathematical models including compartment models, non-compartment models, and physiological-based models. We do not intend to have a detailed discussion on pharmacokinetics in this chapter. For further reading on pharmacokinetic principles, we refer the readers to Gibaldi and Perrier, and Rowland and Tozer. Pharmacodynamics describes the time course and the magnitude of pharmacological response of drugs. Based on the classic receptor-occupancy theory, after drug molecules reach the target biophase, it binds to the receptors to form the drug–receptor complex to exert pharmacological response.

Ariens introduced the concept that the pharmacological response is directly proportional to the concentration of drug–receptor complex. Pharmacological responses can generally be categorized into two groups: continuous response (e.g., blood pressure and fasting blood glucose) and discrete categorical response. The latter can be further subcategorized into dichotomous response (e.g., response vs. no response), ordered categorical response (e.g., Likert pain rating scale where higher numbers represent greater pain), count response (e.g., number of seizures per month), and time-to-event response (e.g., survival, time to deferverscence).

Pharmacokinetic/pharmacodynamic modeling relates the dose or concentration (exposure) of a drug provided by the kinetic model to its observed pharmacological effects (response) by establishing an exposure–response relationship.

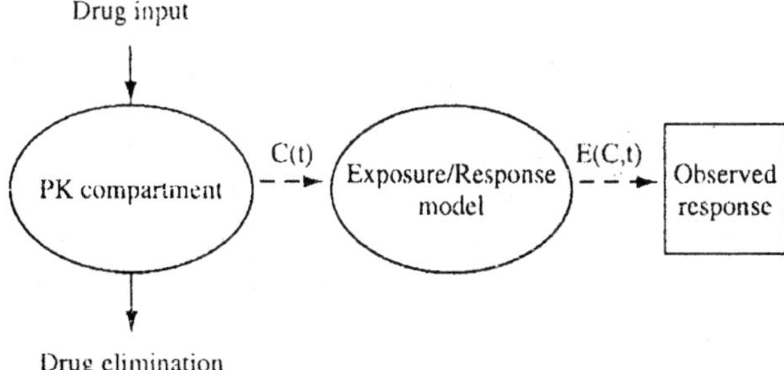

Fig. 9.2. Conceptualization of pharmacokinetic and pharmacodynamic diagram.

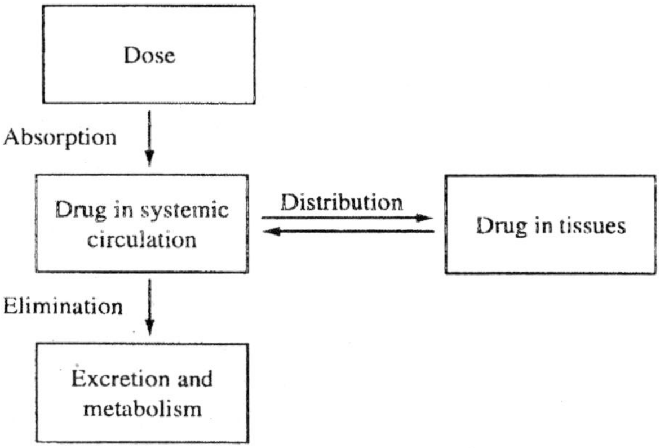

Dose
Absorption
Drug in systemic circulation
Distribution
Drug in tissues
Elimination
Excretion and metabolism

Fig. 9.1. Schematic representation of the relationship between absorption, distribution, and elimination kinetics of a drug.

PK/PD Models

Many PK/PD models have been developed to characterize the exposure–response relationship for a variety of classes of drugs. In the following section we provide a brief discussion on some simple direct effect models that assume a rapid equilibrium between plasma and biophase concentrations (steady-state) and time-invariant pharmacodynamics, as well as some more advanced non-steady-state and time-dependent models.

Simple direct effect models

Linear model

In the simplest case, the observed effect (E) is directly related to drug concentrations (C) that can be described by the linear function

$$E = S * C \qquad \text{...(1)}$$

where S is the slope parameter. If there is a baseline effect (E_0) when drug is absent, then the model may be expressed as

$$E = E_0 + S * C \qquad \text{...(2)}$$

The linear model is the special case of the E_{max} model (discussed later) when the observed concentrations are much lower than EC_{50}. However, one should be aware that the assumption of a direct proportionality between effect and concentration is only valid within a limited linear range of the effect–concentration curve.

Log-linear model

If the effect is measured over a large concentration range, the relationship between effect and concentration may appear curvilinear. The log-linear model is given in Eq. (3)

$$E = E_0 + S * \log C \qquad \text{...(3)}$$

where S and E_0 have the same interpretation as in the linear model. One obvious limitation of this model is that the pharmacologic effect cannot be estimated when the concentration is zero because of the logarithmic function.

Emax model

E_{max} model was originally derived from the classic drug–receptor occupancy theory. It is an empirical function for describing a non-linear concentration–effect relationship with the general form:

$$E = E_{max} * C/(C + EC_{50}) \qquad ...(4)$$

where the effect E is a function of E_{max}, the maximum effect due to drug, C, the drug concentration, and EC_{50}, the concentration required to achieve 50% of the maximum effect. The E_{max} model describes the hyperbolic shape of the response vs. drug concentration curve.

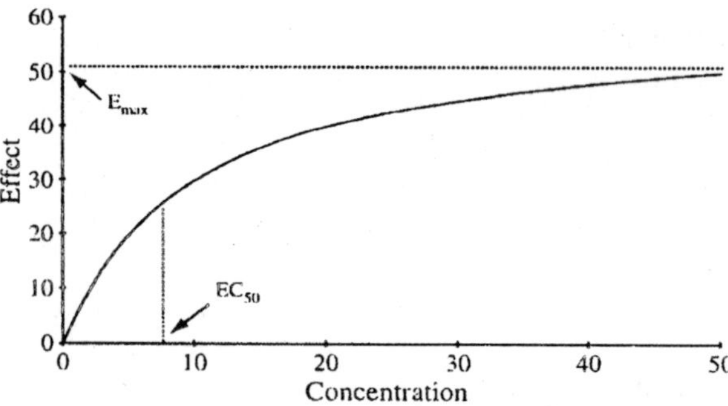

Fig. 9.3. Effects vs. concentration for the E_{max} model.

In many cases, the baseline pharmacologic effect (E_0) exists when the drug is absent, and the equation can be modified as follows:

$$E = E_0 + E_{max} * C=(C + EC_{50}) \qquad ...(5)$$

Sigmoidal E_{max} model

The sigmoidal E_{max} model, originally derived based on oxygen–hemoglobin dissociation kinetics, is a generalization of the E_{max} model. It describes the response vs. drug concentration curve for many drugs that appear to be S-shaped (sigmoidal) rather than hyperbolic as described by the simple E_{max} model.

$$E = E_{max} * C^{\gamma}/(C^{\gamma} + EC^{\gamma}_{50}) \qquad ...(6)$$

where γ represents a sigmoidicity factor or the steepness of the curve: $\gamma = 1$ for the hyperbolic curve; $\gamma > 1$ for a steeper curve; and $\gamma < 1$ for the smoother curve. The sigmoidal E_{max} model is generally flexible in describing the concentration–effect relationship for many drugs with simple direct and reversible action.

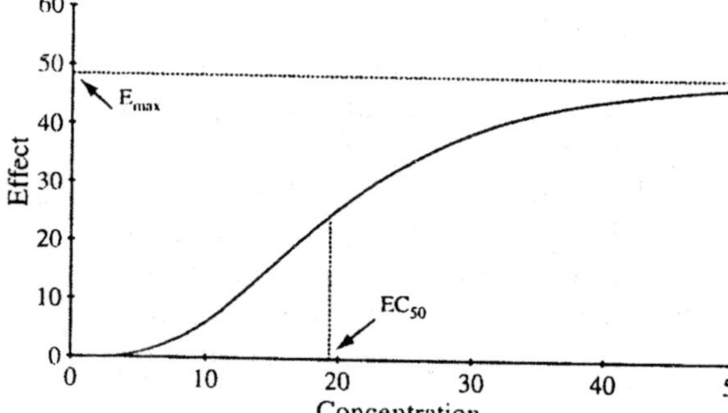

Fig. 9.4. Effect vs. concentration for the sigmoidal E_{max} model.

Nonsteady and time-dependent models

An important assumption associated with the above- mentioned simple direct effect models is that a rapid equilibrium exists between plasma and effect site concentrations. Accordingly, maximum effects are predicted to occur simultaneously with peak drug concentrations. For many drugs, however, there is a temporal dissociation between the time course of concentration and the time course of effect, a phenomenon resulting in hysteresis observed in plots of effect vs. concentration.

This temporal displacement may be related to a slow biophase distribution process between plasma and effect concentrations, and the specific mechanism of drug action, such as an indirect effect or a signal transduction process. Several models that have been developed to account for this phenomenon are discussed below.

Biophase distribution model

Drug distribution to the effect site may represent a rate-limiting step for drugs in exerting their pharmacological effect. Holford and Sheiner introduced a hypothetical effect–compartment, and proposed that a drug must first enter this effect compartment from either the central or the peripheral pharmacokinetic compartment before its pharmacological response is exerted.

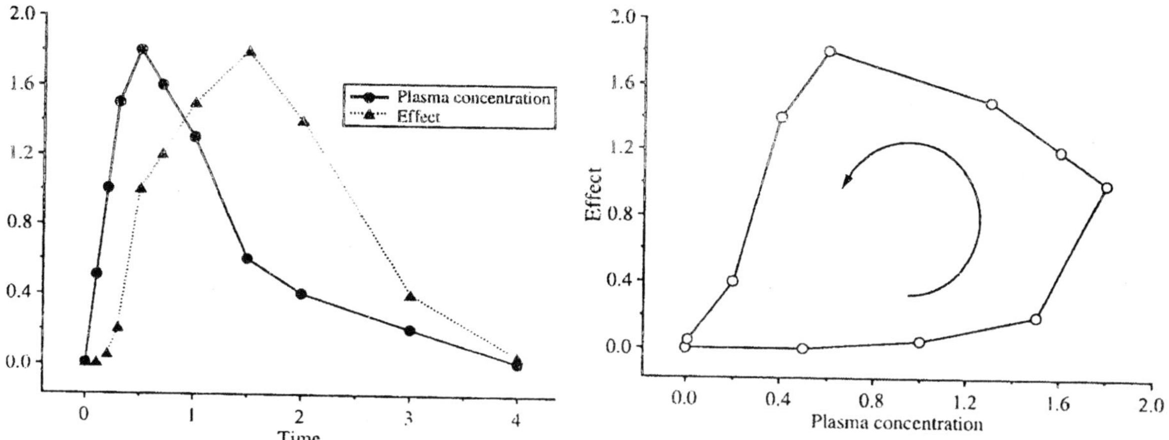

Fig. 9.5. Schematic presentation of delay between plasma concentration and effect resulting in counterclockwise hysteresis.

Additionally, the drug influx into the effect compartment (C_e) from the pharmacokinetic compartment (C_p) is assumed to follow a first-order process, but with negligible mass transfer as described below:

$$dC_e/dt = K_e * C_p - K_{e0} * Ce \quad \ldots(7)$$

where K_{le} and K_{e0} are the first-order distribution rate constants. Concentrations in the effect compartment are then directly related to response through an exposure–response model (e.g., linear or E_{max} model). The effect compartment model has been successfully used to characterize the PK/PD of several drugs, including pancuronium, midazolam, and alprazolam. In- depth reviews of the effect compartment model are readily available.

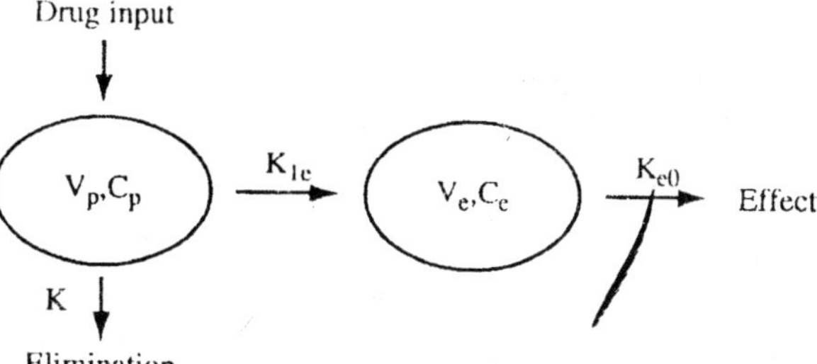

Fig. 9.6. Schematic presentation of biophase distribution model.

Mechanism-based indirect response model

Aside from the distribution process, temporal dissociation between the time courses of concentration and effect might also be caused by an indirect response mechanism. Indirect response modeling was first introduced by Nagashima et al. for the anticoagulant effect of warfarin. Dayneka et al. later proposed four basic models for indirect pharmacodynamic response. The indirect response model is based on the premise that the drug response is indirectly mediated by either inhibition or stimulation of the factors controlling either the production (K_{in}) or the dissipation of response (K_{out}).

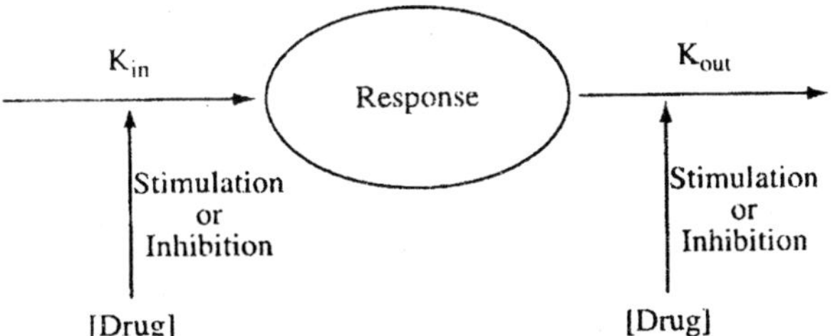

Fig. 9.7. Schematic presentation of indirect response model.

In the absence of drug, the rate of change in response over time (*dR/dt*) can be described by a differential equation as follows:

$$dR/dt = k_{in} - k_{out} * R \quad \ldots(8)$$

where k_{in} represents the zero-order constant for the production of response and k_{out} represents the first-order rate constant for the dissipation of response. Depending on whether k_{in} or k_{out} is either inhibited or stimulated by the drug, the following four basic models have been developed in which the drug effect is mediated by an E_{max}-like model:

$$dR/dt = k_{in} * I(t) - k_{out} * R \quad ...(9)$$

for the inhibition of k_{in}

$$dR/dt = k_{in} - k_{out} * I(t) * R \quad ...(10)$$

for the inhibition of k_{out}

$$dR/dt = k_{in} * S(t) - k_{out} * R \quad ...(11)$$

for the stimulation of k_{in}

$$dR/dt = k_{in} - k_{out} * S(t) * R \quad ...(12)$$

for the stimulation of k_{out}

where $S(t)$ and $I(t)$ denote stimulation and inhibitory functions, respectively, which can be described as Emax models.

Indirect response modeling has been used successfully to describe the pharmacodynamics of many drugs, especially in cases where endogenous mediators are involved in the expression of the observed response. These models may be appropriate for various classes of drugs, including histamine H2-receptor antagonists (such as cimetidine) that inhibit gastric acid secretion, and oral hypoglycemic agents (such as tolbutamide) that lower blood glucose level by stimulating insulin secretion.

Signal transduction model

The pharmacological effects of drugs may be mediated by a time-dependent signal transduction process, which involves multiple steps. Sun and Jusko proposed a signal transduction model to account for the delayed effect of pharmacodynamic responses. This model has been used to characterize the parasympathomimetic activity of scopolamine and atropine in rats.

Tolerance model

For some drugs, pharmacodynamic parameters like E_{max} and EC_{50} may appear to vary over time, resulting in changes in pharmacological response despite the presence of constant concentrations at the effect site. Tolerance is characterized by a reduction in pharmacological response after repeated or continuous drug exposure. The complex mechanism of tolerance may involve receptor pool depletion, decrease in receptor affinity, and up- or down-regulation.

The development of tolerance can have a significant impact on the exposure response relationship and, if not recognized, can contribute to poor clinical outcome. Pharmacokinetic/pharmacodynamic modeling can be a very useful tool to characterize the time course and magnitude of tolerance development. Jonkers et al. modeled the time course of hypokalema and β2-adrenoreptor agonist terbutaline concentrations and noted an increase in EC_{50} over time, which is likely attributed to a decrease in the receptor number in the presence of spare receptors. Mathot and Geus characterized the development of tolerance to the acid inhibitory effect of ranitidine. The derived model indicated that ranitidine developed tolerance with increased EC_{50} by 100% within 6–10 hr after prolonged IV administration.

Pharmacokinetic/pharmacodynamic modeling techniques

Pharmacokinetic/pharmacodynamic modeling is a complex, iterative process involving multiple steps. Once data are collected, exploratory graphic analyses of the raw data are usually carried out to (1) detect outliers; (2) explore distribution of variables; and (3) assess

correlation between variables for hidden structure and/or relationships. Subsequently, data are fitted to a selected mathematical model by optimizing an objective function that quantifies the variation between data and model. Once the parameter estimates associated with an optimal objective function are achieved, a number of diagnostic assessments have to be performed to ensure that the estimates are reasonable. Questionable diagnostic results may call for reevaluation of model assumptions, and/or investigation of alternative models. At last, model evaluation on the final model is performed to assess its goodness-of-fit, reliability, stability, and/or predictive performance.

Population PK/PD modeling has been accepted as a useful tool during drug development. One of the major objectives of population PK/PD modeling is the characterization of interindividual variability in PK/PD parameters. This includes the search for covariates such as patient weight, age, renal function, and disease status that may significantly contribute to interindividual variability, thereby affecting drug PK/PD relationship. The detection and quantification of covariate effects may influence the dosage regimen design.

A variety of methods have been proposed for the characterization of population PK/PD of drugs. The choice of method is generally dependent on the data type and the study objectives. The learning-oriented studies during the early phases of clinical development usually involve small homogenous groups of subjects, often consisting of healthy volunteers. In general, these studies are well controlled with extensive data taken from each subject, which allows the characterization of individual (PK/PD) profile. In contrast, confirmatory studies in the later phases of clinical development often involve large numbers of heterogenous patient populations. Study control is often difficult: usually multicenter trials involving outpatients. Furthermore, only a few samples can be taken per subject (sparse data), which does not allow the characterization of individual profile. Accordingly, PK/PD modeling technique is also shifted from traditional analysis of rich data sets in individuals to more sophisticated population analysis approach to handle the sparse, unbalanced, and fragmented data.

Two-stage approach

The standard two-stage approach can be used to estimate population model parameters. In the first stage, individual parameters are estimated for each subject. Using these estimates, in the second stage, population mean values and inter- individual variability of parameters are calculated. The obvious advantage of the standard two-stage approach is in its simplicity. However, this approach requires extensive sampling for each individual in order to estimate individual parameters. Further, it has been shown from simulation studies that the standard two- stage approach tends to overestimate parameter dispersion. Other modified two-stage approaches are available, including the global two-stage approach, the iterative two-stage approach, and the Bayesian two-stage approach.

Naive pooled approach

The naive pooled approach, proposed by Sheiner and Beal, involves pooling all the data from all individuals as if they were from a single individual to obtain population parameter estimates. Generally, the naïve pooled approach performs well in estimating population pharmacokinetic parameters from balanced pharmacokinetic data with small between-subject variations, but tends to confound individual differences and diverse sources of variability, and it generally performs poorly when dealing with imbalanced data. Additionally, caution is warranted when applying the naïve pooled approach for PD data analysis because it may produce a distorted picture of the exposure–response relationship and thereby could have safety implications when applied to the treatment of individual patients.

Hierarchical non-linear mixed-effects modeling

Unlike the traditional approaches mentioned above, which require data from extensive sampling, the hierarchical non-linear mixed-effects model approach can handle both sparse and intensive sampled data, making it a powerful tool to study PK/PD in special populations, such as neonates, the elderly, and AIDS patients, where the number of samples to be collected per subject is limited due to ethical and/or medical concerns. The hierarchical non-linear mixed-effects models analyze the data of all individuals at once, estimating individual and population parameters, as well as the interindividual, intraindividual residual, and interoccasion variabilities. It also allows the evaluation and quantification of potential sources of variability in pharmacokinetics and pharmacodynamics in the target population. For example, the influence of patient demographics (e.g., weight, gender, âge, etc.) and pathophysiological factors (e.g., hepatic function, renal function, disease status, etc.) on drug PK and PD disposition may be assessed through modeling. This information is very important for the design of dosing regimens and therapeutic drug monitoring.

The non-linear mixed effects model is the most widely used method and has proven to be very useful for continuous measures of drug effect, categorical response data, and survival-type data. The nonlinear mixed-effects modeling software (NONMEM) introduced by Sheiner and Beal is one of the most commonly used programs for population analysis. A detailed review of software for performing population PK/PD analysis is available.

Simulation

Pharmacokinetic/pharmacodynamic modeling is more than an analytical tool for characterizing the exposure– response relationship; it can also be used as a predictive tool for exploring the exposure–response relationship under various dose regimens, as well as for optimizing further clinical trial designs. Given the critical importance of efficient and informative clinical study design (e.g., number of dose levels, number of subjects, number of samples per subject, sampling times, number of subject per subpopulation, and distribution of covariates) during the drug development process, clinical trial simulation has emerged as an important extension of PK/PD-based simulations. It provides a way to integrate uncertainties into the design process by answering "what if'' question(s). To date, clinical trial simulation has been predominantly applied in Phase 2–Phase 4 clinical trials, but there has also been an increase in the application of this methodology in Phase 1 studies.

One key element involved in trial simulation is the simulation model development. In general, a simulation model consists of three components: a covariate distribution model, an input–output model, and a trial execution model. The covariate distribution model defines the expected distribution of demographic covariates (e.g., age, weight, gender, and renal function) in the target trial population. The input–output model incorporates scientific knowledge about the drug and disease collected during the preclinical and various clinical development phases. This may include the PK/PD model, the disease progression or placebo effect model, and the covariate model relating covariates to typical parameter values. A trial execution model describes any deviation in the simulated clinical trial design from the nominal clinical trial design due to uncontrollable factors during the execution of the study, such as patient dropouts, compliance, mistimed observation, and missing samples.

Once the models are defined, simulation can be carried out using a specific computer program that incorporates the study design parameters along with the simulation models. These virtual, in numero trials may be repeated many times to provide probability distributions for trial performance evaluations. By varying the trial design parameters and assumptions (e.g., study design, dosing regimen, and patient selection), stochastic simulations may reveal the impact of those parameters and assumptions on trial outcome and performance, and ultimately provide critical information that helps select a design best suited to meet the study objectives. The value of simulation in drug discovery and development has not only attracted the attention of the pharmaceutical industry, but also of the regulatory agencies. A consensus document is available to describe principles and good practice for modeling and simulation of clinical trials, covering the areas of planning, conduction, analysis, and reporting.

Applications of PK/PD Modeling and Simulations in Drug Development

The paradigm in drug development is sequentially divided into several phases starting with preclinical assessment. After selection of a drug candidate based on preclinical studies, clinical Phase 1 studies are initiated to characterize the safety, tolerability, biomarker, and pharmacokinetic profiles of the candidate, typically in healthy subjects. Phase 2 studies test the drug efficacy hypothesis in patients and explore dose range, and Phase 3 studies aim to demonstrate efficacy in the intended patient population in a statistically robust manner.

Historically, this well-established approach often relies on empirical decision-making, in which decisions are made in a semiquantitative manner based on the series of study results. As opposed to this, Sheiner has advocated a novel approach to clinical trial design that incorporates two successive "learning–confirming" cycles. He describes the drug development as an information gathering process. The first cycle addresses the question of whether therapeutic benefit can be reasonably expected with the candidate. It comprises of learning safety, tolerability, and pharmacokinetic profile of the candidate and confirming that the candidate has some desired, measurable pharmacological response at a tolerable dose. A confirmative answer in the first cycle provides the justification for a larger second learning–confirming cycle. The learning step of the second cycle aims at learning what is an appropriate drug regimen to achieve acceptable benefit/risk ratio, whereas the confirming step aims at demonstrating acceptable benefit/risk in a statistically robust manner.

Pharmacokinetic/pharmacodynamic modeling and simulation are vital tools in applying this learning-confirming approach in drug development. The following sections describe how PK/PD modeling and simulation can be applied in each stage of drug development. In addition, an example using docetaxel is provided to illustrate how these approaches can be prospectively utilized throughout the entire drug development process for one particular candidate.

Preclinical Phase

The incredible advances in discovery technology and lead optimization over the past few years have enabled the industry to generate more compounds than ever to be tested in clinical investigations. With this rush of new compounds for evaluation, PK/PD modeling and simulation touch various aspects of the preclinical phase of drug development.

One of the major benefits that PK/PD modeling can offer in the preclinical phase of drug development is assisting with the identification of potential surrogates or biomarkers for a particular mechanism of action. This can expedite the decision-making steps to get to the clinical phase, and also allow an early read on the drug candidate's performance in the clinical phases of drug development, especially when clinical effects of a new drug are not easily measurable or are slow to develop. One good example of this is the identification and utilization of C_{max}/MIC or AUC_{24}/MIC as an efficacy surrogate of fluoroquinolone antibiotics.

Pharmacokinetic/pharmacodynamic modeling can also assist in identification of the appropriate animal model in which to evaluate the mechanism of action. Cox and his colleagues have developed a tooth pulp evoked potential (TPEP) rat model in order to investigate the analgesic effects of opioid drugs. The authors utilized a population sigmoidal E_{max} pharmacodynamic model to characterize the relationship between alfentanil exposure and TPEP effect in rats that resulted in similar PD parameter estimates as previously observed in humans. Therefore, the TPEP rat model was identified as an appropriate animal model to develop future analgesics.

Development of mechanism-based PK/PD models for efficacy and toxicity early in the drug development process is very useful and preferred over the development of empirical models. Unlike empirical models, mechanism-based PK/PD models take into account the physiological processes behind the observed pharmacological response, likely making it more "*predictive*" for future study outcome. For example, Zuideveld and his colleagues successfully developed and evaluated a semimechanistic set-point model in rats for the characterization of 5-HT1A receptor agonists such as R- and S-8-OH-DPAT, buspirone and its metabolite, flexinoxan, WAY-100,635, and WAY-100,135, using the hypothermic effect as a PD marker. Later, the investigators further developed this semimechanistic model into a full mechanistic model by replacing the empirical Hill equation portion of the model with the operational model of agonism. The Hill equation has only limited applicability as a model to predict the expression of agonism, because the parameters from this empirical equation depend on both "*drug-specific*" and "*system-related*" properties, complicating the extrapolation and prediction from in vitro to in vivo systems. With a fully mechanistic model, Zuideveld was better able to predict the in vivo affinity and efficacy of 5-HT1A receptor agonists from in vitro receptor binding assay.

Understanding and developing the PK/PD relationship early in the discovery stage can also provide a quantitative way of selecting the best candidate. In the anticancer area, a typical way of selecting the most potent candidate within a series of anticancer drug candidates is to measure tumor volumes from in vivo evaluation of the antitumor effect. Simeoni et al. points out how this approach utilizes only partial information by neglecting the time course of the tumor growth and the selection is limited to a series of compounds using the same dosing regimen. The authors emphasize the use of a PK/PD model to link the dosing regimen of a candidate and tumor growth dynamics in developing a signal transduction model. This model predicted the tumor response from different dosing regimens of different test compounds providing the quantitative evidence to support the compound selection as well as the dosing selection in future trials.

Furthermore, for initial dose selection and the subsequent escalation scheme in Phase 1 studies, there are many examples in which PK/PD models enabled the successful extrapolation of preclinical results in order to predict the effective and toxicologic drug concentrations for clinical investigations. Gomeni and his colleagues discuss one emerging technology called computer-assisted drug development (CADD), which integrates mathematical modeling and simulation from preclinical data to design clinical trials. Illustrating how clinical trials can be rationally and informatively designed, the specific examples they list resulted in the recommendation of a dose range of 1–60 mg in the first-in-human study and a dose regimen of 30–60 mg once a day for a week for the proof of concept study of a new CNS compound based on a collection of preclinical data and simulation, including in vitro receptor affinity in rhesus monkey, projected human and rhesus monkey PK parameters using allometric scaling, PK/PD modeling results from rodents, a positron-emission tomography study in rhesus monkey, and PD simulation. In another example, the use of PK/PD modeling from a conscious dog model predicted a better safety/efficacy profile of fiduxosin in human as a new α1-adrenoceptor antagonist for the treatment of benign prostatic hyperplasia (BPH). When fiduxosin's potency was compared to that of three other α_1-adrenoceptor antagonists, terazosin, doxazosin, and tamsulosin using IC_{50} values from the sigmoidal E_{max} model of intraurethral pressure (IUP) and mean arterial pressure, the findings showed that fiduxosin could effectively treat BPH in human with reduced cardiovascular side effects. Last, PK/PD modeling has been successfully applied in assessing and predicting drug–drug interaction potential as well as formulation development.

Phase 1

The major objectives of Phase 1 studies are to determine the PK profile, investigate the initial safety and tolerability, and assess the PD or biomarker response of the drug candidate that may provide an early read of activity/efficacy. Typically, Phase 1 starts with dose- escalating studies in normal volunteers with rigorous sampling. In addition, one may establish an initial dose–concentration–effect relationship that offers the opportunity to predict and assess drug tolerance and safety in early clinical development. Based on the nature of studies that are conducted in Phase 1, this is generally categorized as a learning phase of drug development, but it can also be a confirming phase for predictions that were made in the preclinical phase, especially with regard to PK. The knowledge gained in this phase can be communicated back to the preclinical phase in order to facilitate a more informed selection of the next generation of drug candidates.

Phase 1 trials, as early as the first-in-human study, can be viewed as a critical point for assessing the therapeutic effectiveness of a drug and deciding whether to invest further in the development process. Parasrampuria and colleagues demonstrated how the first-in-human study of RWJ 67657, a p38 mitogen-activated protein kinase inhibitor in potential treatment of arthritis and Crohn's disease, was utilized to garner a preliminary assessment of the potential efficacy of a novel drug from PD measurement.

Further results were used to guide dose selection for future trials via a PK/PD modeling. This example also utilized biomarkers—cytokines—as PD measurements for an early read on the therapeutic benefit in a diseased area that is mediated by these cytokines. Zannikos and colleagues illustrated how the application of PK/PD modeling in a Phase 1 study can identify issues or concerns, besides the potential efficacy, that should he considered for further drug development. Their Phase 1 study evaluated the PK of ARA, an adenosine receptor agonist as well as the mean percent change in plasma free fatty acid (FFA), and led to the development of an E_{max}-based tolerance model. This exercise demonstrated that ARA, which is able to reduce circulating levels of FFA, should be examined more carefully for potential desensitization of adenosine receptor-mediated inhibition of lipolysis in human before pursuing further development as an antilipolytic agent.

Additionally, quantitative dose–concentration–effect relationships generated from PK/PD modeling in Phase 1 can be utilized in Phase 2 study design. Bouillon et al. described their work on propofol, which is commonly used for anesthesia and conscious sedation in spontaneously breathing patients. An informative study design in healthy volunteers enabled the authors to investigate the ventilatory depression induced by propofol. Using the indirect response model, the authors identified the optimal propofol dosage regimen to reduce the risk of significant ventilatory depression for future clinical trials. Bos et al. presented another example of a population PK analysis of Phase 1 study data that was used to derive the optimal sampling strategy for estimating the PK parameters most accurately in future Phase 2 trials for a novel anthracycline analog. This effort not only reduced the costs of determining drug concentrations, but also reduced the inconvenience for patients and staff.

Pharmacokinetic/pharmacodynamic modeling can also help explain or predict the clinical outcome respective to gender differences or special populations such as the renally or hepatically impaired. A PK/PD study of morphine-6-glucuronide (M6G), a metabolite of morphine and a μ-opioid agonist, conducted in healthy volunteers, addressed the effect of gender and renal impairment on M6G-induced analgesia via modeling and simulation, respectively. Previous animal and human studies have reported the existence of gender differences in opioid-induced analgesia. This study, using PK/PD modeling, showed that M6G formation from morphine was independent of gender, and that gender differences observed in morphine analgesic or respiratory effect, therefore, were not related to the metabolism of morphine. Through the simulation, the investigators also showed that the influence of impaired renal clearance was significant on M6G concentration, thus affecting its analgesic contribution after morphine administration.

Pharmacokinetic/pharmacodynamic modeling is an important tool in assessing drug–drug interaction potential. Sale, Sadler and Stein described how NONMEM analysis and Monte Carlo simulation, based on data from previous PK drug interaction studies, were used to predict amprenavir concentrations for different dosing regimen combinations of amprenavir and ritonavir. Mertens et al. assessed the influence of alfentanil on propofol pharmacokinetics using mixed-effects modeling and simulations, showing that heart rate is an important parameter in determining the PK of propofol. In both studies, the failure to demonstrate efficacy in a certain regimen combination was explained by simulation based on the PK or the identification of important parameters that impacted the PK of combined drug yet are beyond the scope of a typical PK interaction study.

Dosage form improvements often occur based on the PK properties of the drug candidate. Hoffman and his colleagues, however, emphasized the importance of considering PK, PD, and the PK/PD relationship in dosage form preparation. As an example candidate, they chose amoxicillin, a beta-lactam antibiotic, and showed how a review of the PK/PD relationship helped optimize the dosing regimen by prolonging the "time over MIC × 4," a clinically relevant parameter. Lotsch and colleagues performed population PK and PK/PD modeling to explain the advantage of fast onset formulation of diclofenac over the conventional tablet for treatment of acute mild to moderate pain. The highly variable PK of the tablet form, with a short delay between the PK and PD effects, guided the program to recommend the fast release formulation for its better predictability with fast onset of therapeutic effect, which is especially important for a pain medication.

Phase 2

Phase 2 trials are typically divided into two stages, each with some specific objectives. The major objective of the first stage, Phase 2A, is to test the efficacy hypothesis of a drug candidate, demonstrating the proof of concept. This stage ends the first learning-comfirming cycle according to Sheiner. The confirmed positive output from this stage gives a justification for the drug candidate to advance to the next cycle starting with Phase 2B.

One of the major objectives of Phase 2B is to develop the concentration–response relationship in efficacy and safety by exploring a large range of doses in the target patient population. The PK/PD relationship that has evolved from the preclinical phase up to Phase 2B is used to assist in designing the Phase 3 trial.

Magner et al., using PK/PD modeling, identified some important parameters that contribute to the intersubject variability observed in glycoprotein IIb/IIa antagonist abciximab, a narrow therapeutic index drug. They developed an integrated PK/PD model based on the principles of target-mediated drug disposition, successfully describing the free plasma abciximab concentrations and ex vivo pharmacodynamics collected from patients undergoing percutaneous transluminal coronary angioplasty. More specifically, the final model predicted that maximum receptor density and drug sensitivity were important parameters that may contribute to intersubject variability. This information adds value to future clinical trial design and optimizing the dose individualization. Cox et al. described the population PK and PK/PD modeling of argatroban in combination with a platelet glycoprotein IIb/IIIa receptor antagonist in patients undergoing percutaneous coronary intervention. The population PK parameters of argatroban in the patients were comparable with the values reported from a previous healthy volunteer study, but the relationship between argatroban concentration and its effect, activating clotting time, was best described by a sigmoidal E_{max} model, while the relationship in healthy volunteers, as previously reported, was linear. This is a good example of how modeling can help update the information for a drug in development, as data in the target patient population are added to that from healthy subjects.

Burger and his colleagues have illustrated an example of bridging different populations with PK/PD modeling to assess the dose adjustment need. They compared the PK/PD relationships of indinavir, a human immunodeficiency virus protease inhibitor, with or without ritonavir, in HIV-infected Thai patients to those in Caucasian patients, and recommended no dose adjustment despite the general lower body weight in the Thai population.

As an example of establishing a concentration– response relationship in Phase 2 studies, Pillai and his colleagues utilized a "*kinetics of drug action*" model and simulation to recommend a novel intermittent oral and IV ibandronate regimen for the treatment of osteoporosis. The model characterized the relationship between an ibandronate dose and the change of μCTX, a sensitive biomarker of bone turnover, as a PD response, and adequately described the time-course of μCTX change. In that paper, utility of biomarkers was demonstrated when clinical outcome is slow to come.

Although clinical trial simulation efforts can start as early as the discovery stage with in vitro and preclinical data, simulating the confirmatory phase of a program—Phase 3 trials based on data accumulated from all of the previous learning phases, discovery, Phase 1, and Phase 2 trials—can often answer some important questions in optimizing study design even more efficiently, such as questions regarding adjustment of drug dosage for patient subgroups, optimal administration regimen, need for a new formulation, and effect of inclusion/exclusion criteria. Pfister and colleagues utilized PK/PD modeling and simulation for a vasopeptidase inhibitor, which inhibits both angiotensin-converting enzyme and neutral endopeptidase 24.11, using combined Phase 1 and Phase 2 data to give guidance on dose regimen for future clinical trials. In this exercise, they also utilized biomarkers such as plasma ACE activity, plasma rennin activity, angiotensin II/ angiotensin I ratio, bradykinin, urine ANP, and cGMP as the PD responses, making this study another good example of utilizing biomarkers to make decisions in drug development where the measurement of clinical outcome might be difficult or inconvenient (in this case, hypertension, heart failure, and renoprotection). In another example, Lockwood et al. used clinical trial simulation to evaluate the distribution of outcome from two Phase 2 trials with pregabalin, a GABA-agonist for the treatment of neuropathic pain, and used the simulation results to select the appropriate dose for Phase 3 trials. Work by Drusano et al. also described how population PK modeling of three different doses of GW 420867X, a new non-nucleoside reverse transcriptase inhibitor, and Monte Carlo simulation based on the results of the population PK modeling helped choose a rational dose for further clinical trials.

Phase 3

The major objective of Phase 3 studies is to provide confirmatory evidence that demonstrates an acceptable benefit/risk in a large target patient population. This period provides the ideal condition for final characterization of the PK/PD in patients as well as for explaining the sources of interindividual variability in response, using population PK/PD approaches.

In order to understand the factors leading to pharmacokinetic and pharmacodynamic variability that impinge upon drug safety and efficacy, it is critical to establish comprehensive patient profiles in Phase 3 studies. The study populations should be representative of the target patient population with respect to demographics (such as gender, age, and weight), environmental, and pathophysiological characteristics. The final outcome of the PK/PD message provides supportive evidence of efficacy and safety, as well as dosing information for drug labeling.

Prior to launching large expensive Phase 3 clinical trials, the drug development team must select the best dose(s) and regimen(s) for evaluation in Phase 3. In many cases, the best dose is not the dose that gives the maximal beneficial effect. Safety must also be considered. The net benefit to the patient is the beneficial response minus the adverse response, in other words, the benefit to risk ratio. It is critical to investigate the best compromise between efficacy and safety when facing dose selection decisions for Phase 3 trials. Chabaud et al. provided an example of how PK/PD modeling and simulation can be utilized in choosing the best regimen for a future Phase 3 trial of a bradycardic agent with a potential indication in stable angina pectoris. The authors conducted Monte Carlo simulations using a PK/PD model as well as a physiopathologic mechanistic model developed based on Phase 1 data and literature references. The findings from this model development and simulation process permitted the prospective evaluation of dosing regimens, and the number of patients to include in future clinical trial and resulted in a conclusion that a daily dose of 20 mg could be used safely and efficiently in a future Phase 3 trial, and that it is necessary to include 200 patients per group in order to meet the therapeutic target.

Aside from providing supportive evidence of efficacy and safety, PK/PD modeling also provides dosing information for drug labeling. Based on population PK/PD modeling, Minto, Schnider and Shafer identified age and lean body mass as significant covariates for the clearance of short-acting opiod remifentanil, and developed a formula to relate remifentanil clearance to age and body weight. For clinicians' convenience, this relationship could be translated into a nomogram for dose individualization. Based on this PK/PD model, the authors conducted a series of simulations and concluded that bolus doses should be halved and the infusion rate decreased to one-third in the elderly as compared to young patients.

Selecting a clinical trial design is a rather complex task. Gieschke, Reigner and Steimer presented an example of how simulation can be used to improve decision-making in drug clinical development. The authors applied PK/PD-based simulation for an oral anticancer agent to determine the optimal study design and to evaluate the consequences of dose adaptation rules on efficacy and adverse events. The findings of this simulation predicted that both continuous and intermittent dosage regimens lead to comparable efficacy, whereas continuous treatment is likely to cause a greater risk of adverse effects. Accordingly, only an intermittent dosage regimen was considered for future study.

NDA Review and Postmarketing Phase

The application of PK/PD modeling can be beneficial during the life cycle of a drug; namely, during the preparation and review of regulatory documents for New Drug Application (NDA) submission, and during post marketing surveillance.

Pharmacokinetic/pharmacodynamic modeling plays an important role during the NDA submission and review phase by integrating information from the pre-clinical and development phases. Existence of a well- defined PK/PD model furthermore enables the reviewer to perform PK/PD simulations for various scenarios. This ability helps the reviewer gain a deeper understanding of the compound and provides a quantitative basis for dose selection. Thus, PK/PD modeling can facilitate the NDA review process and help resolve regulatory issues.

In addition to meeting current regulatory requirements, as a postmarketing strategy, population modeling approaches can provide the clinician with relevant information regarding dose individualization by characterizing the variability associated with PK and PD and by identifying subpopulations with special needs, thus leading to safer and more efficacious drug use. The concept of one dose fits all is an ideal but rarely attainable goal. The same dose administered to a variety of patients is likely to produce a range of responses due to interpatient, intrapatient, and interoccasion variability. The development of a population PK/PD model permits the application of a Bayesian feedback approach to obtain improved estimates of individual PK/PD parameters in the light of observed response via therapeutic drug monitoring. This Bayesian adaptive control approach is especially useful for drugs used for life- threatening diseases with a proven PK/PD relationship, a narrow therapeutic index, or large interpatient variability. For example, the use of the population approach has been advocated for antibiotic dose regimen individualization.

Docetaxel Example

The clinical development of antineoplastic agent, docetaxel (Taxotere) provides an excellent example of how modeling and simulation approach can be implemented prospectively in the clinical development and play a key role in developing the dosing recommendation for labeling. Throughout the various phases of docetaxel clinical development, PK/PD modeling and simulation were used to optimize the design of the subsequent studies and to derive relevant information from the collected data. Based on the data from Phase 1 studies, a preliminary population PK model of docetaxel was developed and used to design a sparse sampling strategy for Phase 2 studies. This sampling design, which involved four randomized sampling schedules, was then prospectively implemented in 24 Phase 2 studies. The influence of covariates on PK variability was studied in a large number of patients. Subsequent PK/PD analyses, performed using the individual Bayesian PK parameter estimates derived from the developed model showed that base-line levels of alpha-1-acid glycoprotein (AAG) were inversely correlated with clinical response and that patients with a higher baseline AAG had a shorter survival. Subsequently, trial simulations for Phase 3 studies were performed to assess whether patients with high AAG would benefit from a higher dose. The simulations showed that survival was somewhat longer in the higher-dose treatment arm, but the difference was only significant in 6 out of 100 simulated trials. Thus, higher doses were no further studied in the high-AAG population. This exemplified the use of simulations for dose optimization. Moreover, PK/PD analyses demonstrated that the variability in clearance was a significant predictor of several safety end points. A subset of patients with clinical chemistry suggestive of liver impairment (SGOT and/or SGPT $>1.5 \times$ ULN concomitant with alkaline phosphatase $>2.5 \times$ ULN) had a reduced docetaxil clearance, which resulted in an increased risk of febrile neutropenia.

Last, the findings of these PK/PD analyses were fully integrated into the regulatory documents and resulted in the following label information for docetaxel worldwide. In the European "Summary of Product Characteristics" under the heading "Special Population," it states: "Patients with liver impairment: Based on pharmacokinetic data, in patients who have both elevations of transaminases values (ALT and/or AST) greater than 1.5 times the upper limit of the normal range (ULN) and increases in alkaline phosphatase greater than 2.5 times the ULN, the recommended dose of docetaxel is 75 mg/m^2." The recommended dose is 100 mg/m2 in patients with normal liver functions.

Today, a PK/PD modeling and simulation approach in drug development has increasingly gained recognition by the pharmaceutical industry, regulatory agencies, and academic institutions, as a valuable tool to stream-line the drug development process. Application of PK/PD modeling in the preclinical stage allows a better understanding of the mechanism and intrinsic potency of drug candidates, providing an opportunity for candidate selection in a quantitative manner, as well as facilitating successful extrapolation of preclinical results to clinical investigations. In clinical drug development, PK/PD modeling and simulation can potentially impact both internal and regulatory decisions in drug development. PK/PD analyses on the data from Phase 1 studies assist in characterizing PK, safety, and tolerability of the drug candidate and provide information for the rational design of all subsequent clinical trials. In Phases 2 and 3, population PK/PD modeling and simulation are frequently applied to assess the concentration–response relationship in the target patient population, identify and quantify the sources of interindividual variabilities in PK and PD, and optimize the clinical trial design. The information from these modeling and simulation efforts can influence the final labeling decisions, as well as dose individualization for optimal therapeutic outcome to balance risk/benefit. In summary, PK/PD modeling and simulations are valuable tools that can improve decision-making at all stages of drug development, thereby contributing to a more efficient drug development process.

10

Drug Administration and Elimination

Pharmacokinetics is the study of the way that the body deals with pharmacologic compounds. In other words, what does the body do to the drug? This includes the manner in which the drug is administered, absorbed, distributed, and eventually eliminated from the body. These topics are discussed in this chapter and the next.

Routes of Administration

In general, drugs can be administered via two primary routes: through the alimentary canal (*enteral administration*) or through nonalimentary routes (*parenteral administration*). Each major route has several variations, and each offers distinct advantages and disadvantages. The primary features of some of the major routes are discussed here.

Enteral

Oral

The primary way that drugs are given enterally is through the oral route. This is the most common method of administering medications and offers several distinct advantages. Oral administration is the easiest method of taking medications, especially when self-administration is necessary or desired. The oral route is also relatively safe because drugs enter the system in a fairly controlled manner. This avoids the large, sudden increase in plasma drug levels, which can occur when the drug is administered by other methods such as through intravenous injection. Most medications that are administered orally are absorbed from the small intestine, thus utilizing the large surface area of the intestinal microvilli to enhance its entry into the body.

Several disadvantages may preclude drugs from being given orally. Drugs that are administered by mouth must have a relatively high degree of lipid solubility in order to pass through the gastrointestinal mucosa and into the bloodstream. Large, nonlipid-soluble compounds are absorbed very poorly from the alimentary canal and will eventually be lost from the body in the feces. Absorption of some nonlipid-soluble substances (peptides, small proteins) can be enhanced to some extent by encapsulating these agents in lipid vesicles (liposomes); this technique was recently developed to enable the oral administration of drugs that were formerly administered only through injection or some other parenteral route. Other drawbacks to the oral route include the fact that certain medications may irritate the stomach and cause discomfort, vomiting, or even damage to the gastric mucosa. The acidic environment and presence of digestive proteases in the stomach may also cause various compounds to be degraded and destroyed prior to absorption from the gastrointestinal tract. Drugs that are given orally are subject to a phenomenon known as the *first-pass effect*. After absorption from the alimentary canal, the drug is transported directly into the liver via the portal vein, where a significant amount of the drug may be metabolized and destroyed prior to reaching its site of action. The dosage of the orally administered drug must be sufficient enough to allow an adequate amount of the compound to survive hepatic degradation and to eventually reach the target tissue. Some drugs—such as nitroglycerin—undergo such extensive inactivation from the first-pass effect that it is usually preferable to administer them through nonoral routes.

A final limitation of the oral route is that the amount and rate at which the drug eventually reaches the bloodstream tends to be somewhat less predictable with oral administration compared with more direct routes, such as injection. Factors that affect intestinal absorption (intestinal infection, presence of food, rate of gastric emptying, amount of visceral blood flow, and so on) can alter the usual manner in which a drug is absorbed into the body from the gastrointestinal tract.

Sublingual and buccal

Drugs are administered sublingually by placing the drug under the tongue. Buccal administration occurs when the drug is placed between the cheek and gums. A drug that is administered sublingually or buccally is then absorbed through the oral mucosa into the venous system that is draining the mouth region. These veins eventually carry blood to the superior vena cava, which in turn carries blood to the heart. Consequently, a drug administered sublingually or buccally can reach the systemic circulation without being subjected to first-pass inactivation in the liver. This provides an obvious advantage for drugs such as nitroglycerin that would be destroyed in the liver when absorbed from the stomach or intestines. These routes also offer a means of enteral administration to people who have difficulty swallowing or to patients who cannot be given drugs rectally. The restrictions of the sublingual and buccal routes are that the amount of drug that can be administered is somewhat limited, and the drug must be able to pass easily through the oral mucosa in order to reach the venous drainage of the mouth.

Rectal

A final method of enteral administration is via the rectum. Many drugs are available as rectal suppositories to allow administration through this route. This method is less favorable because many drugs are absorbed poorly or incompletely, and irritation of the rectal mucosa may occur. Rectal administration does offer the advantage of allowing drugs to be given to a patient who is unconscious, or when vomiting prevents drugs from being taken orally. However, the rectal route is used most often for treating local conditions such as hemorrhoids.

Parenteral

All methods of drug administration that do not use the gastrointestinal tract are termed *parenteral*. Parenteral administration generally allows the drug to be delivered to the target site more directly, and the quantity of the drug that actually reaches the target site is often more predictable. Also, drugs given parenterally are not usually subject to first-pass inactivation in the liver. Other advantages and disadvantages of various par- enteral routes are discussed further on in this section.

Inhalation

Drugs that exist in a gaseous or volatile state, or that can be suspended as tiny droplets in an aerosol form, may be given via inhalation. Pulmonary administration is advantageous because of the large (alveolar) surface area for diffusion of the drug into the pulmonary circulation and it is generally associated with rapid entry of the drug into the bloodstream. This method is used extensively in administering the volatile general anesthetics (e.g., halothane) and it is also advantageous when applying medications directly to the bronchial and alveolar tissues for the treatment of specific pulmonary pathologies. The pulmonary route may also be a potential way to administer larger nonlipid-soluble agents such as peptides, small proteins (including insulin), and DNA.

One limitation of the inhalation route is that the drug must not irritate the alveoli or other areas of the respiratory tract. Also, some patients have trouble administering drugs by this route, and drug particles tend to be trapped by cilia and mucus in the respiratory tract. Both of these factors tend to limit the ability to predict exactly how much of the drug eventually reaches the lungs. Efforts continue to advance the use of inhaled drugs by improving the physicochemical properties of these drugs, and also by improving the devices used to deliver these drugs (i.e., inhalers). Technological advancements in inhaled drugs will be addressed in more detail when respiratory medications are addressed later in this text.

Injection

Various types of injection can be used to introduce the drug either systemically or locally. If sterility is not maintained, all types of injection have the disadvantage of possible infection, and certain types of injection are more difficult; if not impossible, for the patient to self-administer. Specific types of injection include the following routes.

Intra-venous

The bolus injection of a medication into a peripheral vein allows an accurate, known quantity of the drug to be introduced into the bloodstream over a short period of time, frequently resulting in peak levels of the drug appearing almost instantaneously in the peripheral circulation and thus reaching the target site rapidly. This occurrence is advantageous in emergency situations when it is necessary for the medication to exert an immediate effect. Of course, adverse reactions may also occur because of the sudden appearance of large titers of the drug in the plasma. Any unexpected side effects or miscalculations in the amount of the administered drug are often difficult to deal with after the full dose has been injected. In certain situations, an indwelling intravenous cannula (IV "line") can be used to allow the prolonged, steady infusion of a drug into the venous system. This method prevents large fluctuations in the plasma concentration of the drug and allows the dosage of drug to be maintained at a specific level for as long as desired.

Intra-arterial

The injection of a drug directly into an artery is understandably a difficult and dangerous procedure. This method permits a large dose of the medication to reach a given site, such as a specific organ, and may be used to focus the administration of drugs into certain tissues. Intra-arterial injections are used occasionally in cancer chemotherapy to administer the anticancer drug directly to the tumor site with minimal exposure of the drug to other healthy tissues. This route may also be used to focus the administration of other substances such as radiopaque dyes for various diagnostic procedures.

Subcutaneous

Injecting medications directly beneath the skin is used when a local response is desired, such as in certain situations requiring local anesthesia. Also, a slower, more prolonged release of the medication into the systemic circulation can be achieved in situations where this is the desired effect. A primary example is insulin injection in a patient with diabetes mellitus. Subcutaneous administration provides a relatively easy route of parenteral injection that can be performed by patients themselves, providing they are properly trained.

Some limitations are that the amount of drug that can be injected in this fashion is fairly small and that the injected drug must not irritate or inflame the subcutaneous tissues. The subcutaneous route can also be used when certain types of drug preparations are implanted surgically beneath the skin, so that the drug is slowly dispersed from the implanted preparation and then absorbed into the bloodstream for prolonged periods of time. A common example of this form of subcutaneous administration is the use of implanted hormonal contraceptive products (e.g., Norplant).

Intra-muscular

The large quantity of skeletal muscle in the body allows this route to be an easily accessible site for parenteral administration. Intramuscular injections can be used to treat a problem located directly in the injected muscle. For example, botulinum toxin and other substances can be injected directly into hyperexcitable muscles to control certain types of muscle spasms or spasticity. Alternatively, intramuscular injection can be used as a method for a relatively steady, prolonged release of the drug into the systemic circulation to control conditions such as psychosis, or to administer certain vaccines.

Intramuscular injection offers the advantage of providing a relatively rapid effect (i.e., within a few minutes), while avoiding the sudden, large increase in plasma levels seen with intravenous injection. The major problem with intramuscular administration is that many drugs injected directly into a muscle cause significant amounts of local pain and prolonged soreness, tending to limit the use of this route for repeated injections.

Intrathecal

Intrathecal injections are given by injecting the medication within a sheath, and frequently refer to injections within the spinal subarachnoid space (i.e., the space between the arachnoid membrane and the pia mater that help form the meninges surrounding the spinal cord). This particular type of intrathecal route allows drugs such as narcotic analgesics, local anesthetics, and antispasticity drugs to be applied directly to an area adjacent to the spinal cord, thereby allowing these drugs to gain better access to the cord. Also, intrathecal injections allow certain drugs—such as antibiotics and anticancer drugs—to bypass the blood-brain barrier and reach the central nervous system. Other intrathecal injections include administration of the drug within a tendon sheath or bursa, which may be used to treat a local condition such as an inflammation within those structures.

Topical

Drugs given topically are applied to the surface of the skin or mucous membranes. Most medications applied directly to the skin are absorbed fairly poorly through the epidermis and into the systemic circulation and are used primarily to treat problems that exist on the skin itself. Common examples of topical administration include the use of antibiotics to treat cutaneous infections, application of anti-inflammatory steroids to reduce skin inflammation, and the use of various topical products to promote wound healing. Topical application to mucous membranes is also used frequently to treat problems on the membrane itself. Significant amounts of the drug, however, can be readily absorbed through the mucous membrane and into the bloodstream. Topical application of drugs to mucous membranes can therefore provide a fairly easy and convenient way to administer drugs systemically. Certain medications, for example, can be administered to the nasal mucosa (via nasal spray), to the occular membranes (via eye drops), or to other mucous membranes to facilitate systemic absorption and treat disorders throughout the body. Nonetheless, the potential for adverse systemic effects must also be considered if large amounts of topically administered drugs are absorbed inadvertently into the body.

Transdermal

Unlike topical administration, transdermal application consists of applying drugs directly to the surface of the skin with the intent that they will be absorbed through the dermal layers and into either the subcutaneous tissues or the peripheral circulation. A transdermally administered drug must possess two basic properties: (1) it must be able to penetrate the skin, and (2) it must not be degraded to any major extent by drug-metabolizing enzymes located in the dermis. Absorption may be enhanced by mixing the drug in an oily base or in some other chemical enhancer, thus increasing solubility and permeability through the dermis. Transdermal administration provides a slow, controlled release of the drug into the body that is effective in maintaining plasma levels of the drug at a relatively constant level for prolonged periods of time. Drugs that can be administered transdermally are often delivered through medicated "*patches*" that can be adhered to the skin much like a small adhesive bandage. This method has been used for some time to allow the prolonged administration of drugs such as nitroglycerin and some antimotion sickness medications such as scopolamine. The use of transdermal patches has been expanded recently to include other medications such as hormonal agents (estrogen, testosterone) and opioid analgesics (fentanyl). Likewise, transdermal nicotine patches have received a great deal of attention for their use in helping people to quit smoking cigarettes. Researchers continue to explore the use of the transdermal route, and the use of transdermal patches continues to gain acceptance as a safe and effective method of administering many medications.

The transdermal route also includes the use of iontophoresis and phonophoresis to administer the drug. In iontophoresis, electric current is used to "drive" the ionized form of the medication through the skin. Phonophoresis uses ultrasound waves to enhance transmission of the medication through the dermis. Both phonophoresis and iontophoresis are often used to treat pain and inflammation by transmitting specific medications to a subcutaneous tissue such as a muscle, tendon, or bursa. These forms of transdermal administration are important in a rehabilitation setting since they are often administered by a physical therapist following a prescription written by a physician. Specific medications that can be administered via iontophoresis or phonophoresis are listed in Appendix A. For a more detailed description of how these transdermal routes are employed, the reader is referred to several additional sources.

Drug Absorption and Distribution: Bioavailability

Although several routes exist for the administration of drugs, merely introducing the drug into the body does not ensure that the compound will reach all tissues uniformly or that the drug will even reach the appropriate target site. For instance, oral administration of a drug that affects the myocardium will not have any pharmacologic effect unless the drug is absorbed from the gastrointestinal tract into the bloodstream. The extent to which the drug reaches the systemic circulation is referred to as *bioavailability*, which is a parameter expressed as the percentage of the drug administered that reaches the bloodstream. For instance, if 100 g of a drug is given orally, and 50 g eventually make it into the systemic circulation, the drug is said to be 50 percent bioavailable. If 100 g of the same compound were injected intravenously, the drug would be 100 percent bioavailable by that route.

Consequently, bioavailability depends on the route of administration as well as the drug's ability to cross membrane barriers. Once in the systemic circulation, further distribution into peripheral tissues may also be important in allowing the drug to reach the target site. Many drugs must eventually leave the systemic capillaries and enter other cells. Thus, drugs have to move across cell membranes and tissue barriers to get into the body and be distributed within the body. In this section, the ability of these membranes to affect absorption and distribution of drugs is discussed.

Membrane Structure and Function

Throughout the body, biologic membranes act as barriers that permit some substances to pass freely, while others pass through with difficulty or not at all. This differential separation serves an obvious protective effect by not allowing certain substances to enter the body or by limiting the distribution of the substance within the body. In effect, the body is separated into various "compartments" by these membranes. In the case of pharmacotherapeutics, there is often the need for the drug to cross one or more of these membrane barriers to reach the target site.

The ability of the membrane to act as a selective barrier is related to the membrane's normal structure and physiologic function. The cell membrane is composed primarily of lipids and proteins. Membrane lipids are actually *phospholipids*, which are composed of a polar, hydrophilic "head" (which contains a phosphate group) and a lipid, hydrophobic "tail". The phospholipids appear to be arranged in a bilayer, with the hydrophobic tails of the molecule oriented toward the membrane's center and the hydrophilic heads facing away from the center of the membrane. Interspersed throughout the lipid bilayer are membrane proteins, which can exist primarily in the outer or inner portion of the membrane or can span the entire width of the cell membrane.

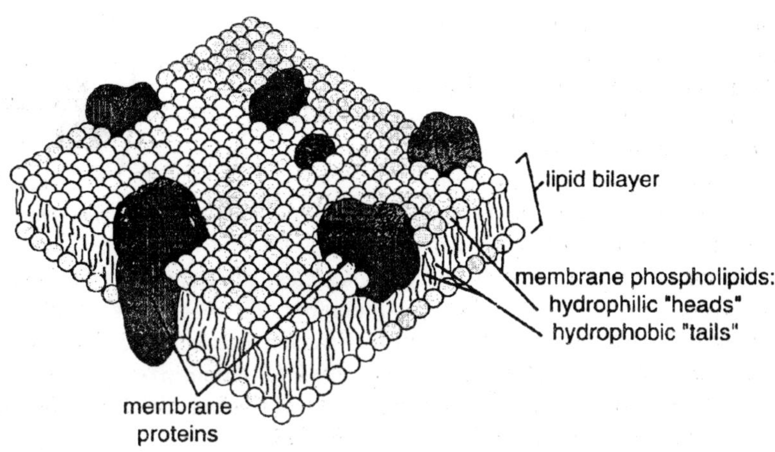

Fig. 10.1. Schematic diagram of the cell membrane.

Recent evidence also suggests that the distribution of phospholipids and proteins within the cell membrane is not random, but that certain areas of the cell membrane are organized into special regions or "domains." In particular, certain domains appear to consist primarily of lipids such as cholesterol and sphingolipids. These lipid domains are often described as lipid "rafts" that move freely about the cell membrane and these lipid rafts appear to be important in controlling various cell functions including cell signaling, endocytosis, and ion channel function. Future research will help further define the role of the lipid rafts and other specific domains within the cell membrane.

The lipid bilayer that composes the basic structure of the cell membrane acts as a water barrier. The lipid portion of the membrane is essentially impermeable to water and other nonlipid-soluble substances (electrolytes, glucose). Lipid-soluble compounds (including most drugs) are able to pass directly through the membrane by becoming dissolved in the lipid bilayer. Nonlipid-soluble substances, including water, may be able to pass through the membrane because of the presence of membrane pores. Small holes or channels appear to exist in the membrane, thereby allowing certain substances to pass from one side of the membrane to the other. These channels are believed to be formed by some of the membrane proteins that span the width of the membrane. The ability a substance has to pass through a specific pore depends primarily on the size, shape, and electrical charge of the molecule. Also, in excitable membranes (nerve, muscle) some of these pores are dynamic in nature and appear to have the ability to "open" and "close," thus regulating the flow of certain ions in and out of the cell. These dynamic ion channels are especially important in pharmacology because many drugs can affect their ability to open and close, thus altering cell excitability by regulating the movement of ions across the cell membrane.

Movement Across Membrane Barriers

Drugs and other substances that pass through biologic membranes usually do so via passive diffusion, active transport, facilitated diffusion, or some "special" process such as endocytosis. Each of these mechanisms is discussed here.

Passive Diffusion

Drugs and other substances will pass through a membrane by way of diffusion providing two essential criteria are met. First, there must be some type of difference or "gradient" on one side of the membrane compared to the other. A concentration gradient, for example, occurs when the concentration of the substance differs on one side of the membrane compared to that on the other side. When this gradient occurs, the diffusing substance can move "downhill" from the area of high concentration to that of low concentration. In addition to a concentration difference, diffusion can also occur because of the presence of a pressure gradient or, in the case of charged particles, an electrical potential gradient. The rate of the diffusion is dependent on several factors, including the magnitude of the gradient, the size of the diffusing substance, the distance over which diffusion occurs, and the temperature at which diffusion occurs. The term *passive diffusion* is often used to emphasize the fact that this movement occurs without expending any energy. The driving forces in passive diffusion are the electrical, chemical, and pressure differences on the two sides of the membrane.

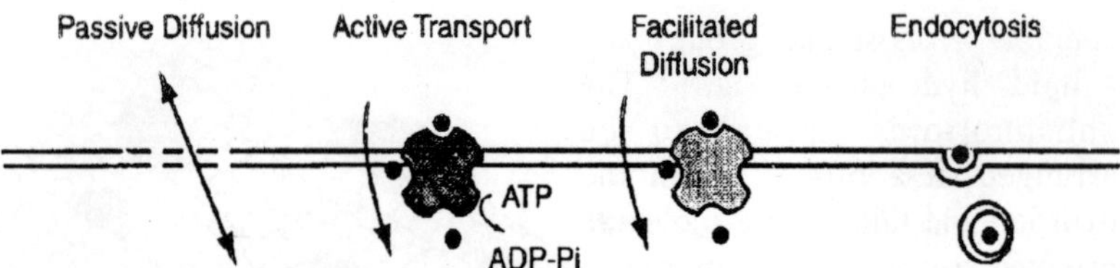

Fig. 10.2. Schematic diagram summarizing the ways in which substances may cross the cell membrane.

For passive diffusion through a membrane to occur, the second essential factor is that the membrane must be permeable to the diffusing substance. As mentioned earlier, nonlipid-soluble compounds can diffuse through the membrane via specific pores. Some nonlipid-soluble drugs such as lithium are small enough to diffuse through these pores. Many drugs, however, are able to diffuse directly through the lipid bilayer; hence, they must be fairly lipid soluble. Passive lipid diffusion is nonselective, and a drug with a high degree of lipid solubility can gain access to many tissues because of its ability to pass directly through the lipid portion of the cell membrane. As indicated earlier, certain non-lipidsoluble substances—including some proteins—can be encapsulated in lipid vesicles, thereby enhancing their lipid solubility and increasing their ability to cross lipid membranes by passive diffusion.

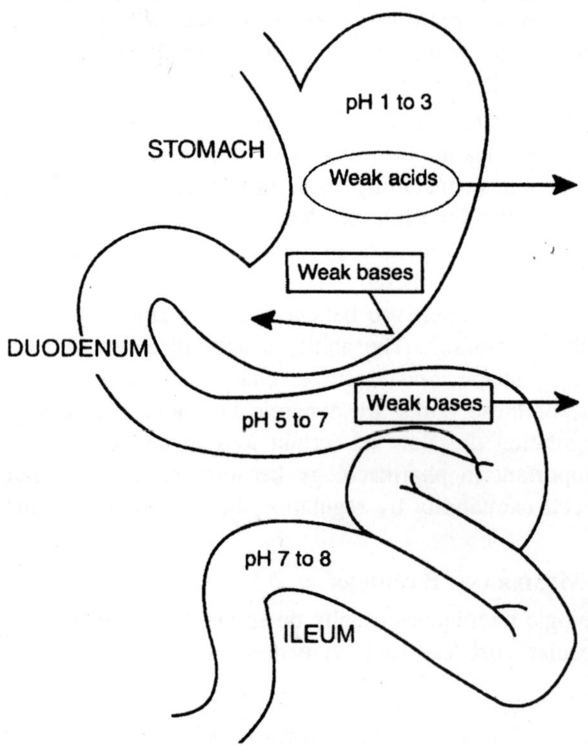

Fig. 10.3. Effect of pH and ionization on absorption of drugs from the gastrointestinal tract.

Effect of ionization on lipid diffusion

Passive lipid diffusion of certain drugs is also dependent on whether or not the drug is ionized. Drugs will diffuse more readily through the lipid layer if they are in their neutral, nonionized form. Most drugs are weak acids or weak bases, meaning that they have the potential to become positively charged or negatively charged, depending on the pH of certain body fluids. In the plasma and in most other fluids, most drugs remain in their neutral, nonionized form because of the relatively neutral pH of these fluids. In specific fluids, however, a drug may exist in an ionized state, and the absorption of the drug will be affected because of the decreased lipid solubility associated with ionization. For instance, when a weak acid is in an acidic environment (e.g., gastric secretions of the stomach), it tends to be in its neutral, nonionized form. The same drug will become positively charged if the pH of the solution increases and becomes more basic (e.g., the digestive fluids in the duodenum). A weak acid such as aspirin will be nonionized and will therefore be absorbed fairly easily from the stomach because of its lipid solubility. This same drug will be poorly absorbed if it reaches the basic pH of the duodenum and becomes ionized. Conversely, a drug that is a weak base will be ionized and poorly absorbed from the acidic environment of the stomach. The same drug will be nonionized and will therefore be lipid soluble when it reaches the duodenum, allowing it to be absorbed from the proximal small intestine.

Diffusion trapping

Changes in lipid solubility caused by ionization can also be important when the body attempts to excrete a drug in the urine. Here the situation becomes slightly more complex because the urine can sometimes be acidic and at other times basic in nature. In either situation, it is often desirable for the drug to remain ionized while in the urine so that the drug will be excreted from the body. If the drug becomes nonionized while in the nephron, it may be reabsorbed back into the body because of its increased lipid solubility. An ionized form of the drug will remain "trapped" in the nephron and will eventually be excreted in the urine. Thus, if the urine is basic, weak acids will become trapped in the nephron and will be excreted more readily. Weak bases will be excreted better if the urine is acidic.

Diffusion between cell junctions

So far, the diffusion of drugs and other substances through individual cell membranes has been discussed. Often, groups of cells will join together to form a barrier that separates one body compartment from another. In some locations, cells form "*tight junctions*" with each other and do not allow any appreciable space to exist between adjacent cells. In these cases, the primary way that a drug may diffuse across the barrier is by diffusing first into and then out of the other side of the cells comprising the barrier. Such locations include the epithelial lining of the gastrointestinal tract and the capillary endothelium of the brain (one of the reasons for the blood-brain barrier). In other tissues such as peripheral capillaries, there may be relatively large gaps between adjacent cells. Here, relatively large substances with molecular weights as high as 30,000 may be able to diffuse across the barrier by diffusing between adjacent cells.

Osmosis

Osmosis refers to the special case of diffusion where the diffusing substance is water. In this situation, water moves from an area where it is highly concentrated to an area of low concentration. Of course, permeability is still a factor when osmosis occurs across a membrane or tissue barrier. During osmosis, certain drugs may simply travel with the diffusing water, thus crossing the membrane by the process of "*bulk flow.*" This is usually limited to osmosis through the gaps between adjacent cells because membrane pores are often too small to allow the passage of the drug molecule along with the diffusing water.

Active Transport

Active or carrier-mediated transport involves using membrane proteins to transport substances across the cell membrane. Membrane proteins that span the entire membrane may serve as some sort of carrier that shuttles substances from one side of the membrane to the other. Characteristics of active transport include the following:

1. *Carrier specificity.* The protein carrier exhibits some degree of specificity for certain substances, usually discriminating among different compounds according to their shape and electrical charge. This specificity is not absolute, and some compounds that resemble one another will be transported by the same group of carriers.
2. *Expenditure of energy.* The term *active* transport implies that some energy must be used to fuel the carrier system. This energy is usually in the form of adenosine triphosphate (ATP) hydrolysis.

3. *Ability to transport substances against a concentration gradient.* Carrier-mediated active transport may be able to carry substances "uphill"—that is, from areas of low concentration to areas of high concentration.

The role of active transport in moving drugs across cell membranes has some important implications. Essentially, the drug can use one of the body's active transport systems if the drug resembles some endogenous substance that is routinely carried by the transport system. Thus, drugs that resemble amino acids and small peptides can be absorbed from the gastrointestinal (GI) tract via active transport proteins that normally absorb these substances into the body. Active transport systems in the kidneys, liver, brain, intestines, and placenta are likewise responsible for the movement of organic ions, peptides, and other substances across cell membranes, and these transport systems play an important role in the disposition of certain drugs within these tissues. Conversely, some drugs may exert their effect by either facilitating or inhibiting endogenous transport systems that affect cellular homeostasis. For example, some of the drugs used to treat excess gastric acid secretion (e.g., famotidine, ranitidine) inhibit the active transport of hydrogen ions into the stomach, thus reducing the formation of hydrochloric acid within the stomach. Hence, medications can interact with the body's active transport systems in several ways and researchers continue to develop new methods to enhance a drug's effects by using or modifying active transport pathways.

Facilitated Diffusion

Facilitated diffusion, as the name implies, bears some features of both active transport and passive diffusion. A protein carrier is present in facilitated diffusion, but no net energy is expended in transporting the substance across the cell membrane. As a result, in most cases of facilitated diffusion there is an inability to transport substances uphill against a concentration gradient. The entry of glucose into skeletal muscle cells via facilitated diffusion is probably the best example of this type of transport in the body. As in active transport, the movement of drugs across membranes through facilitated diffusion is fairly infrequent, but certain medications may affect the rate at which endogenous facilitated diffusion occurs.

Special processes

Certain cells have the ability to transport substances across their membranes through processes such as endocytosis. Here the drug is engulfed by the cell via an invagination of the cell membrane. Although limited in scope, this method does allow certain large, nonlipid-soluble drugs to enter the cell.

Distribution of Drugs Within the Body

Factors Affecting Distribution

Following administration, the extent to which a drug is uniformly distributed throughout the body or sequestered in a specific body compartment depends on several factors:

Tissue permeability

As discussed earlier, the ability to pass through membranes radically affects the extent to which a drug moves around within the body. A highly lipid-soluble drug can potentially reach all of the different body compartments and enter virtually every cell it reaches. A large nonlipid-soluble compound will remain primarily in the compartment or tissue to which it is administered. Also, certain tissues such as the brain capillary endothelium have special characteristics that limit the passage of drugs. This so-called blood-brain barrier limits the movement of drugs out of the bloodstream and into the central nervous system tissue.

Blood flow

If a drug is circulating in the bloodstream, it will gain greater access to tissues that are highly perfused. More of the drug will reach organs that receive a great deal of blood flow—such as the brain, kidneys, and exercising skeletal muscle—than will other, less active tissues such as adipose stores. Similarly, diseases that reduce blood flow to specific tissues and organs will result in less drug being delivered to those tissues.

Binding to plasma proteins

Certain drugs will form reversible bonds to circulating proteins in the bloodstream such as albumin. This fact is significant because only the unbound or "free" drug is able to reach the target tissue and exert a pharmacologic effect. Basically, the fraction of the drug that remains bound to the circulating proteins is sequestered within the vascular system and not available for therapeutic purposes in other tissues and organs.

Binding to subcellular components

In a situation similar to plasma protein binding, drugs that are bound within specific cells are unable to leave the cell and be distributed throughout other fluid compartments. Several drugs, for example, bind to subcellular organelles such as the lysosome, thus trapping the drug within the cell. Examples of this type of subcellular binding include certain antidepressants, antipsychotics, and other drugs with a relatively high pH that are attracted by the acidic environment found inside the lysosome.

Volume of Distribution

The distribution of a given drug within the body is often described by calculating the *volume of distribution* (V_d) for that drug. V_d is the ratio of the amount of drug administered to the concentration of drug in the plasma:

$$V_d = \text{amount of drug administered} \div \text{concentration of drug in plasma}$$

V_d is used to estimate a drug's distribution by comparing the calculated V_d with the total amount of body water in a normal person. A normal 70 kg man has a total body fluid content of approximately 42 L (5.5 L blood, 12.0 L extracellular fluid, 24.5 L intracellular fluid). If the calculated V_d of a drug is approximately equal to the total amount of body water, then the drug is distributed uniformly throughout all of the body's fluids. If the V_d of the drug is far less than 42 L, then the drug is being retained in the bloodstream due to factors such as plasma protein binding. A V_d much greater than 42 L indicates that the drug is being concentrated in the tissues. It should be noted that V_d is not a "real" value; that is, it does not indicate the actual amount of fluid in the body, but is merely an arbitrary figure that reflects the apparent distribution of a drug using total body water as a reference point.

Drug Storage

Storage Sites

Following administration and absorption, many drugs are "stored" to some extent at certain locations in the body; that is, prior to drug elimination, the drug may be sequestered in its active form in a relatively inert tissue that may be different from the target site of the drug. Some storage sites include the following:

Adipose

The primary site for drug storage in the body is adipose tissue. Because many drugs are lipid soluble, fat deposits throughout the body can serve as a considerable reservoir for these compounds. In some individuals, the amount of fat in the body can reach as high as 40 to 50 percent of body weight, thus creating an extensive storage compartment. Once drugs have been stored in adipose tissue, they tend to remain there for long periods of time because of the low metabolic rate and poor blood perfusion of these tissues. Examples of drugs that tend to be stored in fat include highly lipid- soluble anesthetics such as the barbiturates (thiopental) and inhalation anesthetics (halothane).

Bone

Bone acts as a storage site for several toxic agents, especially heavy metals like lead. Also, drugs such as the tetracyclines, which bind to and form molecular complexes with the crystal components within the skeletal matrix, are stored within bone.

Muscle

Binding of drugs to components within the muscle may create the long-term storage of these compounds. Various agents may be actively transported into the muscle cell and may form reversible bonds to intracellular structures such as proteins, nucleoproteins, or phospholipids. An example is the antimalarial drug quinacrine.

Organs

Drugs are often stored within certain organs such as the liver and kidneys. As in muscle cells, the drug may enter the cell passively or by active transport and then form bonds to subcellular components. Examples include antimicrobial aminoglycoside agents (such as gentamicin and streptomycin), which accumulate in renal proximal tubular cells.

Adverse Consequences of Drug Storage

High concentrations of drugs, drug metabolites, and toxic compounds within tissues can cause local damage to the tissues in which they are stored. This event is particularly true for toxic compounds that are incorporated and stored in the matrix of bone or that are highly concentrated within specific organs. Lead poisoning, for example, causes several well-known and potentially devastating effects when this metal accumulates, in the CNS, bone, GI tract, and several other tissues.

Exposing various organs to high concentrations of therapeutic drugs can also result in myriad problems. Actaminophen, for example, is normally metabolized in the liver to form several highly reactive by-products or metabolites. When normal doses of acetaminophen are metabolized in a reasonably healthy liver, these metabolites are rapidly inactivated in the liver and subsequently excreted by the kidneys. Very high doses of acetaminophen, however, result in the formation of excessive amounts of a toxic metabolite that can react with hepatic proteins and cause severe liver damage. Hence, organs such as the liver and the kidneys are often subjected to local damage when these organs must deal with high concentrations of therapeutic and toxic agents.

Another problem with drug storage occurs when the storage site acts as a reservoir that "*soaks up*" the drug and prevents it from reaching the target site. For instance, a highly lipid-soluble drug such as a general anesthetic must be administered at a sufficient dose to ensure that there will be enough drug available to reach the CNS, despite the tendency for much of the drug to be sequestered in the body's fat stores. Storage sites may also be responsible for the redistribution of drugs. This occurrence is seen when the drug begins to leak out of the storage reservoir after plasma levels of the drug have begun to diminish. In this way, the drug may be reintroduced to the target site long after the original dose should have been eliminated. This redistribution may explain why certain individuals experience prolonged effects of the drug or extended adverse side effects.

NEWER TECHNIQUES FOR DRUG DELIVERY

Controlled-Release Preparations

Controlled-release preparations, also known as *timed-release*, *sustained-release*, *extended-release*, or *prolonged-action preparations*, are generally designed to permit a slower and more prolonged absorption of the drug from the gastrointestinal tract and other routes of administration. This technique may offer several advantages such as decreasing the number of doses needed each day, preventing large fluctuations in the amount of drug appearing in the plasma, and sustaining plasma levels throughout the night. This type of preparation has been used successfully with several types of drugs, including cardiovascular medications (beta blockers, calcium channel blockers), narcotic analgesics such as morphine, and anti-Parkinson medications that contain L-dopa. Controlled- release preparations will probably continue to gain popularity as a means for administering these and other medications in the future.

Implanted Drug Delivery Systems

Several techniques have been developed whereby a type of drug "*reservoir*" is implanted surgically within the body and is then released in a controlled fashion from the implanted reservoir. These drug reservoirs typically consist of a small container placed under the skin in the abdomen. The containers are often programmed to allow a small, measured dose of the drug to be released periodically from the reservoir. Alternatively, the reservoir can be controlled electronically from outside of the body through the use of small, remote-controlled devices, thus allowing the patient to regulate release of the drug as needed. In some cases, the drug reservoir may be connected by a small cannula to a specific body compartment—such as the subarachnoid space or epidural space—so that the drug can be delivered directly into that space. This type of system appears to be very helpful in applying certain drugs such as analgesics, anesthetics, and muscle relaxants into the spinal cord.

Another type of implantable system has been developed recently that incorporates the drug into some type of biodegradable or nonbiodegradable substance such as a polymer matrix or gel. The drug-polymer complex is then implanted in the body and the drug is slowly released into surrounding tissues (*nonbiodegradable*), or is released as the matrix gradually dissolves (*biodegradable*). This type of system is probably best known for administering contraceptive hormones such as progesterone; these implants have also shown promise in delivering other medications such as local anesthetics, insulin, and vaccines.

Hence, implantable drug delivery systems are being considered as a potential means of administering several drugs including analgesics, muscle relaxants, and hormones. Improvements in the technology of this type of drug delivery will hopefully permit increased clinical applications of these systems in the near future. The use of implantable drug delivery systems with specific types of medications will be discussed in more detail when these medications are addressed in subsequent chapters in this book.

Targeting Drug Delivery to Specific Cells and Tissues

Some very innovative approaches have been attempted on a molecular level to try to target the drug specifically to the cells that require treatment. For instance, specific types of antibodies (monoclonal antibodies) can be synthesized and attached to certain drugs such as the cytotoxic agents often used in cancer chemotherapy. The antibodies are then attracted to antigens located on the surface of the tumor cells. This offers the distinct advantage of focusing the drug more directly on the cancerous cells rather than on healthy human tissues. Other cellular techniques have been investigated that could also help direct the drug to the affected tissues. It may be possible, for example, to link a drug to a modified virus so that the virus transports and helps insert the drug directly into specific cells; the virus, of course, must be modified so that it will not cause viral infection. Other nonviral techniques include encapsulating the drug in a certain type of fat particle (liposome) or attaching the drug to certain proteins that will be attracted to the surface receptors of specific cells. These viral and nonviral techniques have been particularly important in helping deliver DNA to specific cells in order to modify the genetic regulation of those cells (gene-based therapy).

Drugs can also be targeted to specific sites by capitalizing on unique physiologic properties of various tissues and organs. Certain drugs, for example, might be activated by enzymes that are found only in the kidneys, thereby targeting these drugs specifically to the kidneys. Abnormal tissues, including some tumors, might also have specialized enzymes that could be used to activate certain drugs only after the drugs reach these tissues. Various techniques can also be used to modify a drug so that it is activated only after reaching the colon. This action will allow the drug to be administered orally, but remain inactive as a "prodrug" until it reaches the colon, where it will then become activated to treat local problems or be absorbed into the systemic circulation.

The idea of targeting drugs to specific tissues through various cellular and chemical mechanisms is still relatively new. These techniques have shown considerable promise, however, and may ultimately be extremely useful in increasing the effectiveness of certain drugs while decreasing side effects. In order for any drug to be effective, it must be able to reach specific target tissues. The goal of drug administration is to deliver the drug in the least complicated manner while still allowing sufficient concentrations of the active form of the drug to arrive at the desired site. Each route of administration has certain advantages and disadvantages that will determine how much and how fast the drug is delivered to specific tissues. In addition to the route of administration, the distribution of the drug within the body must be taken into account. Simply introducing the drug into certain body fluids such as the bloodstream does not ensure its entry into the desired tissues. Factors such as tissue permeability and protein binding may influence how the drug is dispersed within the various fluid compartments within the body. Finally, some drugs have a tendency to be stored in certain tissues for prolonged periods of time. This storage may produce serious toxic effects if high concentrations of the compound damage the cells in which it is stored.

Drug Elimination

All drugs must be eliminated from the body eventually to terminate their effect and to prevent excessive accumulation of the drug. Drugs are usually eliminated by chemically altering the original compound while it is still in the body so that it is no longer active (*biotransformation*), by excreting the active form of the drug from the body (*excretion*), or by a combination of biotransformation and excretion.

Biotransformation

Drug metabolism, or *biotransformation*, refers to chemical changes that take place in the drug following administration. Enzymes that are located within specific tissues are responsible for catalyzing changes in the drug's structure and subsequently altering the pharmacologic properties of the drug. The location of these enzymes and the reactions involved in biotransformation are discussed later in this chapter.

Biotransformation usually results in an altered version of the original compound known as a *metabolite*, which is usually inactive or has a greatly reduced level of pharmacologic activity. Occasionally, the metabolite has a higher level of activity than the original compound. In these cases, the drug may be given in an inactive, or "prodrug," form that will activate via biotransformation following administration. However, after it has exerted its pharmacologic effect, drug termination is the primary function of biotransformation.

Inactivating a drug and terminating its effects after it is no longer needed are often essential. For instance, the effects of general and local anesthetics must eventually wear off, allowing the patient to resume normal functioning. Although termination of drug activity can occur when the active form of the drug is excreted from the body via organs such as the kidneys, excretory mechanisms are often too slow to effectively terminate any activity within a reasonable time period. If excretion were the only way to terminate drug activity, some compounds would continue to exert their effects for several days or even weeks. Drug biotransformation into an inactive form usually occurs within a matter of minutes or hours, thus reducing the chance for toxic effects caused by drug accumulation or prolonged drug activity.

Cellular Mechanisms of Drug Biotransformation

The chemical changes that occur during drug metabolism are usually caused by oxidation, reduction, hydrolysis, or conjugation of the original compound. Each type of reaction and the location of the enzymes catalyzing the reaction are also discussed here.

1. *Oxidation*. Oxidation occurs when either oxygen is added or hydrogen is removed from the original compound. Oxidation reactions comprise the predominant method of drug biotransformation in the body, and the primary enzymes that catalyze these reactions are known collectively as the cytochrome P450 monooxygenases. These enzymes are primarily located on the smooth endoplasmic reticulum of specific cells and are sometimes referred to as the *drug microsomal metabolizing system* (DMMS).

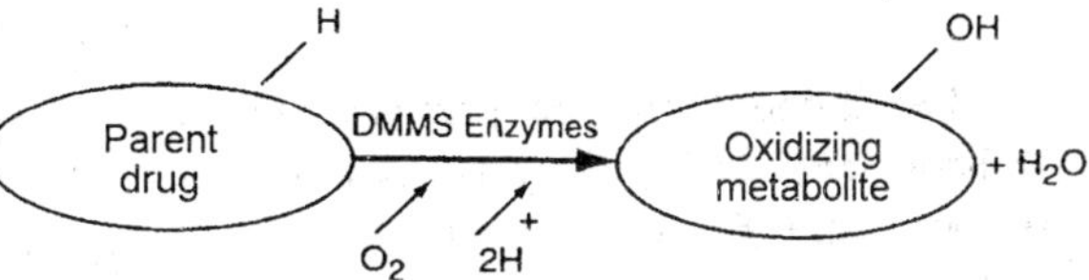

Fig. 10.4. Drug oxidation catalyzed by drug microsomal metabolizing system (DMMS) enzymes.

2. *Reduction*. Reduction reactions consist of removing oxygen or adding hydrogen to the original compound. Enzymes that are located in the cell cytoplasm are usually responsible for drug reduction.
3. *Hydrolysis*. The original compound is broken into separate parts. The enzymes responsible for the hydrolysis of the drug are located at several sites within the cell (i.e., the endoplasmic reticulum and cytoplasm) as well as extracellularly (e.g., circulating in the plasma).
4. *Conjugation*. In conjugation reactions, the intact drug or the metabolite of one of the reactions described earlier, is coupled to an endogenous substance such as acetyl coenzyme A (acetyl CoA), glucuronic acid, or an amino acid. Enzymes catalyzing drug conjugations are found in the cytoplasm and on the endoplasmic reticulum.

The chemical reactions involved in drug biotransformation are also classified as either phase I or phase II reactions. Phase I reactions consist of those using oxidation, reduction, or hydrolysis. Phase II reactions involve conjugation of the parent drug or the metabolite of a drug that was already metabolized using a phase I reaction.

Regardless of the type of chemical reaction used, biotransformation also helps in metabolite excretion from the body by creating a more polar compound. After one or more of the reactions just described occurs, the remaining drug metabolite usually has a greater tendency to be ionized in the body's fluids. The ionized metabolite is more water soluble, thus becoming transported more easily in the bloodstream to the kidneys. Upon reaching the kidneys, the polar metabolite can be excreted from the body in the urine.

Organs Responsible for Drug Biotransformation

The primary location for drug metabolism is the liver. Enzymes responsible for drug metabolism, such as the cytochrome P450 enzymes, are abundant on hepatic smooth endoplasmic reticulum; liver cells also contain other cytoplasmic enzymes responsible for drug reduction and hydrolysis. Other organs that contain metabolizing enzymes and exhibit considerable drug transformation abilities include the lungs, kidneys, gastrointestinal epithelium, and skin. Drug metabolism can be radically altered in conditions where these tissues are damaged. For instance, inactivation of certain drugs may be significantly delayed in the patient with hepatitis or cirrhosis of the liver. As expected, dosages in these patients must be adjusted accordingly to prevent drug accumulation and toxicity.

Enzyme Induction

A frequent problem in drug metabolism is the phenomenon of *enzyme induction*. Prolonged use of certain drugs "induces" the body to be able to enzymatically destroy the drug more rapidly, usually because either more metabolizing enzymes are being manufactured or less are being degraded. Enzyme induction may cause drugs to be metabolized more rapidly than expected, thus decreasing their therapeutic effect. This may be one reason why *tolerance* to some drugs occurs when it is used for extended periods (tolerance is the need for increased drug dosages to produce the same effect). Long-term ingestion or inhalation of other exogenous compounds such as alcohol, cigarette smoke, or environmental toxins may also cause enzyme induction. When this occurs, medicinal drugs may be more rapidly metabolized even when they are first administered because of the preexisting enzyme induction.

Drug Excretion

The kidneys are the primary sites for drug excretion. The functional unit of the kidney is the nephron, and each kidney is composed of approximately 1 million nephrons. Usually, the metabolized or conjugated version of the original drug reaches the nephron and is then filtered at the glomerulus. Following filtration, the compound traverses the proximal convoluted tubule, loop of Henle, and distal convoluted tubule before reaching the collecting ducts. If a compound is not reabsorbed while moving through the nephron, it will ultimately leave the body in the urine. As discussed earlier, biotransformation plays a significant role in creating a polar, water-soluble metabolite that is able to reach the kidneys through the bloodstream. Only relatively polar drugs or their metabolites will be excreted in significant amounts by the kidneys because the ionized metabolite has a greater tendency to remain in the nephron and not be reabsorbed into the body. Non-polar compounds that are filtered by the kidneys are relatively lipophilic and can easily be reabsorbed back into the body passively by diffusing through the wall of the nephron. However, the polar metabolite is relatively impermeable to the epithelium lining, and the metabolite tends to remain "trapped" in the nephron following filtration, where it will eventually be excreted in the urine.

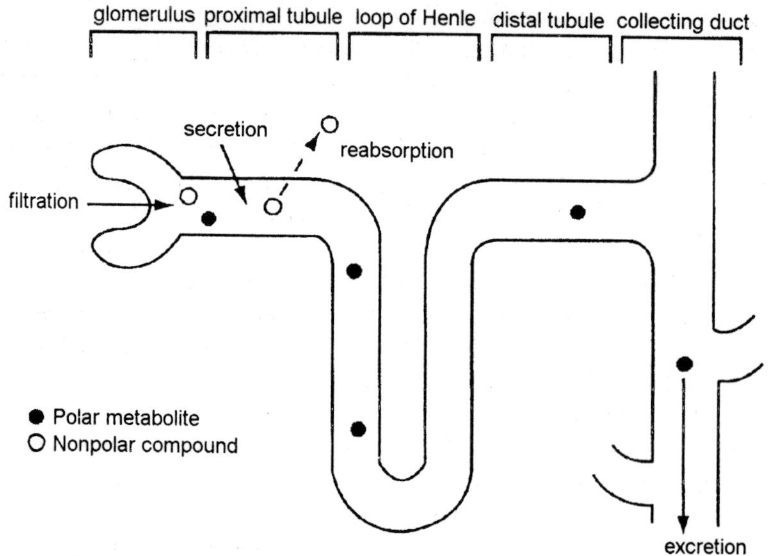

Fig. 10.5. Drug excretion at the nephron.

In addition to filtration, some drugs may be secreted into the nephron by active transport mechanisms located in the proximal convoluted tubule. Several distinct types of transport proteins have been identified that secrete substances such as organic cations (e.g., uric acid), organic anions (e.g., choline, histamine), prostaglandins, conjugated drug metabolites, and a variety of other compounds. Certain drugs can also be transported by one of these carrier systems so that they are actively secreted into the nephron. For example, penicillin G is actively secreted via the transport system for organic acids, and morphine is secreted by the organic base transport system. In these cases, elimination of the drug is enhanced by the combined effects of tubular secretion and filtration in delivering the drug to the urine.

Other routes for drug excretion include the lungs and gastrointestinal tract. The lungs play a significant role in excreting volatile drugs, that is, drugs that are usually administered by inhalation. Consequently, the lungs serve as the route of both administration and excretion for drugs such as gaseous anesthetics. The gastrointestinal tract usually plays only a minor role in drug excretion. Certain drugs can be excreted by the liver into the bile and subsequently reach the duodenum via the bile duct. If the drug remains in the gastrointestinal tract, it will eventually be excreted in the feces. However, most of the secreted bile is reabsorbed, and drugs contained in it are often reabsorbed simultaneously.

Other minor routes for drug excretion include the sweat, saliva, and breast milk of lactating mothers. Although drugs excreted via lactation are considered a relatively minor route with regard to loss from the mother, the possibility that the infant may imbibe substantial concentrations of the drug does exist. Careful consideration for the welfare of the nursing infant must always be a factor when administering medications to the lactating mother.

Drug Elimination Rates

The rate at which a drug is eliminated is significant in determining the amount and frequency of the dosage of the drug. If a drug is administered much faster than it is eliminated, the drug will accumulate excessively in the body and reach toxic levels. Conversely, if elimination greatly exceeds the rate of delivery, the concentration in the body may never reach therapeutic levels. Several parameters are used to indicate the rate at which a drug is usually eliminated so that dosages may be adjusted accordingly. Two of the primary measurements are *clearance* and *half-life*.

Clearance

Clearance of a drug (CL) can be described either in terms of all organ's and tissue's ability to eliminate the drug (systemic clearance) or in terms of a single organ or tissue's ability to eliminate the drug. To calculate clearance from a specific organ, two primary factors must be considered. First, the blood flow to the organ (Q) determines how much drug will be delivered to the organ for elimination. Second, the fraction of drug removed from the plasma as it passes through the organ must be known. This fraction, termed the *extraction ratio*, is equal to the difference in the concentration of drug entering (Ci) and exiting (Co) the organ, divided by the entering concentration (Ci). Clearance by an individual organ is summarized by the following equation:

$$CL = Q \times [(Ci - Co) \div Ci].$$

The calculation of clearance using this equation is illustrated by the following example. Aspirin is metabolized primarily in the liver. Normal hepatic blood flow (Q) equals 1500 mL/min. If the blood entering the liver contains 200 μg/mL of aspirin (Ci) and the blood leaving the liver contains 134 μg/mL (Co), hepatic clearance of aspirin is calculated as follows:

$$CL_{hepatic} = Q \times [(Ci - Co) \div Ci]$$
$$= 1500 \text{ mL/min X } [(200\ \mu\text{g/mL} - 134 \text{ pg/mL}) \div 200 \text{ pg/mL}]$$
$$= 495 \text{ mL/min}.$$

This example illustrates that clearance is actually the amount of plasma that the drug can be totally removed from per unit time. As calculated here, the liver would be able to completely remove aspirin from 495 mL of blood each minute. Tetracycline, a common antibacterial drug, has a clearance equal to 130 mL/min, indicating that this drug would be completely removed from approximately 130 mL of plasma each minute.

Clearance is dependent on the organ or tissue's ability to extract the drug from the plasma as well as the perfusion of the organ. Some tissues may have an excellent ability to remove the drug from the bloodstream, but clearance is limited because only a small amount of blood reaches the organ. Conversely, highly perfused organs may be ineffective in removing the drug, thus prolonging its activity.

In terms of drug elimination from the entire body, systemic clearance is calculated as the sum of all individual clearances from all organs and tissues (i.e., systemic CL = hepatic CL + renal CL + lung CL, and so on). Note that the elimination of the drug includes the combined processes of drug loss from the body (excretion) as well as inactivation of the drug through biotransformation.

Half-Life

In addition to clearance, the *half-life* of the drug is important in describing the duration of activity of the compound. Half-life is defined as the amount of time required for 50 percent of the drug remaining in the body to be eliminated. Most drugs are eliminated in a manner such that a fixed portion of the drug is eliminated in a given time period. For example, a drug such as acetaminophen with a half-life of 2 hours indicates that in each 2-hour period, 50 percent of the acetaminophen still in the body will be eliminated.

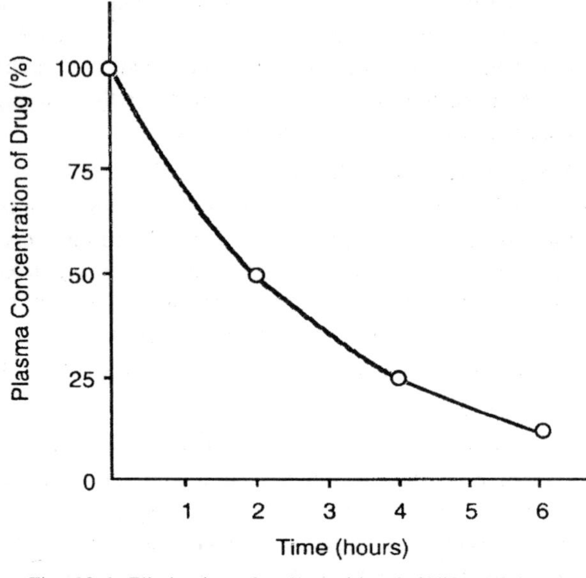

Fig. 10.6. Elimination of a drug with a half-life of 2 hours.

Half-life is a function of both clearance and volume of distribution (V_d); that is, the time it takes to eliminate 50 percent of the drug depends not only on the ability of the organ(s) to remove the drug from the plasma, but also on the distribution or presence of the drug in the plasma. A drug that undergoes extensive inactivation in the liver may have a long half-life if it is sequestered intracellularly in skeletal muscle. Also, disease states that affect either clearance or V_d will affect the half-life of the drug, so dosages must be altered accordingly.

Dosing Schedules and Plasma Concentration

With most medications, it is desirable to bring plasma concentrations of the drug up to a certain level and maintain it at that level. If the drug is administered by continuous intravenous administration, this can be done fairly easily by matching the rate of administration with the rate of drug elimination (clearance) once the desired plasma concentration is achieved. In situations where the drug is given at specific intervals, the dosage must be adjusted to provide an average plasma concentration over the dosing period. The dosing interval is relatively long (e.g., 12 hours), the dose must be considerably large to provide the same relative plasma concentration that would exist in a shorter dosing interval (e.g., 8 hours). Note also that larger doses given further apart result in greater plasma fluctuations; that is, greater maximum and minimum plasma levels over the dosing period. Giving smaller doses more frequently provides an equivalent average concentration without the extreme peaks and valleys associated with longer intervals.

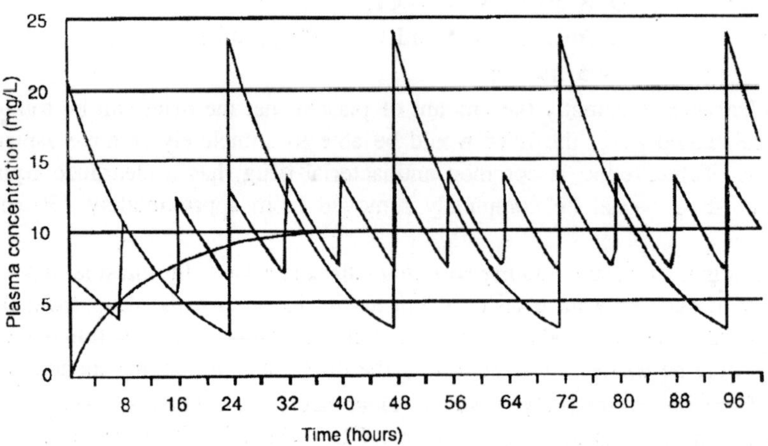

Fig. 10.7. Relationship between dosing interval and plasma concentrations of the antiasthmatic drug theophylline.

Variations in Drug Response and Metabolism

The fact that different people react differently to the same relative drug dosage is an important and often critical aspect of pharmacology. Two patients who are given the same drug may exhibit different magnitudes of a beneficial response as well as different adverse effects. Several primary factors that are responsible for variations in the response to drugs are discussed below.

Genetic factors

Genetic variability can result in altered drug pharmacokinetics in certain individuals. In extreme cases, genetic variations may result in abnormal or absent drug-metabolizing enzymes. This deficiency can be harmful or even fatal if the drug is not metabolized and begins exerting toxic effects due to accumulation or prolonged pharmacologic activity. For example, some individuals lack the appropriate plasma cholinesterase to break down circulating acetylcholine and acetylcholine-like compounds. Succinylcholine is a neuromuscular blocking agent that is usually administered during general anesthesia to ensure muscular relaxation during surgery. Normally, the succinylcholine is quickly degraded by plasma cholinesterase; however, individuals lacking the appropriate form of cholinesterase may suffer respiratory paralysis because the succinylcholine exerts its effect much longer than the expected period of time. In addition to the extreme case described above, we now realize that many people have subtle but important differences in the genes controlling the synthesis of many drug-related proteins. These differences—know as genetic polymorphisms—will result in the production of proteins that are somewhat different in structure and function. From this, various aspects of drug disposition and response will be affected. For example, differences in proteins that transport drugs across membranes will result in altered absorption, distribution, and excretion of drugs using these transport systems. Differences in the genetic control of drug metabolizing proteins (enzymes) will likewise result in altered metabolism and biotransformation of specific drugs. Finally, differences in the proteins that function as drug receptors on specific cells and target tissues might cause variability in the tissues' responses.

The potential influence of genetic variability on drug responses and metabolism has actually evolved into a branch of genetics known as pharmacogenetics, or pharmacogenomics. Research in pharmacogenetics will continue to expand as more details emerge about human genetic make-up (i.e., the human genome project). We can tailor drug therapy more specifically for patients by realizing how specific genetic differences might influence drug responses. That is, doses can be adjusted to account for genetic differences in drug disposition, and certain drugs can be avoided altogether in people who lack the appropriate enzymes for these drugs. Drug regimens that take into account genetic variability will ultimately result in better drug effects with fewer side effects.

Disease

Structural or functional damage to an organ or tissue responsible for drug metabolism or excretion presents an obvious problem in pharmacology. Diseases initiating change in tissue function or blood flow to specific organs like the liver and kidneys can dramatically affect the elimination of various drugs. Certain diseases may also impair the absorption and distribution of the drug, further complicating the problem of individualized response. The significance of disease in affecting the patient's response is crucial since response to a medication may be affected by the very same pathology that the drug is being used to treat. For instance, renal excretion of antibiotics, such as the aminoglycosides, is altered radically in many types of bacterial infection, but these drugs are typically administered to treat the same infections altering their own excretion. Consequently, great care must be taken to adjust the dosage accordingly when administering medications in conditions where drug disposition might be altered by various diseases.

Drug interactions

When two or more drugs are present in the body at the same time, the chance exists that they may interact and alter each other's effects and metabolism. The majority of drug-drug interactions are insignificant and do not result in any clinically meaningful adverse effects. Likewise, certain drug combinations and interactions can be beneficial because two or more compounds might act synergistically to produce a cumulative effect that is greater than each drug would produce alone. Several drugs, for example, are often administered simultaneously so that they augment each other when treating conditions such as hypertension, cancer, and human immunodeficiency virus infection. However, certain combinations can lead to serious adverse effects and interactions. For example, two or more drugs can have additive effects that cause an adverse response, even if each drug is given in a nontoxic dose. For instance, taking two central nervous system (CNS) depressants simultaneously (e.g., barbiturates and alcohol) may cause such severe CNS inhibition that the additive effects are lethal.

In contrast to an additive effect, drugs with opposite actions may essentially cancel each other out, thus negating or reducing the beneficial effects of one or both medications. A drug that causes bronchodilation (i.e., for the treatment of asthma) will be negated by an agent that constricts the bronchioles.

Some of the most serious problems occur during drug interactions because one drug delays the biotransformation of the other. If a second compound inhibits the enzymes that normally metabolize a drug, the original drug will exert its effect for prolonged periods, possibly leading to toxic effects. For instance, the antiulcer drug cimetidine (Tagamet) inhibits the hepatic metabolism of oral anticoagulants such as warfarin (Coumadin). Taking these two drugs together tends to cause elevated plasma levels of the anticoagulant, which may prolong blood clotting and lead to a possible hemorrhage. Another type of interaction occurs when two or more drugs alter each other's absorption and distribution, and can occur when they compete for the same active transport carrier or bind to the same plasma proteins. An example is the interaction between aspirin and methotrexate, a drug used to treat cancer and rheumatoid arthritis. Aspirin can displace methotrexate from its binding site on plasma proteins, thus allowing relatively high amounts of unbound or "free" methotrexate to exist in the bloodstream. The increased levels of free methotrexate may lead to toxic effects.

Considering the large number of drugs on the market, it is well beyond the scope of this text to discuss all of the clinically relevant drug interactions. The prescribing physician and pharmacist, however, must carefully evaluate the potential for drug interactions. Likewise, physical therapists, occupational therapists, and other individuals dealing with patients taking medications must be alert for any abnormal symptoms or untoward effects because they may indicate a possible drug interaction.

Age

In general, older patients are more sensitive to drugs. Drugs are usually not metabolized as quickly in the elderly, primarily because of decreases in liver and kidney function that typically accompany the aging process. Decreased drug elimination therefore results in higher plasma levels in older adults than those occurring in younger adults given equivalent doses. Older adults also suffer more illnesses, and consequently receive more drugs than younger adults; this fact further increases their vulnerability to altered drug responses. Various other age-related changes in physiology (increased body fat, decreased cardiovascular function, and so forth) can affect pharmacokinetics and pharmacodynamics in older adults.

Children are also subject to problems and variability in drug metabolism. Because liver and kidney function is immature, newborns may be deficient in specific drug-metabolizing enzymes, thus prolonging the effects of drugs. Infants also differ from adults in several other key factors affecting drug disposition including differences in membrane function, plasma proteins, regional blood flow, and body composition (i.e., percentage of body fat and total body water). Hence, drug absorption, distribution, and elimination will be altered in infants, and these alterations will be especially problematic in infants who are born prematurely.

Diet

Diet is shown to affect the absorption, metabolism, and response to many drugs. Animal and human studies indicated that the total caloric input as well as the percentage of calories obtained from different sources (carbohydrates, proteins, and fats) influence drug pharmacokinetics. Specific dietary constituents such as cruciferous vegetables and charcoal-broiled beef can also alter drug metabolism.

Fortunately, most food-drug interactions are not serious and will not alter the clinical effects of the drug. There are, however, a few well- known food-drug combinations that should be avoided because of their potentially serious interaction. For example, it was recently discovered that grapefruit juice inhibits the enzymes that metabolize certain drugs as they are absorbed from the gastrointestinal (GI) tract. As a result, taking these drugs orally with grapefruit juice will result in *increased* drug bioavailability because more of the drug's active form will reach the bloodstream. This increased bioavailability will result in plasma levels that are higher than expected, thereby increasing the risk of side effects and adverse reactions.

Another important food-drug interaction involves certain foods such as fermented cheese and wine. These foods contain high amounts of tyramine, which stimulates the release of catecholamines (norepinephrine, epinephrine) within the body. Hence, these foods should not be ingested with drugs that inhibit the monoamine oxidase enzyme (MAO inhibitors). MAO-inhibiting drugs work by suppressing the destruction of catecholamines, thus allowing higher levels of norepinephrine and epinephrine to occur. (MAO inhibitors are frequently used in the treatment of depression) Consequently, when MAO inhibitors are taken with tyramine-containing foods, excessive levels of catecholamines may develop, leading to a dangerous increase in blood pressure (hypertensive crisis). A number of other potential food-drug interactions occur, but it is beyond the scope of this text to discuss all of them. These interactions are addressed in more detail elsewhere. Clinicians should therefore be aware of these well-known interactions and be on the alert for others as new drugs arrive on the market.

Sex

Men and women may have distinct differences in the way that certain drugs are absorbed, distributed, and metabolized. This idea makes sense when one considers that sex-related differences in body composition, gastrointestinal function, enzyme activity, and various other systems can potentially affect pharmacokinetic variables. Drug disposition may also be influenced in women by the cyclic hormonal variations occurring during the menstrual cycle, whereas men do not typically undergo such routine hormonal fluctuations. Pharmacokinetics can clearly differ between men and women, and future research is needed to determine how sex-related differences affect the therapeutic outcomes of specific drugs.

Other factors

A number of additional factors may alter the predicted response of the patient to a drug. As discussed earlier, environmental and occupational hazards may produce certain toxins that alter drug absorption and metabolism. Factors such as cigarette smoking and alcohol consumption have been shown to influence the metabolism of specific compounds. Drug distribution and metabolism may be altered in the obese patient, or in response to chronic and acute exercise. Individuals with spinal cord injuries have a decreased ability to absorb certain drugs from their gastrointestinal tract, presumably because of a general decrease in gastrointestinal motility. Conversely, patients with extensive burn injuries may have increased gastrointestinal absorption and therefore increased bioavailability of certain drugs, although the reason for this effect is not clear.

There are many factors that influence the way each individual responds to a medication, and these factors must be taken into account whenever possible. Clinicians should also realize that these factors are not mutually exclusive. For example, a premature infant with genetic polymorphisms might present an extremely complex pharmacologic dilemma because of the combination of very young age and genetic variability. In older adults, the combined effects of old age and disease can likewise increase the complexity of pharmacokinetic variability. Hence, special care must be taken in prescribing appropriate dosages in any situation where the predicted responses to drug therapy might be altered by one or more of the factors described. Drug elimination occurs because of the combined effects of drug metabolism and excretion. Elimination is essential in terminating drug activity within a reasonable and predictable time frame. Various tissues and organs (especially the liver and kidneys) are involved in drug elimination, and injury or disease of these tissues can markedly alter the response to certain drugs. In cases of disease or injury, dosages must frequently be adjusted to prevent adverse side effects from altered elimination rates. Many other environmental, behavioral, and genetic factors may also alter drug metabolism and disposition, and possible variability in the patient's response should always be a matter of concern when selecting the type and amount of the drug.

Drug Absorption

For a drug to exert the desired pharmacological effect, therapeutic concentrations of the drug need to be available at the cellular sites of action. In practice, systemic concentrations are measured and this systemic bioavailability is used as an indicator of whether adequate concentrations of the drug are achieved at the final site of action. Absorption from the site of administration is one of the foremost hurdles that a drug molecule encounters before it can reach systemic circulation. Depending on the route of drug administration, several anatomical barriers to drug absorption and resultant systemic bioavailability exist. The ability of a drug to cross these barriers depends not only on the physicochemical properties of the drug molecule and the formulation characteristics (drug product design), but also on various physiological processes at the site of absorption. In addition, interactions between drug–drug, drug–food, drug–disease, as well as the presence of various drug-metabolizing enzymes, uptake and efflux transport proteins at the membrane barriers, influence drug absorption. Knowledge of factors influencing drug absorption is critical for choosing an appropriate route of administration and development of an optimal dosage form. In this chapter we will discuss the basics of drug absorption from a biopharmaceutical perspective, that is, those factors whether physiological or physicochemical that may influence the ability of a drug to get absorbed from the site of administration into the systemic circulation.

Routes of Drug Administration

Choosing an optimal route for drug administration is one of the most important decisions in drug development, as this choice may influence several end points that include:

1. Drug stability
2. Size and frequency of dosing
3. Rate and extent of drug absorption
4. Time for onset of therapeutic response
5. Duration and magnitude of the therapeutic response
6. Adverse event profile
7. Patient compliance and convenience

Commonly employed routes of drug administration intended for systemic effect of the drug include:

1. Parenteral (intravenous, intramuscular, subcutaneous, intra-arterial)
2. Enteral (buccal, sublingual, oral, rectal)
3. Percutaneous (or transdermal)
4. Inhalation
5. Intranasal

The parenteral routes of drug administration are associated with high bioavailability due to the absence of (intravenous) or limited (intramuscular) barriers to drug absorption. Bioavailability from extravascular routes is usually lower and also highly variable. This results from the presence of significant barriers to drug absorption and also a complex interplay of multiple drug and physiological factors.

Parenteral

Intravenous route is the fastest and most predictable route of drug administration as it avoids the rate-limiting absorption phase associated with other routes. The onset of the desired pharmacological effect is prompt and is, therefore, especially beneficial in case of emergencies. However, because of the rapid appearance of peak drug concentrations in systemic circulation, this route of drug administration can also be risky. Several drugs are administered by intravenous routes including analgesic, anesthetic, antibiotic, anticancer, and antiepileptic drugs. Intravenous infusions are particularly desirable when peak drug concentrations need to be avoided and the drug concentrations in blood need to be controlled within a desirable range to maximize therapeutic benefit and to minimize toxicity.

Typically drug absorption from the subcutaneous and intramuscular routes depends on the solubility of drug in surrounding fluids and the blood flow to the site of administration. Absorption is usually rapid compared to oral route or can be modified to achieve a sustained release when desired (e.g., intramuscular depot injection of Leuprolide).

Oral

Drug absorption from the gastrointestinal (GI) tract is determined by transport across both the GI epithelial membrane as well as the endothelial membrane of the capillary walls. Drug absorption across the epithelial barriers typically occurs via passive diffusion. For some drugs such as L-dopa and 5-fluorouracil, drug absorption across intestinal epithelial cells involves transport by endogenous carrier proteins. In general, drug absorption from the GI tract is influenced by several factors including:

1. Physicochemical properties of the drug: particle size, lipophilicity, solubility, polymorphism, etc.,
2. Physiological variables of the gastrointestinal tract: gastric emptying, small intestinal transit time, pH, presystemic elimination, drug efflux, etc., and
3. Propensity for drug-, food-, or disease-related interactions.

Therefore, the net bioavailability of a drug as well as therapeutic effectiveness is highly variable compared to parenteral routes. However, due to high safety, patient convenience, compliance, and low cost, it is still by far the most preferred route.

Transdermal

This route of administration makes use of the readily accessible surface of human skin for achieving drug delivery into systemic circulation. The drug products typically are multi-layered patches that include either a layer of the active drug separated from the skin by a layer of rate-controlling polymer (membrane or reservoir-type) or where the active drug is dispersed in a matrix of rate-controlling material (matrix-type). This route of administration allows a noninvasive, zero-order drug input that delivers drug to the body at a constant rate with minimal fluctuations in the resultant serum drug concentrations. In addition, bioavailability via this route is improved compared to oral route, as it avoids the firstpass metabolism and drug instability in the GI environment. Patient compliance due to the noninvasive and less frequent nature of drug administration is another advantage. However, drug absorption may become erratic when the skin integrity is compromised due to an infection, injury, or in cases where the patch itself might become damaged. Contraceptives, hormone replacement therapies, analgesics, and smoking-cessation products are some of the commonly delivered treatments by means of this route. While most patches employ passive transdermal technology, i.e., drug delivery across a concentration gradient, due to the high dependence of this pathway on the physicochemical properties of the molecule including its molecular size and polarity, the number of molecules that are amenable to this route are limited. Use of active transdermal technologies that employ external driving forces to deliver a molecule through the skin, makes it feasible to achieve transport of large molecules such as peptides, proteins, and drugs with unfavorable physicochemical properties, which otherwise could not penetrate intact skin. Examples include the use of sonophoresis, iontophoresis, electroporation, heat or thermal energy.

Inhalation

This route is primarily used to treat diseases of the respiratory tract (e.g., bronchodilators and corticosteroids) and for the administration of anesthetics. It allows localized delivery of drugs for a faster onset of action and reduced systemic toxicity. Systemic absorption can also occur readily from the lungs due to the large surface area of the alveoli and can be employed for systemic drug therapy. It is also a noninvasive alternative for delivery of macromolecules such as peptides and proteins. Absorption from this route is also dependent upon the adaptability of a drug molecule to formulation processes critical for maximizing the inhalation and deposition. These include:

1. Particle size reduction,
2. Dispersability to form a fine aerosol,
3. Compatibility with excipients including solvents, suspending agents, permeation enhancers, polymers to achieve sustained release, and
4. Drug stability during formulation development and upon inhalation.

Intranasal

The intranasal route is commonly employed to achieve local therapeutic benefit for conditions such as allergic rhinitis, asthma (e.g., nasal decongestants, antihistamines, corticosteroids) or for local anesthetic effect (e.g., lidocaine). However, drugs administered into the nasal cavity can also be absorbed into the systemic circulation by means of the richly perfused and large surface area of the nasal mucosa. Absorption by this route bypasses the first pass metabolism, thereby allowing greater drug absorption to occur compared to the oral route for certain drugs. Because of the potential for improved bioavailability and a rapid onset of therapeutic effect, several drugs are administered via this route. These include selective 5-hydroxytryptamine receptor agonists for migraine relief, desmopressin for nocturia, insulin for diabetes, calcitonin for osteoporosis, and live influenza virus vaccine. Lipophilic drugs in general are readily absorbed through the nasal mucosa with bioavailability approaching close to that from an intravenous injection.

Absorption of polar drugs as well as large molecular weight peptides and proteins from nasal mucosa may be a challenge due to their low membrane permeability and also due to the rapid mucociliary clearance mechanism. Absorption enhancers such as surfactants, bile salts, phospholipids, cyclodextrins, chitosan, mucoadhesive agents have been demonstrated to improve the uptake of such therapeutic agents due to their varying effects on the nasal mucosa. Such effects include changes in the integrity of phospholipid bilayers, effects on the tight intercellular junctions of the epithelial membrane, inhibition of enzymatic activities, or simply by prolonging the residence time of the drug in the nasal cavity to promote absorption. In recent years, nasal route has also been explored as a pathway to achieve therapeutic drug concentrations in the brain, which may benefit treatment of central nervous system indications such as Parkinson's and Alzheimer's diseases. Some of the disadvantages of this route include the need for instilling small concentrated volumes of the drug, a smaller residence time, and irritation of the nasal mucosa.

Buccal and Sublingual

Drugs can be absorbed from the sublingual (floor of the mouth) and buccal (cheeks) mucosal membranes of the oral cavity because of the high permeability of these linings and their ability to retain a drug for prolonged duration. Drug absorption occurs directly from the oral cavity, bypassing the firstpass metabolism and can result in rapid achievement of therapeutic concentrations in the plasma and prompt therapeutic benefits. Nitroglycerin therapy for acute angina pectoris is a popular example of a drug that is benefited from this route of administration, resulting in pharmacological benefit after only one to two minutes. Other drugs that demonstrated benefit by means of this route include morphine, verapamil, nifedipine, captopril, and 17-beta estradiol.

Rectal

Rectal mucosa can be used for achieving systemic delivery of drugs such as antiemetics, antiepileptics, pain relievers, sedatives, and anesthetics. Although absorption from this route can be quite erratic, it is nevertheless a beneficial route for use in pediatric patients and for patients who are unable to swallow or retain an oral dosage form. The absorption from this route is influenced by several factors including:

1. Formulation characteristics
2. Drug concentration
3. Site of drug delivery
4. Temperature and pH of the rectal cavity
5. Presence of stools in the rectum
6. Retention of the dosage form and
7. Differences in venous drainage of the rectum

Drug Transport Across Biological Barriers

Physiological barriers to drug absorption exist in the form of membrane structures that prevent the cellular uptake of most charged, hydrophilic, large lipophilic molecules, or molecules attached to protein structures. Drug absorption from the site of administration into the systemic circulation as well as drug absorption from the systemic circulation to the sites of action is regulated by the presence of these cellular membranes.

The Fluid-Mosaic model describes the cell membrane as a fluid, dynamic structure comprised of phospholipids, proteins, and carbohydrates. In this model the phospholipids molecules are hypothesized to be arranged in a bilayer, with the polar groups in each layer oriented away from the center forming the inner and outer surfaces of the membrane, and the hydrocarbon chains of each layer aligned in the middle to form the core hydrophobic domain. This central hydrophobic domain represents the primary barrier to absorption of water-soluble molecules including drugs across cellular structures. While small, lipophilic molecules are able to diffuse easily through this lipophilic cell membrane, the presence of pores within the membrane allows the passage of essential molecules including water into and out of the cell. In addition, presence of interspersed transmembrane protein structures, either partially or completely embedded within the bilayer, enables the transport of some essential hydrophilic molecules. The presence of peripheral protein structures provide for structural integrity of the membrane.

In general, passage of drugs across cell membranes may involve transcellular (movement across the cell) or paracellular (movement between the cells) processes. Paracellular process is passive (not requiring external energy) and depending only on the size and shape of the drug molecule. Transcellular uptake processes can be passive, active, or facilitated, and are responsible for the membrane permeability of most drugs with a molecular weight above 200 daltons. Passive diffusion or simple diffusion is the most common mechanism of drug uptake across cell membranes. It is a nonenergy dependent, nonsaturable, concentration gradient-dependent spontaneous movement of drug molecules across cell membranes. As described by Fick' s Law of Diffusion, which states that the rate of diffusion, or flux

J of a species is proportional to the concentration gradient, movement of drug molecules occurs from a high concentration region to a low concentration region, and is influenced by various factors inherent to the drug molecule and the membrane such as the lipid solubility of the drug, the surface area, and thickness of the exposed barrier, as defined by the following equation:

$$J\ 1 = -DAK/L(C_o - C_i)$$

where J is the rate of diffusion, i.e., rate of solute flux from C_o to C_i, which represents the concentration difference between the outside and inside of the membrane structure across which the diffusion occurs; D is the diffusion coefficient (i.e., speed with which a molecule can move across the membrane as influenced by its size and shape); A is the surface area of the membrane (larger the surface area, greater is the amount of drug that passes through); K is the lipid-water partition coefficient, i.e., a measure of lipid solubility, one of the major determinant of the pharmacokinetic characteristic of drugs (K increases with increasing lipid solubility; because the cell membranes are lipophilic in nature, lipid-soluble drugs diffuse more freely than relatively lipid-insoluble drugs); and L is the membrane thickness (as thickness increases, rate of diffusion decreases); the term DAK/L is collectively known as the permeability constant "P," which is the number of molecules crossing the membrane per unit area in unit time. As the value of the permeability constant increases, the rate of drug equilibration across membranes increases.

Facilitated diffusion is a nonenergy dependent (passive), saturable process that is mediated by carrier proteins or ion channels (voltage-gated or ligandgated) that allow transport of selective molecules or ions down a concentration gradient. Because of the involvement of protein structures and hydrophilic channels this process is selective for a closely related group of molecules and is subject to competitive inhibition. Facilitated diffusion allows for the cellular passage of highly polar or ionized molecules such as glucose, sodium and chloride ions, and so on. The uptake of excess glucose from the blood and storage in the liver cells following a high carbohydrate meal as well as release of stored glycogen into the systemic circulation during hypoglycemic conditions involves facilitated diffusion by transporters across the hepatic cell membranes.

Vesicular transport involves the engulfing of fluid or small particulate (pinocytosis) and large particulate (phagocytosis) material by vesicles and vacuoles, which then fuse with the cell membranes to either transport/store (endocytosis) or release (exocytosis) molecules into and out of the cells. The release of insulin by pancreatic cells is a classic example of exocytotic vesicular transport.

Ion pairing occurs when highly charged ions, which are otherwise not permeable across cell membranes, form lipid-soluble complexes with oppositely charged ions. This results in the formation of a neutral molecule that has a polarity and hydrophobicity more suitable for partitioning into lipid phase of the membranes, than each ion by itself.

Active transport is an energy-dependent saturable process facilitating drug transport against concentration gradient. Transporters such as P-glycoprotein, organic anion transport protein, OATP, and System L transporters are known to affect absorption of endogenous and exogenous chemicals, including drugs from GI tract. P-glycoprotein (P-gp or MDR1) is a member of the efflux transporter classified as the ATP-binding cassette transporters. It is present in the brush border membrane of small intestine enterocytes and its efflux transport activity is responsible for low systemic absorption of a number of drugs. Its expression and efflux activity is also noted in liver, kidney, and endothelial cells of the blood-brain barrier and placenta. OATP subtype A, is expressed in the intestine and its uptake activity is responsible for absorption of drugs. Since P-gp and OATP are coexpressed in the intestine and share specificity for a variety of substrate drugs, coordinate activity of the efflux and uptake activities might determine the extent of drug absorption. System L consists of several basolateral membrane transporters, which mediate Na^+-independent transport of large neutral amino acids through the epithelial cells of blood-tissue barriers [blood- brain barrier (BBB) and placenta], small intestine, and renal proximal tubules. For example, gabapentin, a gamma amino butyric acid (GABA) analogue, is a substrate for this transporter and its absorption is limited at higher doses as explained by the saturation of this low capacity transporter activity.

Factors Influencing Drug Absorption

Physicochemical Factors Affecting Drug Absorption

Drug absorption is primarily a function of drug dissolution and membrane permeability of the dissolved drug. For hydrophilic or polar drugs, membrane permeability usually is the rate-limiting step for drug absorption, while for those drugs (small lipophilic or uncharged) that can easily penetrate the membrane barriers, drug dissolution in the aqueous GI fluids may be rate limiting. Therefore, physicochemical formulation as well as physiological factors of the GI tract that alter drug dissolution and permeability will ultimately influence the dose absorbed from the administration site into the systemic circulation. The Noyes-Whitney equation, which is an extension of the Fick' s First Law of Diffusion, suggests that the rate of dissolution of a drug in the GI tract is driven by its solubility in the GI contents and the surface area of the drug exposed to lumenal fluids. Factors that can influence drug solubility in the GI fluids include the drug's polymorphism, lipophilicity, and pKa in relation to the pH profile of the GI tract.

Polymorphism

Polymorphism is the ability of a substance to exist in more than one crystalline form, each differing in their arrangements and/or conformations of the molecules within the crystal lattice. Due to differences in their energies, polymorphs usually differ in physico-chemical properties including solubility and therefore may result in varying dissolution rates. A very large number of pharmaceuticals are shown to exhibit polymorphism, with solubility being affected by the nature of the polymorph for several drugs including diflunisal, chloramphenicol palmitate, glibenclamide, ketorolac, ranitidine, and ritonavir. Characterization of these polymorphs and understanding their potential for interconversion during the manufacturing or storage of a pharmaceutical is important to produce a pharmaceutical product of consistent bioavailability and biological effectiveness.

pKa and pH

According to the pH-partition theory, uncharged or neutral molecules are able to pass biological membranes (i.e., undergo passive diffusion) more efficiently due to their greater lipid solubility compared to ionized molecules that are not lipid soluble. Because most drugs are either weak acids or bases, the rate of permeation of these drugs is largely governed by the relative concentrations of their ionized and unionized species at the cell membrane. This in turn is dependent on the pKa of the drug as well as the pH of the environment as described by the Henderson– Hasselbalch equations.

For a weak acid that dissociates in presence of water by donating a proton to form an ionized species, Henderson–Hasselbalch equation is defined as

$$pH = pKa + \log[\text{ionized/unionized}],$$

where Ka is the dissociation constant of the weak acid (lower the pKa, stronger is the acid). Therefore, for a weak acid as pH increases, the concentration of unionized species decreases.

For a weak base that acts as a proton acceptor to form its molecular (unionized) species, Henderson–Hasselbalch equation is defined as

$$pH = pKa + \log[\text{unionized/ionized}],$$

where Ka is the dissociation constant of the weak base in presence of water (i.e., higher the pKa, stronger is the base). Therefore for a weak base as the pH increases, the concentration of the unionized species also increases. These equations facilitate the calculation of the relative concentrations of ionized and unionized (lipid-soluble) species of a drug at any given pH, provided Ka of the drug is known.

Particle Size

Decreasing the particle size of drugs may enhance the rate of solubilization by increasing the effective surface area of the drug that is exposed to the dissolution medium. Therefore, for those drugs with limited aqueous solubility, particle size plays an important role in determining the rate and extent of drug absorption. Examples of some drugs that demonstrate varying drug absorption with particle size include griseofulvin, phenacetin, digoxin, and nitrofurantoin. The gastrointestinal absorption of ultramicrocrystalline griseofulvin, a fungistatic agent is reportedly 1.5-fold greater than that of the microsize griseofulvin. Increased absorption due to a reduction in the particle size allows for the administration of lower doses with the ultramicrocrystalline compound (500 mg vs. 375 mg, once daily for the microsize griseofulvin).

Physiological and Pathological Factors Affecting Drug Absorption

Physiological factors at the site of administration also influence the drug absorption from a given dosage form. Dissolution of drugs into the surrounding medium and permeation across biological membranes represent the primary factors guiding the rate and extent of drug absorption.

pH profile of the gastrointestinal tract

The pH of the GI tract varies across its length, ranging from acidic (pH 1-3) in the stomach to alkaline (pH 7-8) in the large intestine. Drug absorption preferentially occurs in the slightly alkaline pH (6.5) of the small intestine. As explained earlier, most drugs are either weak acids or bases. The unionized or neutral form of the drug is preferentially absorbed across the lipophilic intestinal barriers. Depending on the pKa of the drug and the pH of the surrounding environment, the degree of unionized drug available for membrane transport varies. Therefore a small change in the pH of the environment is likely to cause a significant change in the percentage of unionized drug available for absorption. However, presence of even a small fraction of unionized drug is usually sufficient to allow absorption. This is because of the continual existence of equilibrium between the ionized and unionized forms that allows formation of more unionized drug whenever some of it is absorbed. In addition to its effect on ionization, the pH of the GI tract may also affect the absorption of a drug due to its potential influence on the stability and solubility of the drug.

Gastric emptying rate

Because most drugs are primarily absorbed from the small intestine, their absorption from the GI tract is influenced by the gastric emptying rate, which refers to the release of stomach contents into the first segment of the small intestine (i.e., duodenum). Increased or decreased gastric emptying may impact the stability, dissolution, as well as the rate and extent of absorption of a drug from the GI tract. For example, a direct correlation has been found between gastric emptying rate and systemic absorption of acetaminophen, a drug that has negligible absorption from the stomach. Prolonged residence of certain drugs like aspirin may irritate the stomach mucosa if the gastric emptying is delayed. For some drugs such as L-dopa, penicillin, the acidic pH of the stomach may result in loss of stability in the case where gastric emptying is prolonged. For some drugs with poor aqueous solubility, longer residence time in the stomach may aid in increased dissolution. Several factors have been shown to have varying influences on the gastric emptying rate: quality of ingested meals (volume, viscosity, temperature, pH, and composition), diurnal variations, age, presence of diseases or conditions (gastric ulcers, diabetes, peritoneal irritation, pregnancy, surgery, pain, and emotional stress), body posture, coadministration of alcohol, and drugs (anticholinergics, antihistamines, opioid analgesics, anesthetics, antacids, dopamine D2-receptor agonists, and antagonists).

Intestinal transit time

For maximal systemic absorption from the GI tract, a drug should reside at its intestinal site of absorption for an adequate amount of time before it undergoes elimination in the feces. Factors that influence the intestinal motility and thereby alter the transit time may therefore contribute to incomplete absorption of the drug from a dosage form. Presence of solid food in the small intestine delays the transit time, however, the net effect on absorption is variable due to the potential influences of the nutritional contents and viscosity of the food on drug dissolution at the site of absorption. Also, coadministered medications as well as presence of disease conditions such as dehydration or diarrhea may influence the net transit time and intestinal absorption of drugs from the GI tract.

Blood flow to the gastrointestinal tract

Ample blood flow to the small intestine is one of the factors responsible for the faster absorption rates from this region. Factors that may influence the blood flow to the GI tract such as presence of food in the gut, cardiac disease, exercise, and so on may therefore have an impact on the net absorption of drugs.

Effect of food on drug absorption

Presence of food in the GI tract may alter the rate and/or the extent of systemic absorption of a drug. The outcome of a food–drug interaction can be a delayed, reduced, or increased absorption and may depend on the physicochemical properties of the drug, the formulation excipients, and the degree to which these may influence the stability, disintegration, release, and dissolution of the drug in the GI tract. In addition, the volume and nutritional content of the coingested food as well as the time of food administration relative to drug intake also influence the food effect outcome due to their varying effect on the GI physiology. The largest food-effect is often observed with foods that are high in fat content and for this reason, the food-effect bioavailability and fed bioequivalence studies are often conducted in presence of high-calorie and high-fat meals.

Various intrinsic mechanisms may be involved in the observed effect of food on bioavailability of drugs, including postprandial changes in the gastrointestinal motility, gastric pH, biliary secretions, and blood flow that alter the GI residence time, solubility, intestinal permeability, and, ultimately, the systemic bioavailability of drugs. On the other hand, certain foods may induce or inhibit certain drug metabolizing enzymes in the GI tract (e.g., grapefruit juice), thereby altering the extent of presystemic metabolism of coadministered drugs and their resultant systemic bioavailability. While, an understanding of the type and magnitude of food-effect on the systemic absorption of a drug is often adequate to enable optimal dosage recommendations, knowledge of the mechanisms leading to the observed effect may prove beneficial; for example, when attempting to address the food-effect of a novel or altered formulation.

Delayed drug absorption (i.e., a prolonged T_{max}) in the presence of food may not usually warrant dosage adjustments as long as the extent of absorption is unaffected. In the case of NSAIDs (ibuprofen, ketoprofen, flurbiprofen, naproxen, etc.) a delayed absorption can be useful to avoid GI side effects of these drugs. Reduced drug absorption (i.e., lower AUC_{inf}) in presence of food may require that the drug be taken on an empty stomach (e.g., trospium chloride, rifampin). However, in some cases when the extent of decrease is not significant in terms of clinical outcome, dosage recommendations may not be needed. Increased drug absorption in presence of food, may have varying implications depending on the therapeutic index of the drug and the clinical utility or potential risk of an increased systemic drug exposure. While in some drugs increased drug absorption with food may be utilized to achieve maximal systemic bioavailability (e.g., itraconazole, ritonavir, saquinavir), for drugs with narrow therapeutic indices concomitant food intake may not be recommended due to increased frequency of adverse events (e.g., efavirenz).

Presence of high-fat food in the GI tract may increase the bioavailability of certain poorly soluble drugs as a consequence of their enhanced solubility in bile (e.g., griseofulvin, troglitazone, halofrantine). In addition to meals, many beverages including water, milk, juices, carbonated drinks, alcohol as well as nutrients such as iron, magnesium, calcium, and certain vitamins have been shown to influence the GI absorption of drugs due to their varying effects on rates of drug dissolution, gastric emptying, gastric pH, stability of the drug, as well as presystemic metabolism.

Drug–Excipient Interactions

The choice of excipients for use with an active ingredient in a formulation may impact the stability, solubility as well as bioavailability of the drug. Most interactions result in decreased stability of the drug (e.g., ascorbic acid and penicillin G, bisulfite and epinephrine, edetate salts and insulin, thiomerosal, amphotericin, hydralazine HCl, meta-cresol and chlorpromazine, amlodipine, fluoxetine and lactose, etc.). The absolute bioavailability of ranitidine from an immediate release encapsuled pellet formulation containing the excipients PEG 400 was found to be significantly reduced (from 51% to 35%). PEG 400 also affected the absorption rate of ranitidine as demonstrated via major differences observed in the T_{max} and C_{max}, suggesting that it adversely influences the GI absorption of ranitidine.

Presystemic Metabolic Enzymes and Transporters

Peptide drugs, such as insulin and heparin, are usually indicated for chronic conditions, requiring daily injections for a long-term treatment. Gastric digestive enzymes, in addition to acidic environment and bacterial degradation present a major hurdle in oral delivery of peptide drug molecules. Contribution of drug metabolizing enzyme expression and activity in GI tract as a major component of the first pass metabolism of drugs has been a subject of interest over the years. Some enzymes, particularly Cytochrome P450 (CYP) enzymes, have been extensively studied more so than others. Sufficient evidence is available to indicate the major role of intestinal CYP3A4 and CYP1A2 in the metabolism of drugs even before reaching systemic circulation.

Active transport mechanisms in GI tract, as discussed earlier, play an important role by themselves and also in conjunction with the drug metabolizing enzymes. For example, several researchers have noted the coexpression of drug metabolizing enzyme, CYP3A4, and drug efflux-transporter, P-glycoprotein, in the GI tract. Their co-expression is believed to limit the absorption of xenobiotics including a variety of drugs. Intestinal metabolism may be a major route of clearance for an orally administered CYP3A4 substrate (e.g., midazolam). Systemic absorption is limited due to P-gp mediated efflux for its substrates (e.g., digoxin). A combination of metabolism and efflux may limit the absorption of a CYP3A4 and P-gp substrate (e.g., cyclosporine).

Drug–Drug Interactions

Changes in drug absorption may occur because of physiological or physicochemical factors that are altered by precipitant drug. Some of the factors previously discussed, such as pH of gastric contents, gastric emptying time, presystemic metabolic enzymes, and transporters, might be altered due to the presence of another drug. Drugs that reduce gastric pH (antacids, H_2-antagonists, proton- pump inhibitors, etc.) might alter the solubility of a coadministered drug. Opioid drugs are known to cause delay in gastric emptying time. Depending on the physicochemical parameters, these physiological changes could result in changes in C_{max}, AUC or T_{max} of target drug. Oral clearance of drugs metabolized in intestine could be increased or decreased when coadministered with inhibitors or inducers of metabolic enzymes.

Drug–Disease Interaction

With regards to oral administration, GI diseases resulting in pH changes, gastric emptying time changes and, GI resection would potentially affect the absorption of drugs. However, the changes, to the distribution, and clearance of drugs due to celiac and inflammatory bowel diseases must be considered before attributing abnormal serum concentrations of drugs to malabsorption. GI disease may slow gastric emptying and delay the complete absorption of drugs when their rate of absorption depends on gastric emptying time. Other inflammatory GI diseases such as graft-versus-host disease (GVHD) of the gut, Behcet's syndrome, and scleroderma involving the GIT may directly reduce absorption of drugs such as acetaminophen, amitriptyline, certain anticonvulsants, benzodiazepines, and cyclosporine. Surgical resection drastically changes the anatomy of the GIT and alters important variables in the absorption process. Diminished small bowel surface area is shown to reduce the extent of absorption of phenytoin, digoxin, cyclosporin, aciclovir, hydrochlorothiazide, and certain oral contraceptives. The underlying cause of the reduction is unknown. When gastric emptying time or pH is altered by surgery, the rate of drug absorption appears to be reduced. However, it is not clear which variable is more important in determining therapeutic effects.

Tools for Assessing Drug Absorption

Use of drug absorption models early on in the drug development process increases the probability of success by identification of drug candidates with good absorption potential. Systemic bioavailability of drugs is a composite of processes that favor and inhibit absorption such as active/passive/facilitated uptake processes, removal via efflux transporters such as P-gp, degradation via drug metabolizing enzymes such as CYP450s. Therefore, early assessment of the relative contributions of each of these components to drug absorption is useful to eliminate potential "problem" drugs and identify those molecules that have good pharmacokinetic profile to go hand in hand with their biological effectiveness. Several in vitro and in vivo methods with a range of throughputs and predictabilities, as well as computational methods have been used with varying rates of success to predict drug absorption potential.

Cell Culture Models

The use of human colon adenocarcinoma-derived Caco-2 cell cultures as a model to mimic the morphological and functional characteristics of the mature enterocyte is well established and is routinely used for screening the intestinal permeability of discovery compounds. When grown on membrane filter supports, cultures differentiate into intestinal cell-like structures with morphological features such as microvilli, carrier-mediated transporters, tight junctions, efflux proteins, and enzymes. Drug transport from the donor compartment, across the monolayer-bearing membrane to the acceptor compartment is measured as the apparent permeability coefficient, P_{app}. While the physicochemical compatibility of the drugs for undergoing passive diffusion is understood by this method, due to the expression of efflux proteins such as P-gp and drug metabolizing enzymes such as CYP450s in these cells, the contribution of these processes to the overall drug delivery is also understood. Several improvements serve to enhance the in vitro prediction capabilities of Caco-2 cultures. These include novel high-throughput and automated techniques, isolation of more homogenous populations of clones to reduce heterogeneity, transfection of cells to improve the expression of specific transport proteins or drug metabolizing enzymes, and identification and standardization of culture-conditions to reduce variability in the morphology (growth media, type of membrane support, seeding density, etc.).

The Madin Darby canine kidney (MDCK) cell line is another model that mimics intestinal epithelium and is particularly suitable to evaluate the passive diffusion of drugs across membranes due to the low expression of transport proteins and drug metabolizing enzymes. The time for establishing a confluent culture and initiating the transport studies is also smaller (7–14 days) compared to Caco-2 cell line (21 days). In addition, MDR1-MDCK cells formed by the transfection of the MDCK cell line with the mdr1-gene are a useful model to screen potential P-gp substrates. Other in vitro cell cultures that mimic small intestine include TC7, LS180, 2/4/A1, HT29-18-C1, as well as cocultures of these cell lines with Caco-2.

Artificial Membranes

Parallel artificial membrane permeation assay or PAMPA is a high throughput tool with potential to screen compounds capable of undergoing transcellular passive diffusion. The methodology involves use of an artificial membrane that is formed by impregnating a mixture of lecithin and an inert organic solvent, into a hydrophobic filter material. The filter is placed in contact with a 96- well microtiter plate completely filled with aqueous buffer solutions and transport studies are initiated by the addition of drug solution on top of the filter plate, to determine its permeability across the artificial membrane. In addition, the effect of pH, phospholipid composition, and effect of surfactants, etc. on the membrane permeability of drugs can also be evaluated. Because this model is devoid of transporters, channels or efflux proteins, it is suitable for a high throughput screening of compounds with transcellular diffusion potential. Therefore, when a drug is classified to have "low" permeability by the PAMPA method, it still needs to be screened for paracellular or active transport, using other in vitro methodologies. Nevertheless, because of its potential to rapidly identify those molecules with "high" permeability under the conditions employed, it could be a very useful tool in early drug development.

Another high throughput technique for characterizing membrane partition coefficients of drugs is the use of IAM or immobilized artificial membrane chromatography. IAMs are chromatographic surfaces prepared by covalently immobilizing cell membrane phospholipids to solid surfaces at monolayer densities to mimic fluid cell membranes. The retention time of a solute on the IAM HPLC column is then measured to determine its membrane partition coefficient.

In Silico Methods

While cell culture-based evaluation of intestinal permeability requires actual synthesis of discovery drugs and is far too time-consuming to be adequately high throughput, in silico or virtual models can allow the absorption screening of thousands of computationally-designed drug-like molecules even before they are synthesized. Such models can predict the solubility and membrane permeability of lead molecules by estimating their physicochemical properties from available structural information alone. Molecules that have been prioritized by such methods can then be synthesized and carried further into drug development. Such computational models can be qualitative or quantitative in nature and are most suited for the screening of drugs absorbed by passive intestinal permeability and may not adequately predict the permeability of compounds that require active transport mechanisms.

Qualitative in silico models are developed by comparing the molecular descriptors of successful drug molecules to those of not-drug-like molecules and identify patterns in drug properties that may contribute to the observed differences. One such example is a model-generated "rule of five" by Lipinski et al., that states that poor absorption or permeation of a drug is more likely when there are more than 5 H-bond donors, 10 H-bond acceptors, the molecular weight is greater than 500, and the calculated Log P is greater than 5. Exceptions to this rule may occur when drugs are predominantly transported by active transport mechanisms.

Several quantitative models to predict intestinal drug absorption have also been developed. These models are derived from vast libraries of drugs and are based on the observed mathematical relationship between the structural features or structurally-derived descriptor parameters for these drugs and their percentage in vivo intestinal absorptions. An external data set containing drugs that are distinct from those used in the learning set is then used to validate these models to determine their reliability in estimating drug absorption potentials. Using such models, the intestinal absorption potential of new molecules and the effect of structural alterations on the intestinal permeability can be reliably estimated to aid in lead optimization.

While the earlier described models predict drug absorption based on the physicochemical properties of the drug and their interaction with the biological membranes, these do not consider the role of physiological factors of the GI tract such as the pH profile, gastric emptying time, intestinal transit time, and so on that could influence the net absorption of drugs. Physiological-based models of drug absorption have been developed that incorporate not only the physicochemical properties of the drug but also the known physiology of the GI tract into the model, thereby improving the prediction of membrane permeability.

Other techniques available for studying drug absorption include the in vitro techniques such as the everted rat intestinal sac model, use of Ussing-chambers, as well as in situ and in vivo perfusion of rat intestines. Although these methods are useful for obtaining information on the behavior of a drug in the GI environment, each comes with its own limitations including the loss of viability of the various isolated intestinal preparations, as well as the difficulty of extrapolating results obtained in animal models to humans.

In vivo assessment of drug absorption in humans using GI perfusion techniques provides the most thorough information on the role of GI physiology including presence of transporters, efflux proteins, enzymes, as well as physicochemical properties of drugs on their net absorption from the small intestine, although this may not be amenable for a high throughput screening. Catheters can be inserted through oral or nasal cavities of subjects under local anesthesia, for the perfusion of an open or isolated intestinal segment such as jejunum to study drug absorption, permeability and excretion of parent drug, and metabolites into the intestinal lumen. The regional intestinal perfusion is a closed segment approach that involves insertion into the desired region of the intestine, of a perfusion tube equipped with two occluding balloons, which when inflated generate an independent, perfusable intestinal segment. The intestinal segment is then perfused with the drug solution and an intravenous dose of the same drug is administered either simultaneously (using radio-labeled drug) or sequentially, following the perfusion experiment. By comparing the area under the plasma concentration-time curves of parent drug and metabolites for the intraluminal and intravenously administered drugs, it is possible to calculate the GI extraction of the drug.

Knowledge of specific factors affecting drug absorption is pivotal during drug development for making an appropriate choice of route of administration and optimal dosage form. The factors affecting the physiological functions and pathological conditions in humans and physicochemical properties of drugs together determine the fate of the drug. While it is difficult to prescribe the use of a single in vitro technique to predict in vivo drug absorption, use of several models is sure to improve our understanding of the absorption characteristics of a drug, early in development.

11

PHARMACOKINETICS OF NUCLEIC ACID-BASED THERAPEUTICS

Nucleic-acid-based therapies include various forms of gene and antisense therapeutics. Gene therapy encompasses the use of plasmid vectors, retroviral and lentiviral vectors, adeno-associated virus (AAV) and other methods of introducing a gene expression or gene silencing nucleic acid sequence into a target tissue or cell. Gene silencing has been achieved with ribozymes, small interfering double-stranded RNAs (siRNAs), and synthetic antisense oligonucleotides (ASOs), whether these are unmodified or chemically modified DNA or RNA structures. Additional chemically synthesized, but not natural, oligonucleotides include DNA-like peptide nucleic acids (PNAs) and phosphorodiamidate morpholino oligonucleotides (PMOs). Some nucleic-acid-based therapeutics are designed to influence the splicing of pre-mRNA to modify or alter the protein produced, rather than to silence the gene expression entirely. Many gene therapy and antisense approaches have unique applications based on local delivery, which limits the distribution of the therapeutic in the body and precludes considerations of their pharmacokinetics (PK).

Most PK studies of nucleic-acid-based therapies are, in fact, devoted to description of the PK properties of ASOs. Many academic and industry researchers have chosen to focus on the use and development of synthetic ASOs as therapeutics. RNA- and DNA-based ASOs designed against a large number of targets have progressed through preclinical stages and into clinical trials. As a consequence, there is a large body of literature describing the PK properties of these ASOs in animals and humans. We will first discuss the various chemical structures of ASOs being developed as therapeutics, and then we will focus on the published animal and human PK data regarding ASOs of two chemistries, exemplified by Genasense (Oblimersen, G3139, targeting the mRNA for the anti-apoptotic protein Bcl-2) and OGX-011 (targeting the mRNA encoding the chaperone protein clusterin).

The second major (and more recent) focus in the literature is on the PK properties of various embodiments of siRNA therapeutics. Excitement has grown recently with our increased understanding of the mechanisms responsible for the endogenous pathways of posttranscriptional gene silencing, also known as RNA interference (RNAi). This understanding has led to design and synthesis of expression vectors, short hairpin RNA (shRNA), and small interfering RNA (siRNA) molecules to reduce or silence expression of target genes. Although use of RNAi technology is widespread in laboratories, therapeutic applications are not yet as far advanced as for ASOs. Studies describing PK properties of siRNA in animal models are limited, and only three siRNA molecules are currently in human clinical trials.

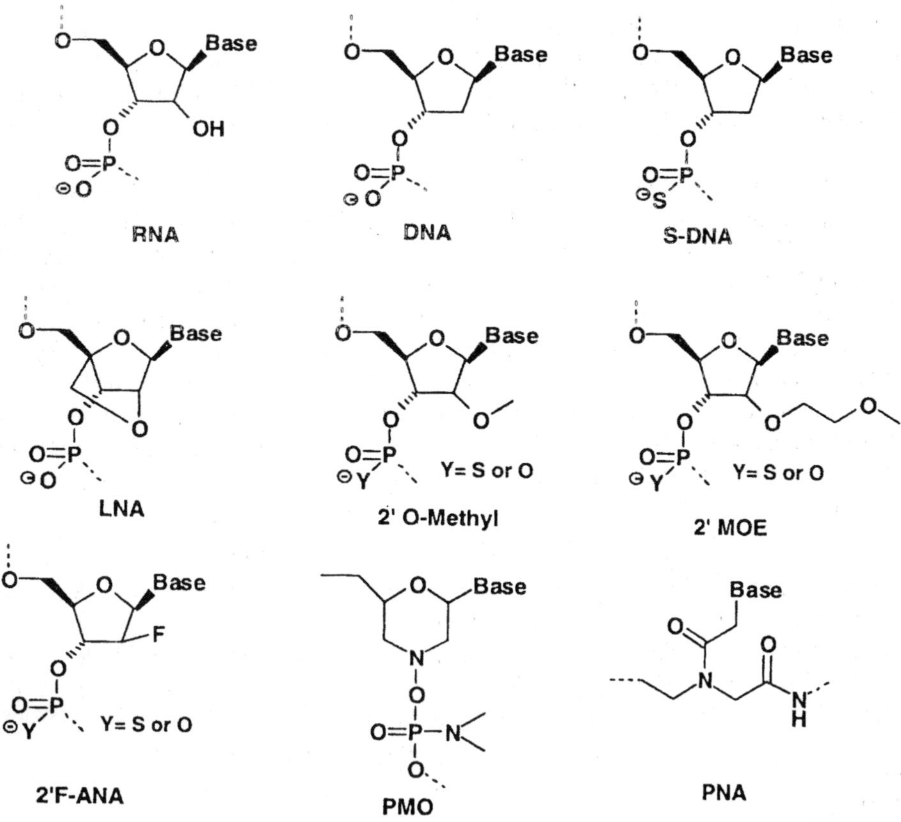

Fig. 11.1.Nucleic acid analogs and artificial backbones commonly used in ASOs and siRNAs.

Antisense Chemistries–Modifications to DNA/RNA Structure

ASOs are designed to reduce expression of a target protein based on double-stranded Watson–Crick base pairing with the mRNA coding for the protein. RNA-based ASOs act by inhibiting translation of the target mRNA, and subsequent normal protein turnover (degradation) results in reduced target protein levels in cells. DNA-based ASOs, also known as oligodeoxynucleotides (ODNs), mediate mRNA degradation by activation of endogenous ribonuclease H and subsequent exonuclease cleavage of the target mRNA. Again, routine protein turnover reduces target protein levels in cells in the absence of the mRNA to provide template for new protein synthesis. Advantages of ASOs over other nucleic-acid-based strategies include ease of delivery into cells and tissues, improved specificity for individual mRNA target molecules, flexibility in target choice and reagent design, and relative ease of chemical synthesis that facilitates large-scale production of pharmaceutical-grade material.

Early studies with unmodified phosphodiester (PD) DNA ASOs revealed various problems, including delivery into target cells and nuclease sensitivity in body fluids and in cells. Since then, numerous chemical modifications to the DNA structure have been incorporated into ASOs. One of the first improvements was inclusion of phosphorothioate internucleotide linkages (PS DNA), where the nonbridging oxygen is replaced with a sulfur atom. This improved stability against endo- and exonucleases inside cells and in body fluids. "Second generation" ASOs were designed to include 2´ methoxyethoxylation (2´-MOE), 2´-O-methyl, or other modifications of the ribose sugar group. These modifications at the 2´ position enhance uptake and stability of antisense ODNs, but they preclude

RNase H activity. ASOs containing 2′ modifications at the 5 or 6 nucleotides on each end, with DNA bases in the central region (called "gapmers"), retain the ability to provide a suitable target for ribonuclease H. Several PS DNA ASOs and gapmer ASOs have progressed through preclinical development stages, including PK and toxicological studies, and many are currently in human clinical trials.

In terms of PK properties, ASOs of the same chemistry but with different nucleotide base sequences seem to behave identically. In contrast, differences in PK profiles depend critically on the ASO chemistry and modifications. That is, ASOs with the same base sequence but having PS versus PD, or DNA versus RNA versus 2′-MOE modifications will have slightly or vastly different PK profiles. Furthermore, separately from PK properties, differences in the nucleotide sequence incorporated into ASOs with identical chemistry do affect physiological responses, including toxicities and off-target effects. For example, ASOs containing CpG dinucleotide motifs often activate particular toxicities and immune responses. Toxicological changes are also dependent on backbone and sugar modifications, such as activation of the complement cascade by ASOs with PS inter-nucleotide linkages but not by those with PD backbones. These toxicological issues are not discussed in detail here, but they have been reviewed recently elsewhere.

Additional Synthetic Chemistries

Several groups of researchers have been pursuing alternative synthetic chemistries to achieve the desirable properties of an ideal ASO. These include locked nucleic acids (LNAs), 2′- fluoroarabinonucleic acids (FANAs), PNAs, and PMOs. Only a limited number of ASOs with these chemistries have progressed to PK studies in rodent models, primate models, or human clinical trials. For brevity and due to the lack of human PK data, we will limit our discussion of these other chemistries.

Methods for Detection of ASOs in Tissues and Fluids

Labeled ASOs

In our work, we have used T4 polynucleotide kinase to end-label ASOs using radioactive [^{32}P]-γ-adenosine triphosphate (ATP). Methods to end-label or synthesize ASOs with biotin, fluorescein, digoxigenin, and so on, are also available. ASOs are amenable to internal labeling with radioactive halogens. Radioactively labeled ASOs are tracked using phospho-imaging, gel electrophoresis, and other techniques. Fluorescence microscopy is used to monitor fluorescently labeled ASOs, whereas detection of biotin-labeled ASOs is done with anti-biotin antibodies or avidin-conjugated enzymes and appropriate substrates.

Nondenaturing Polyacrylamide and Capillary Gel Electrophoresis

Acrylamide gels (15% to 20%) can be used effectively to separate ASOs from longer intact nucleic acids and shorter degradation products. Radio actively labeled ASOs are detected using standard autoradiography or phospho-imaging techniques. Using acrylamide gels cast in capillary tubes, ASOs can also be separated, identified, and quantified after electrophoresis. Absorbance at 260 nm, mass spectrometry, and so on, can be used to detect ASOs as they leave the capillary gels.

Hybridization-Based Approaches

Methods have been developed to detect ASOs in plasma and other biological samples, based on hybridization with labeled complementary probes. The probes are tagged at one end with biotin and the other end with digoxigenin. After hybridization and binding to neutravidin-coated 96-well plates, nuclease S1 is added to degrade unhybridized probe. Anti-digoxigenin antibodies and enzyme- linked secondary antibodies are then added sequentially, followed by enzyme substrate for detection and quantitation.

We have developed a hybridization approach to monitor the intracellular uptake and distribution of ASOs in cell culture experiments. Cells treated with ASOs were fixed in paraformaldehyde and then biotin-labeled complementary oligonucleotides were added in hybridization buffer. Detection was with an avidin–horseradish peroxidase conjugate, which cleaves diaminobenzidine to produce a colored precipitate within the cells. An alternative detection approach uses fluorescein-labeled streptavidin, which is visualized by fluorescence and/or confocal microscopy. We are currently adapting this protocol for use on tissue and tumor sections taken from mice treated systemically with ASOs.

A hybridization-based approach has also been developed to quantitate levels of ribozymes in serum using paired complementary oligonucleotide probes, one labeled with biotin and the other with digoxigenin. The annealed "triplex" is first collected on streptavidin-coated 96-well plates, then an anti-digoxigenin antibody conjugated with alkaline phosphatase is added, followed by addition of the enzyme substrate p-nitrophenyl phosphate, which is cleaved into a soluble colored product that is quantitated by absorbance at 405 nm.

Routes of Administration

As with any drug, the PK profile of nucleic-acid-based therapeutics varies according to the route of administration. Before focusing on the PK properties of ASOs administered intravenously, we briefly discuss the published PK analysis of topical, inhaled, and oral formulations of ASOs. To date, topical administration has not progressed past preclinical animal models, although these include human skin transplanted (grafted) onto immunocompromised mice. The distribution of ASOs applied to the skin is generally limited to epidermis and dermis, and it may be limited in intact skin but more advantageous in conditions that include inflammation or other damage, especially psoriasis. Distinct chemistries of ASOs, such as second-generation versus PMOs, may behave differently when applied topically. Furthermore, the formulation of the application compound and the use of delivery methods such as sonophoresis (ultrasound) may also affect the delivery and PK properties of ASOs applied topically.

Respirable, or inhaled, ASOs have been developed as potential therapeutics for treatment of asthma, allergic rhinitis, and other pulmonary diseases. In animal models including rodents and rabbits, inhaled ASOs are detectable in all cell types in the lungs but only in small amounts (<5–10% of the administered dose) in extra-pulmonary organs, and they exhibit minimal systemic bioavailability of intact, full-length ASO. Less than 5% of the delivered dose was detected in the lung 72 hours after treatment (the elimination half-life is approximately 30 hours). At 72 hours, nearly 70% of the administered dose was excreted in the urine, the major pathway of elimination. ASOs designed and formulated for delivery by inhalation may have particular strengths as potential therapeutics for pulmonary diseases. One ASO, EPI-2010 (targeting the adenosine signaling pathway in asthma), completed phase I and II human trials, but further development was not pursued due to reduced efficacy in important patient markets.

Stability of unmodified DNA ASOs is limited after oral administration, due to degradation in the stomach and small intestine. Although backbone and ribose modifications substantially improved the stability of ASOs administered orally, intestinal permeability of ASOs is limited due to hydrophilicity, high negative charge, and high molecular mass. Formulation of ASOs in sodium caprate further improves stability and intestinal permeability of orally administered ASOs. Oral formulations have progressed to animal studies in rodents, pigs, and dogs, but not yet to human trials.

Lipid delivery vehicles such as stealth liposomes and cationic liposome formulations, and additional vehicles such as polymers of chitosan, are being pursued as potential means to improve uptake and distribution of ASOs. Although these novel formulations and alternative routes of administration might ultimately prove to be more successful, the intravenous route has been the most successful thus far in the development of therapeutic ASOs.

PK of ASOs Administered by Injection

Several routes of administration, including intraperitoneal (i.p.), intravenous (i.v.), intradermal (i.d.), or subcutaneous (s.c.) injection, have been compared in animal models. PK profiles of ASOs in animals correlate well with those observed in human clinical trials, where ASOs are usually administered by i.v. or s.c. injection.

Absorption and Distribution

ASOs are highly bound to albumin and α_2-macroglobulin in the blood, with binding affinities in the micro- to millimolar range. In mice, rats, monkeys, and humans, more than 96% of administered PS ASO was bound to plasma proteins. This high protein binding affinity limits renal clearance, but PS ASOs are rapidly cleared from plasma to tissues. Plasma clearance is dose-dependent, with plasma half-life ranging from 30 to 60 minutes. Widespread systemic distribution of ASOs is observed after i.d. and s.c. injections, but s.c. injection resulted in increased bioavailability and steady-state ASO levels. Minimal differences in distribution were observed when comparing i.p and i.v. injection. In animal models, ASOs accumulated to highest levels in the liver and kidney, followed by spleen and lung, with only minor distribution to the brain and testes. Distribution was independent of ASO length and nucleotide sequence. Subcutaneous tumor xenografts accumulated levels of ASOs similar to spleen and lung. Recent clinical trials of G3139 also measured similar disposition of intact and partially shortened ASO in humans, as discussed below.

Metabolism and Elimination

Metabolism of ASOs occurs primarily through degradation by exonucleases and endonucleases. Degradation products have lower protein binding affinity and higher solubility, facilitating their excretion in urine and exhaled air.

PK Properties of 2′-MOE, PS, and PD ASOs

In a recent study the PK profiles of three distinctly modified ASOs were compared after i.v. injection into monkeys. They compared a PD ASO with 2′-MOE modifications on all nucleotides, a PS ASO with 2′-MOE modifications only on the eight 3′-end residues, and a PS ASO with 2′-MOE modifications on the six nucleotides on each end (i.e., a gapmer). The plasma half-lives of the two PS ASOs were similar (~45 minutes), whereas that of the PD ASO was markedly shorter (~14 minutes). The two PS ASOs also had very similar tissue distribution, with the highest concentrations in kidney, liver, lymph nodes, and spleen. However, the gapmer exhibited a significantly longer tissue half-life, compared with the ASO with only the 3′ MOE modifications (~22 days vs. -5 days). This suggests that the presence of both 5′-end and 3′-end MOE modifications on the gapmer protects the ASO from degradation in tissues and that the position of the modifications could significantly affect biological lifetime and efficacy in a clinical setting. This study confirmed that the chemistry of the ASO contributes to PK behavior and nuclease sensitivity, as suggested by earlier studies. Although the extent of the 2′ -MOE modification did not alter the distribution properties, the presence of this modification is important in the tissue distribution patterns and in determining nuclease resistance within tissues.

PK Analyses from Selected Clinical Trials

Several clinical trials using Genasense (G3139, a PS DNA ASO targeting the anti-apoptotic protein Bcl-2) have included detailed PK analyses. One of the earliest trials of G3139 used a 14-day continuous subcutaneous infusion at doses ranging from 4.6 to 195.8 mg/m^2/day. The mean plasma half-life of G3139 was 7.46 hours. More recent trials measured PK profiles of G3139 administered at 7 mg/kd/ day by continuous i.v. infusion for 8 days, 10 days, or 5 days. All showed similar PK results for plasma clearance, metabolism, and urinary excretion.

The first report of administration into humans of a 2´-MOE gapmer (ISIS 104838, targeting tumor necrosis factor α) included extensive PK analysis of blood and urine samples. This trial also compared i.v. and s.c. dosing regimens. The plasma half-life of the ASO was 1 to 1.8 hours at doses greater than 1 mg/kg. Urinary excretion of full-length ASO during the initial 24 hours postadministration was less than 10%, whereas excretion of 8 to 12 nucleotide metabolites (i.e., degradation products) increased over time thereafter.

Similarly, a recent clinical trial of the 2´-MOE gapmer OGX-011 (targeting the chaperone protein clusterin) in prostate cancer patients indicated dose-dependent PK and pharmacodynamic properties. Plasma distribution half-lives ranged from 0.476 to 3.83 hours, and other plasma PK parameters were similar to the PS ASO G3139. Estimates of ASO concentrations in the target tissue ranged from 1.67 to 4.82 μg/g of prostate tissue, depending on the dose of ASO delivered. Metabolism and elimination were not measured in the study.

Target Downregulation in Tissues of Interest

Drug efficacy for ASOs can be measured in terms of reductions in target mRNA and protein. The outcomes of drug treatment are not formally PK issues, but they are within the realms of pharmacodynamics and toxicology. It is important to consider, however, how the PK profile of a systemically administered ASO affects the pharmacodynamic and toxicological properties of the drug. Many clinical trials of ASOs include some measures of target mRNA and protein in target or surrogate marker tissues. In one of the early trials of the PS DNA ASO G3139 in patients with non-Hodgkin's lymphoma, Bcl-2 mRNA and protein were demonstrably reduced in isolated peripheral blood lymphocytes, but only in 7 of 16 patients. Recent clinical trials have shown similar interpatient variability in target down- regulation. In the case of ASOs targeting clusterin, *in vitro* experiments revealed the improved efficacy of 2´-MOE modified gapmers compared with PS DNA ASOs. Superior target downregulation and increased antitumor activity were also demonstrated in animal models of prostate cancer tumor growth. Dose-dependent reductions in clusterin mRNA and protein in prostate tumor samples were also shown in the phase I clinical trial of OGX-011, indicating that the intended biological activity was achieved in the intended target tissue. This represents a tremendous success for antisense therapeutics and should provide encouragement for others developing ASOs as potential clinically useful drugs.

RNA INTERFERENCE

RNA interference (RNAi) is a cellular regulatory mechanism in which double-stranded RNA (dsRNA) induces the specific degradation of its homologous target mRNA. This process was discovered by Guo et al. who found that injection of both antisense and sense RNAs into *Caenorhabditis elegans* resulted in a decrease of their target mRNA. Several years later, Fire et al. demonstrated that this observation was due to the single-stranded RNA populations containing small amounts of double-stranded RNAs. Using highly purified RNA preparations, they showed that dsRNA injected into *C. elegans* resulted in specific and potent interference of cellular gene expression. This inhibition was much greater than that observed with injection of either the antisense or the sense strands by themselves. The molecular mechanism of RNAi involves cleavage of dsRNAs by an RNase III-like endonuclease termed Dicer into 21–25 nucleotide (nt) dsRNAs. These small interfering dsRNAs (siRNAs) are bound in a multiprotein RNA-induced silencing complex (RISC), which unwinds the siRNA, and one strand is then used as a guide to target complementary mRNAs for degradation.

RNAi gained rapid acceptance as a tool for functional genomics in *C. elegans* and *Drosophila* model systems. It was initially unclear as to whether RNAi existed in mammalian cells, because treatment of mammalian cells with dsRNA results in global degradation of RNAs and repression of protein synthesis. As researchers toiled diligently to understand the detailed molecular mechanisms involved in the RNAi pathway, Elbashir et al. identified 21- to 22-nt dsRNAs as the effector molecules that induce RNAi in *Drosophila* embryos. Additionally, they demonstrated that chemically synthesized siRNAs could be transfected into mammalian cells and induce RNAi without inducing global RNA degradation. Since this discovery, the field of siRNA and related methodologies has grown at an exponential rate. Although siRNAs have competed with ASOs as tools for functional genomic analysis and target validation, one primary interest is to develop siRNAs as thera peutic agents.

siRNA Specificity

One of the most important issues regarding development of new pharmaceuticals is their specificity of effect. The overall intent is to design molecules that inhibit their intended target without undesirable side effects. As with ASOs and other nucleic-acid-based therapies, demonstrating that the observed cellular affects are due to inhibition of the intended mRNA target remains a challenge. Initial studies suggested that one or two mismatches could alleviate the silencing ability of an siRNA. However, recent studies have identified siRNAs with effects on unintended targets with as little as seven complementary nucleotides. Moreover, in addition to the G:U wobble base pair, it has been shown that mismatches formed between adenine (A) and cytosine (C) are well tolerated. Thus, the ability of siRNAs to specifically downregulate predicted targets is being called into question.

Many investigators have turned to microarray analysis to validate the specificity of their siRNAs. This approach may nonetheless provide researchers with a false sense of specificity. Saxena et al. showed that siRNAs with multiple mismatches located in the center of the molecule can function as micro-RNAs that inhibit expression of the target protein through translational arrest and not mRNA degradation. Thus, the microarray patterns from two different siRNAs targeting the same mRNA may be similar, but the siRNAs could still inhibit protein expression through translational inhibition. It remains unclear to what extent each of these potential nonspecific effects may impact their potential therapeutic use. With a more thorough understanding of the RNAi mechanism, new selection guidelines will identify optimal target sites that account for these sequence-based nonspecific effects. Identification of the most active siRNA with limited nonspecific effects will be critical for the success of siRNA molecules as therapeutic agents.

Cell Culture

Since their discovery only a few years ago, many researchers in both academic and industrial settings have used siRNAs to knock down mRNA targets within cultured cells. Unlike ASOs, which can enter cells by themselves when used at high concentrations, siRNAs cannot cross the cellular membrane by themselves due to their two negatively charged phosphate backbones. Cationic lipids such as Lipofectamine 2000 (L2K) and Oligofectamine are commonly used to complex the siRNA and allow uptake into cultured cells. However, a recent publication has demonstrated that cationic lipids can have unintended effects. Fedorov et al. transfected siRNAs into HeLa cells using either L2K or electroporation and performed microarray studies. Although both transfection methods resulted in a similar knockdown of the target mRNA, the number of genes affected by each method differed significantly. Lipid transfection resulted in increased expression of 65 genes, whereas electroporation increased only 11 genes. Over 50% of the upregulated genes could be directly attributed to L2K. Because L2K is also commonly used for transfecting DNA plasmids and ASOs, investigators should thoroughly examine the effect that the transfection reagent has on gene expression patterns. In addition to these lipids, other cationic molecules such as cell-penetrating peptides and polyethyleneimine have also been used to transport siRNAs across the cell membrane. Further studies are needed to determine what affects these transport molecules have on global gene expression.

In vivo Studies with "Naked" siRNAs

Although most siRNA researchers will readily acknowledge that the siRNAs are more potent than the ASOs and result in a more potent and reproducible target suppression, others have shown siRNAs to be equivalent to ASOs. The real difference between these two approaches becomes clear once the nucleic acids are injected into animals. ASOs have therapeutic activity even when they are injected intravenously without any cationic carrier molecule, as discussed in the preceding section. Although most studies show that naked siRNA injections have no effect, some have demonstrated that uncomplexed, unmodified siRNAs can be injected into animals and inhibit the target protein in tissues. Verma et al. intravenously injected approximately 3 μg of a β-catenin-targeted siRNA into the tail vein of tumor-bearing nude mice. After 72 hours, tumors were harvested and significant decreases in β-catenin protein levels could be observed by Western blot analysis. Similarly, Filleur et al. injected intraperitonealy 3 μg of siRNAs targeting either luciferase or vascular endothelcal growth factor (VEGF) and could demonstrate a 50% reduction in luciferase activity and a 70% reduction in VEGF expression. VEGF siRNA injections also delayed the onset of tumors. Furthermore, Duxbury et al. delivered similar amounts of an siRNA targeting ribonucleotide reductase mRNA. After 6 weeks of biweekly tail vein siRNA injections, the levels of target protein in the tumor were suppressed and a small decrease in the tumor growth rate was observed. More importantly, the combination of the siRNA and gemcitabine resulted in a synergistic suppression of tumor growth. The control siRNA did not enhance the antitumor affect of gemcitabine. All of these results using naked siRNAs are surprising because siRNAs are rapidly degraded in plasma with a half-life of about 3 minutes. Given that many investigators have shown that unmodified, uncomplexed siRNAs have little to no activity, it remains unclear as to whether systemic injection of unprotected siRNAs is a viable therapeutic option.

Hydrodynamic High-Pressure "Naked" siRNA Injection

To overcome the problem of siRNA delivery into tissues, several investigators have employed the high-pressure hydrodynamic method. This method involves rapid injection of siRNA in a large volume (1–2 mL) of saline or phosphate-buffered solution (PBS). Surprisingly, the mice can tolerate this harsh administration quite well. Song et al. was able to reduce Fas mRNA and protein levels in mouse liver for up to 10 days after hydrodynamic injection (50 μg siRNA in 1-mL PBS). They also demonstrated that Fas siRNA in-jection could protect mice from fulminant hepatitis. Another group targeted caspase 8 with siRNAs and showed decreased liver expression of caspase 8 and prevented Fas (CD95)-mediated apoptosis after hydrodynamic injection (120-μg siRNA in 2-mL PBS). As with the previous Fas-targeted approach, caspase 8 siRNAs improved the survival of two animal models of acute liver failure. Layzer et al. used quantitative whole-body imaging to demonstrate that hydrodynamic coinjections of luciferase reporter plasmids and luciferase-targeted siRNAs could reduce luciferase expression by 85%. Injection of a nuclease-resistant 2′-F siRNA resulted in a similar reduction in luciferase expression. However, if siRNAs were injected under low pressure, no decrease in luciferase activity was observed. Although the use of hydrodynamic injection in animal models is relatively simple and effective, it is not feasible in the clinical setting. An additional limitation of this methodology is that the liver is the primary organ for siRNA uptake with only limited uptake in other tissues.

Chemically Modified siRNAs

Contrary to the studies demonstrating activity with unmodified siRNAs, the major limitation for the use of nucleic acids as therapeutic agents is their susceptibility to attack from serum and intracellular nucleases. The antisense field has identified a host of ribose ring and phosphate backbone modifications that enhance the stability of ASOs. Extensive analysis has been performed to demonstrate which chemical modifications enhance siRNA stability and still allow for efficient silencing. Altering the phosphate backbone of an siRNA to phosphorothioate reduces its ability to induce RNAi by 50% and increases nonspecific cellular toxicity. Designing siRNAs entirely with 2´-O-methyl moieties improves their nuclease stability dramatically and eliminates their silencing ability. One nucleotide modification that seems to be the most promising is the 2´-fluorine modification on the cytidines and uridine residues. 2´-F-modified siRNAs have plasma half-lives of days instead of minutes and can inhibit their targets with similar potency as the unmodified siRNAs. Researchers at Sirna Therapeutics have developed siRNAs in which all 2´-OH groups have been substituted with deoxy-, 2´-O-methyl-, or 2´- fluoronucleotides, which are termed "short interfering nucleic acid" (siNA). In human serum, siNAs have a half-life on the order of 3 days. Using a hepatitis B viral mouse model, they injected HBV-targeted siNAs by standard low-pressure tail vein injections (60–600-μg siRNA) thrice daily for 2 days. After 24 hours, the levels of serum HBV DNA were significantly reduced in a dose-dependent manner. The inverted control siNA had little to no effect on serum levels of HBV DNA. No significant antiviral activity was observed with unmodified siRNAs at any dose. Although this study demonstrated *in vivo* activity of a fully modified siRNA, it is uncertain whether these siNAs are effectively taken up into tissues by standard intravenous injections. One assumes that lower serum titers are the result of lower viral production from the tissues, but no data were presented regarding decreased HBV tissue expression. Given the high doses required for activity, more studies are needed to validate the therapeutic effectiveness of siNAs.

Ligand-Mediated siRNA Delivery

Another approach to improve tissue delivery of siRNAs is to attach small molecules on the end of the siRNA. Soutschek et al. conjugated a cholesterol molecule on the 3´-end of the sense strand of a partial chemically modified siRNA to generate "chol-siRNA". A chol-siRNA targeting luciferase could reduce luciferase expression in HeLa cells with an IC50 of about 200 nM without any transfection reagents. Upon intravenous injection into animal models, the addition of cholesterol improved the siRNAs pharmacokinetic properties by increasing the elimination half-life and reducing plasma clearance in rodents. Chol-siRNAs, as detected by RNase protection assay, were broadly distributed throughout the tissues of the mouse confirming the improved pharmacological properties. No detectable amounts of unconjugated siRNAs were observed in any tissues. Intravenous injections of a chol-siRNA targeting apolipoptrotein B (1 mg) daily for 3 days resulted in inhibition of apoB mRNA in liver and intestine, decreased serum levels of apoB protein, and a reduction of total plasma cholesterol. Hence, this study demonstrated the importance of conjugating a small molecule to the siRNA that will enhance tissue uptake. However, further optimization is required to identify modifications that will permit more clinically acceptable doses and schedules.

Intranasal siRNA Injection

As an alternative approach to systemic siRNA injections, several groups have demonstrated that intranasal administration of siRNA can be effective for certain disease applications. X. Zhang et al. were the first to demonstrate that unmodified siRNA could be administered intranasally and silence the intended target mRNA without the need for transfection agents. Bitko et al. designed siRNAs targeting the respiratory syncytial virus and parainfluenza virus. A single intranasal siRNA administration (70 μg) provided significant protection against respiratory infection from viral challenge. Two days after intranasal injection, siRNAs could still be detected in the mouse lungs. There are several advantages for this route of administration. It is relatively painless and noninvasive. The risk of potential side effects is also reduced because no cationic carrier molecules are required for cellular uptake. It remains unclear as to the mechanism of cellular uptake after intranasal siRNA administration.

***In vivo* Studies with Encapsulated siRNAs**

An alternative approach for *in vivo* delivery of siRNAs is to encapsulate or complex the siRNA with cationic molecules. These positively charged molecules serve several functions. After interacting with the negatively charged phosphate backbone of the nucleic acid, they condense the nucleic acid into a more compact structure, protect against degradation by plasma nucleases, and enhance tissue uptake. The use of these cationic synthetic molecules is not limited to siRNA delivery. ASOs and DNA plasmid vectors can also be delivered with these molecules. As well, it remains unclear as to whether chemical modifications to the siRNA are necessary if one is using cationic molecules for delivery. In cell culture, lipid- complex siRNAs are protected from degradation by serum nucleases. One benefit of using natural, unmodified siRNAs is that when they actually do degrade, the nucleotides should not have any nonspecific effects of cellular metabolism.

Linear Polyethylenimine

The cationic molecule polyethylenimine (PEI) has been shown to effectively transport nucleic acids into cells in both the *in vitro* and the *in vivo* setting. PEI condenses nucleic acids into 0.2–0.4-nm positively charged particles, is taken up into cells by endocytosis, and then releases the nucleic acid contents into the cytoplasm efficiently via a process called the "*proton sponge*". Urban-Klein et al. demonstrated that PEI complexation of an unmodified siRNA protects the siRNA from nuclease degradation. In cultured ovarian carcinoma cells, they showed that linear low-molecular-weight PEI could transport their HER2-targeted siRNA into cells, inhibit HER2 protein expression by 70%, and reduce colony formation by 50% with a single PEI/siRNA transfection. In a tumor-bearing nude mouse model, intraperitoneal injection of PEI/siRNA resulted in a rapid uptake of the P32-labeled siRNA into the tumor, muscle, liver, and kidney with little uptake into the lungs. No siRNA was observed in the tissues after injection of uncomplexed siRNAs. As they observed no histological changes in the lungs and the absence of visible side effects, intraperitoneal injections of PEI/siRNA seem to avoid systemic PEI-associated toxicity previously reported. Furthermore, they showed that intraperitoneal injections of PEI/HER-2 siRNA (10 μg) two to three times a week significantly reduced growth of tumor xenografts. HER2 mRNA levels were inhibited by 50% by this treatment regimen. As important controls for specificity, injection of either a nonspecific siRNA complexed with PEI or uncomplexed HER-2 siRNA had no effect on tumor growth. However, a recent report demonstrated that tail vein injections of PEI along with other cationic molecules can have antitumor activity by themselves. Although this effect may be cell-line dependent, caution should be used when interpreting the therapeutic effects of siRNAs when cationic molecules are used for delivery.

One main concern with using PEI as a nucleic acid transporter is the lack of tissue specificity. To improve the ability of PEI to target tumors, Schiffelers et al. designed ligand-targeted, sterically stabilized nanoparticles (RPPs) for complexation with siRNAs. These particles comprise branched PEI that is PEGylated with an RGD peptide on the end of the polyethylene glycol (PEG). Once the siRNA is complexed in the nanoparticles, the RGD peptide should preferentially target the tumor neovasculature. One hour after intravenous injection of a fluorescently labeled siRNA complexed with RPP, significant siRNA uptake was observed in the tumor with poor liver and lung accumulation. Conversely, siRNA complexed with only branched PEI did not accumulate in the tumor to any appreciable extent but did accumulate in the liver and lung. To verify whether the siRNA distributed into the tumor was active, they evaluated the expression of luciferase in the tumor and its knockdown by a siRNA specific for luciferase. Thus, luciferase was complexed with either PEI or RPP particles and injected into tumor-bearing mice. Although luciferase levels in the tumor were equivalent for both PEI and RPP particles, only RPP could selectively target the tumor. Two hours after plasmid injections, luciferase siRNA-RPP nanoparticles were injected into the same mice. After 24 hours, the luciferase activity had decreased by 90% demonstrating sequence-specific inhibition. To evaluate whether these nanoparticles have therapeutic potential, siRNAs targeting the VEGF receptor were complexed with RPP and injected into tumor-bearing mice every 3 days at a dose of 40 μg administered in the tail vein. They observed a strong inhibition of tumor growth, a reduction in blood vessel formation around the tumor, and a decrease in the expression of tumor VEGF R2 protein levels. The control siRNA had no effect, demonstrating specificity.

Cationic Lipids

In addition to PEI-related molecules, various cationic lipids have been used for nucleic acid transport *in vivo*. Lipids such as the commercially available DOTAP have been effective in delivering siRNAs into tissues such as kidney and spleen. Others have developed their own delivery lipids. Yano et al. designed a less-toxic cationic liposome (LIC-101) and demonstrated its *in vitro* ability to deliver a Bcl-2-targeted siRNA into four different cell lines and inhibit Bcl-2 protein expression. Furthermore, tail vein injection of LIC-101/Bcl-2 siRNA inhibited tumor growth in two different mouse models. Chien et al. developed a novel cationic liposome based on a synthetic cationic cardiolipin analog (CCLA). They showed their lipid had significantly less-toxic side effects than DOTAP and could suppress tumor growth by >70% in a severe combined immunodeficiency (SCID) mouse xenograft model. Injection of a mismatched siRNA complexed with CCLA had no effect on tumor growth. Morrissey et al., in an attempt to improve delivery of their HBV-targeted siRNA, incorporated their siRNA into a specialized liposome to form a stable nucleic-acid–lipid particle (SNALP). In a mouse model, an unmodified siRNA had a plasma elimination half-life of approximately 2 minutes. Injection of a nuclease-stabilized siRNA improved substantially the elimination half-life to 49 minutes. However, siRNA encapsulation in SNALP improved the plasma pharmacokinetics most dramatically with an elimination half-life of 6.5 hours. They demonstrated that SNALP–siRNA could significantly suppress serum levels of HBV in HBV-challenged mice with much lower doses and reduced dosing frequency than previously shown with uncomplexed siRNA.

siRNAs in Clinical Trials

Although some uncertainly remains for the feasibility and effectiveness of siRNA therapeutics, several companies are rapidly moving ahead with siRNA molecules in clinical trials. In the Fall of 2004, Acuity Pharmaceuticals initiated the first human siRNA clinical trial for treatment of wet age-related macular degeneration (AMD) with their lead compound Cand5, which silences VEGF. Phase I studies showed that intravitreal injections of an unmodified siRNA, Cand5, was safe and well tolerated. Pharmacokinetic analysis revealed that the siRNA was not detected in the plasma of any patient. Lack of systemic exposure due to localized siRNA injection likely prevented the adverse side effects of anti-VEGF therapy. However, given that unmodified siRNAs are very unstable in plasma, it is unclear whether the siRNA could not escape the vitreal cavity or whether it was degraded so rapidly after entry into the bloodstream that it could not be detected in plasma. Acuity Pharmaceuticals has already initiated phase II studies with its lead siRNA candidate. The second siRNA to enter clinical trials was Sirna-027 from Sirna Therapeutics. Although both Cand5 and Sirna-027 are being investigated for treatment of AMD, Sirna-027 targets the VEGF receptor as opposed to VEGF, and is chemically modified to enhance stability. Interim phase I results were recently reported and demonstrated that Sirna-027 seems to be safe and well tolerated. All patients experienced improvement or stabilization of visual acuity, and 23% of the patients showed a clinically significant improvement in visual acuity. A third company (Alnylam Pharmaceuticals) has recently initiated a phase I study with its siRNA (ALN-RSV01), which targets respiratory syncytial virus. Using their Direct RNAi approach, the siRNA will be administered directly to the lungs and silence a key RSV gene, which hopefully will prevent spreading of the viral infection.

Other pharmaceutical companies are also seeking to initiate their own siRNA clinical trials. An Australian company (Benitec) in collaboration with the City of Hope is planning to enter their RNA-based HIV drug into clinical trials sometime in 2006. Unlike Cand5 and Sirna-027, which are siRNA molecules, Benitec specializes in RNAi plasmid and vector expression systems. Patients who have become resistant to HAART therapy would receive a transplant of their own stem cells containing an RNAi expression system targeting HIV to generate HIV resistance. Nucleonics, Inc. also uses RNAi expression systems for gene silencing and expects to file its first IND for hepatitis B and hepatitis C in 2006. CytRx Corporation is rapidly advancing their preclinical siRNA studies for the treatment of obesity, type 2 diabetes, and Lou Gehrig's disease. Thus, many pharmaceutical companies have decided to develop siRNAs as therapeutic agents. However, as with ASOs, the fate of therapeutic siRNAs will be determined from the initial siRNA clinical trials.

Future Directions

Nucleic Acid-Based Therapeutics

Plasmids and viral vectors have been developed to deliver gene therapy in animal models and human clinical trials. These approaches aim to express a gene of interest in target tissue. Many of these approaches use local delivery, and thus, PK analysis is limited to the short-range disposition, metabolism, and excretion of the nucleic acid therapeutic. ASOs and siRNA molecules are being developed as gene therapeutics to reduce the expression of target genes, through double-stranded nucleic acid interactions with target mRNA. Development of orally bioavailable formulations and lipid-encapsulated antisense molecules is being pursued, but most preclinical studies and clinical trials employ intravenous injection to deliver these therapeutics.

PK (ADME) and Toxicology Differences

For ASOs, the differences in PK and toxicology properties depend largely on the chemistry of the backbone and the modifications to the sugars. Thus, the ADME characteristics are independent of nucleotide base sequence and, therefore, do not change significantly according to the gene or protein being targeted. The toxicological properties do depend to a certain extent on the nucleotide sequence, for example, the effects of CpG dinucleotides and G-quartets. Whether these principles will hold for siRNA therapeutics will likely been seen in the next few years, as the development of siRNA with novel chemical modifications progresses.

Relative Clinical Utility of the Different Approaches

The relative effectiveness of ASOs and siRNAs, in terms of target downregulation, have been studied in cell culture and animal experiments. Although it seems that siRNA may be more effective than ASOs in most experimental circumstances, the development of modified ASOs with improved PK properties, including stability to nucleases, uptake into target tissues, and tissue half-life, has progressed much further than for siRNA. Indeed, although many ASOs of various chemistries have progressed into phase II and III clinical trials and thus the PK studies are widely reported, siRNAs are just now entering human clinical trials and their PK properties are not yet fully described or understood. It seems likely that both types of antisense therapeutics will demonstrate clinical utility in a variety of indications in the coming years.

12

Pharmacokinetic Profiling of Drugs

The pharmacokinetic behavior of a drug results from the superposition of its absorption, distribution, biotransformation (metabolism), and excretion in the body. These processes are usually summarized under the acronym of ADME. The pharmacokinetic behavior is mainly determined by the physicochemical characteristics of the compound such as molecular weight, pK_a value, and lipophilicity. Although population studies reveal much inter- and intraindividual pharmacokinetic variability, specific pharmacokinetic core parameters can be defined for each drug in healthy young individuals. All of them can be determined by either in vitro experiments (f_u) or by clinical studies comprising plasma and, in the case of f_e, plasma and urine data.

ADME in vivo Profiling Flow Chart

The pharmacokinetic core parameters can be used to establish a flow chart for the in vivo ADME profiling of compounds. Based on this analysis, predictions can be made on the pharmacokinetic behavior of a drug and its potential interactions at the level of each ADME process. Simplest assumptions are made in a first approach which can be revised at a later stage if necessary. The step-by-step procedure is described below.

Distribution

The distribution of a compound is primarily dependent on its physicochemical parameters and its affinity to plasma and tissue proteins, to receptors, as well as to other components such as nucleic acids and glycosylated proteins and lipids. It has been shown that predictions can be made for the apparent volume of distribution of a new compound by means of empirical equations comprising the apparent partition coefficient under physiological conditions (pH 7.4) and the fraction unbound in plasma. Exceptions to the rule are found with compounds that exhibit affinities to a specific binding site, e.g., digoxin that has a high affinity for Na^+/K^+-ATPase, which leads to a relatively high volume of distribution (ca. 6 l kg^{-1}) as compared to the more-lipophilic digitoxin (ca. 0.6 l kg^{-1}).

To estimate the fraction of unbound drug in tissue (f_{uT}), and thus get an idea on the overall distribution of the compound in the body, a two-compartment model, i.e., plasma and tissue, can be used. This leads to the following relations (Eqns. 1 and 2):

$$V = V_p + V_T\left(\frac{f_u}{f_{uT}}\right) \quad \text{...(1)}$$

$$f_{uT} = \left(\frac{f_u}{V - V_p}\right)V_T \quad \text{...(2)}$$

where V_p represents the plasma volume, which corresponds to ca. 4% of body weight (BW), i.e., ca. 3 l for a 70-kg person. V_T is estimated as the physiological volume of the drug that corresponds to a maximum of the total body water minus plasma volume (ca. 56% BW, i.e., ca. 39 l for a 70-kg person). When a drug is not distributed throughout the body fluids, i.e., when $V < 42$ l, V_T equals ($V - V_p$), and as a consequence f_u equals f_{uT}. Using the mass balance, it can be calculated in percentage of dose to what extent a drug is found in the plasma and tissue, respectively.

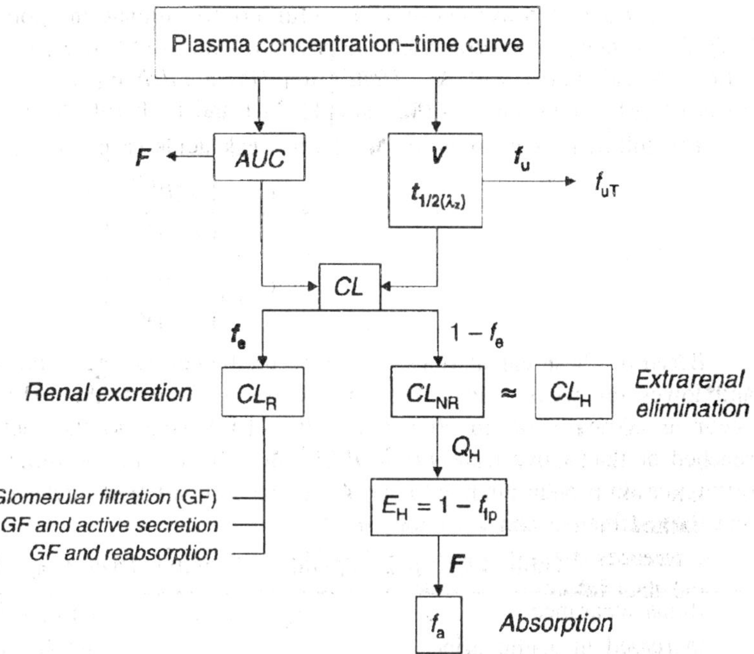

Fig. 12.1. The flow chart of in vivo pharmacokinetic profiling of drugs.

To estimate the risk of displacement from the same binding partner upon comedication with another compound, four points need to be taken into consideration. Significant displacement can be expected if: (a) plasma protein binding is high ($f_u < 0.1$), (b) the apparent volume of distribution is relatively small (<0.2 l kg^{-1}), (c) the therapeutic range of the drug at risk of displacement is narrow, and (d) the molar therapeutic concentration of the displacing drug is in the same range as the molar concentration of the binding partner. Thus, the affinity constant to human serum albumin (HSA) of all acidic drugs is so high that, at therapeutic levels, HSA represents their main binding protein in plasma. Physiological concentrations of HSA are in the range of 500–700 μm. A classical and clinically relevant displacement takes place upon comedication of warfarin (displaced drug, M_r 308.3; association constant $K = 2.1 \times 10^5$ m^{-1}; therapeutic concentration range of 3–32 μm) and salicylic acid (displacing drug, M_r 138.1; association constant $K = 3.8 \times 10^5$ m^{-1}; therapeutic concentration range of 150–2200 μm). Interestingly enough, clinically relevant interactions at the level of protein binding are less frequent than anticipated. This is mainly due to the fact that the unbound fraction of drug is not only relevant for the effect, but also directly influences elimination in the kidneys and liver. An increase in f_u thus leads to an increased clearance and therefore to an internal regulation of the drug level within a short period of time.

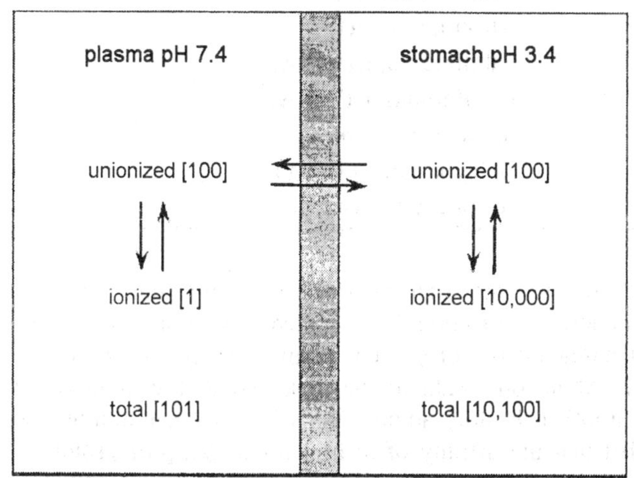

Fig. 12.2. The pH-partition hypothesis: schematic representation of the partitioning of a weak base (pKa 5.4) between two aqueous phases with pH 7.4 (plasma) and pH 3.4 (stomach) at equilibrium.

The pH-partition hypothesis is a useful tool to estimate the potential drug concentrations in different body fluids, being based solely on the physicochemical characteristics of the compound. The concentration ratios are calculated with the *Henderson–Hasselbalch* equation for two aqueous compartments with differing pH values such as plasma (pH 7.4) and milk (pH 6.6), or plasma and stomach (pH 1–3.5).

The following equations are used for weak acids (Eqn. 3) and weak bases (Eqn. 4), respectively:

$$\frac{c_1}{c_2} = \frac{1 + 10^{pH_1 - pK_a}}{1 + 10^{pH_2 - pK_a}} \qquad \text{...(3)}$$

$$\frac{c_1}{c_2} = \frac{1 + 10^{pK_a - pH_1}}{1 + 10^{pK_a - pH_2}} \qquad \text{...(4)}$$

Based on these calculations, it can be predicted that the milk/plasma ratio is higher for weak bases and lower for weak acids. If estimates are made with the pH-partition hypothesis, differences can occur as compared to in vivo data. This can be due to the fact that equilibrium is not necessarily reached or that active transport of drug into milk occurs. Another particularly important aspect is that differences in protein binding between the two compartments under consideration will shift the equilibrium and thus influence concentration ratios.

Table 12.1. pH-Dependent Urinary Excretion of Drugs (selection)

Renal clearance	Drug (pK_a)
increased in acidic urine	amphetamine (9.7 B)
	chloroquine (8.4 B)
	codeine (8.3 B)
	imipramine (9.5 B)
	morphine (8.1 B)
	nicotine (9.7 B)
	procaine (9.0 B)
increased in alkaline urine	amino acids (A)
	barbiturates (A)
	nalidixic acid (6.0 A)
	nitrofurantoin (7.2 A)
	probenecid (3.4 A)
	salicylic acid (3.0 A)
	sulfonamides (A)

Renal Excretion

Kidneys are both regulation and elimination organs. The renal clearance of a drug can comprise different overlapping processes, in particular glomerular filtration (GF), active secretion, passive or active reabsorption, and biotransformation. Depending on the drug, not all of these processes are of equal importance. Thus, GF occurs continuously. About one tenth of the renal blood flow is deviated through the filters of the glomeruli (ca. 120 ml min^{-1} in healthy adults). As with all other elimination processes, only unbound drug is cleared. Provided that the affinity of a drug for a transport protein is high enough, the compound can also be cleared by active secretion. Whether or not a compound is excreted in urine depends on its physicochemical characteristics. Passive reabsorption occurs as a function of the apparent partition coefficient, the pK_a value of the drug, and the urinary pH (pH range of 4.5–8.0). Estimates for the partitioning at equilibrium can be made with the Henderson–Hasselbalch equations.

Renal reabsorption of weak electrolytes by passive diffusion can be influenced by changing the urinary pH. A significant change can be expected when the acidic drug has a pK_a between 3.0 and 7.5 and the basic drug a pK_a between 7.0 and 11.0.

The total clearance, CL, can be calculated from the pharmacokinetic core parameters V and $t_{1/2(\lambda Z)}$, and together with f_e one obtains the renal clearance CL_R. For a drug that is only excreted through GF, CL_R corresponds to the product of the GF rate (GFR) and f_u. When CL_R is larger than the product of GFR and f_u, this indicates that net active secretion occurs. In contrast, when CL_R is smaller than the product of GFR and f_u, net reabsorption can be postulated. Renal insufficiency has a direct impact on the GFR. Dosage adjustments should be considered for compounds with $f_e > 0.3$ when the GFR falls below ca. 25% of the normal rate. For compounds with $f_e < 0.3$, adjustments may be adequate for drugs that are transformed to active metabolites with high f_e.

Nonrenal Elimination

The nonrenal clearance (CL_{NR}) is obtained as the difference between CL and CL_R. In a first approximation, CL_{NR} is assumed to equal CL_H. This is obviously a simplification which has to be verified at a later step of the analysis.

Making use of the physiological or hemodynamic perfusion model, the hepatic extraction ratio $E_{p,H}$ can be calculated from CLH with the help of the hepatic plasma flow Q_H (Eqn. 5):

$$E_{p,H} = \frac{CL_H}{Q_{p,H}} \quad \text{...(5)}$$

Accordingly, the fraction of the absorbed dose remaining systemically available after the first liver passage, f_{fp}, equals $(1 - E_{p,H})$.

Hepatic clearances below ca. 200 ml min^{-1} reflect an extraction ratio of $E < 0.3$ indicative of capacity-limited biotransformation. In this case, the enzyme capacity (also called intrinsic clearance, CL_{int}) of the liver is rate- limiting for elimination. This means that changes in the enzyme capacity through enzyme induction or enzyme inhibition directly affect hepatic clearance. As only the unbound fraction of drug undergoes biotransformation, f_u also has a direct influence on the hepatic clearance (Eqn. 6):

$$\text{For } E_H \rightarrow 0: CL_H \approx f_u\, CL_{int} \quad \text{...(6)}$$

With high extraction compounds (E> 0.7), the enzyme capacity is high and not rate limiting. These are the so-called first-pass drugs. Here, the blood flow represents the limiting factor, whereas changes in enzyme capacity (i.e., enzyme induction or inhibition) do not influence the hepatic clearance (Eqn. 7):

$$\text{For } E_H \rightarrow 1: CL_H \approx Q_H \quad \text{...(7)}$$

First-pass drugs show high inter- and intraindividual variability in plasma concentration–time curves.

When calculations with Eqn. 5 result in $E > 1$, the assumption that the nonrenal clearance is identical to the hepatic clearance has to be revised. In this case, presystemic clearance (e.g., in the intestinal wall and/or the portal vein) has to be assumed in addition to the clearance occurring upon hepatic first passage.

Reduced Bioavailability: Limited Absorption or First-Pass Effect?

In contrast to the other core parameters, bioavailability F is not constant for a given compound but depends on its specific formulation. F results from two contributions, the fraction of the absorbed dose (f_a) and the systemically available fraction of the absorbed dose (f_{fp}) after a possible first-pass extraction (Eqn. 8):

$$F = f_a f_{fp} \quad \text{...(8)}$$

With F known for a specific formulation and E calculated as sketched above, rough estimates can be made whether a reduced bioavailability originates from limited absorption or is the result of a first-pass effect. From the examples, both propranolol and morphine are high-extraction drugs with possible presystemic elimination, whereas penicillin G and sulfasalazine are low-extraction drugs with limited absorption.

Table 12.2. Reduced F – limited absorption or first-pass effect?

Parameter	*Propranolol*	*Morphine*	*Penicillin G*	*Sulfasalazine*
F	0.35	0.4	0.3	0.3
$E_{p,H}$	0.9–1.5	0.25–0.65	0.14	0.24
fa	~1	~1	~0.3	~0.4

Considerations about Dosage Regimens

The pharmacokinetic core parameters are also useful for a rough estimate of the plasma concentration–time curve produced by multiple dosing. For a dosage regimen with constant dose and constant dosing interval, a steady state is reached (>95% of the maximum plasma concentration) after ca. 5 $t_{1/2}$. The average plasma concentration ($c_{ss,av}$) at steady state depends on the dose (D) applied and the dosing interval (τ) in relation to the half-life of the respective drug (Eqn. 9):

$$\frac{FD}{\tau} = CL\,c_{ss,av} = V\frac{\ln 2}{t_{1/2}}c_{ss,av} \qquad \ldots(9)$$

Given the therapeutic concentration range to be reached for a given drug, the appropriate D and τ values can be chosen using its V and $t_{1/2}$ values.

An accumulation ratio, R_{ac}, has been defined that corresponds to the ratio of the maximum plasma concentration at steady state over the maximum plasma concentration after a single dose. R_{ac} depends only on $t_{1/2}$ and τ (Eqn. 10):

$$R_{ac} = \left(1 - e^{-\frac{\ln 2}{t_{1/2}}\tau}\right)^{-1} \qquad \ldots(10)$$

Changes in half-life, e.g., due to renal insufficiency or to enzyme induction or inhibition, directly influence both the time when the steady state is reached and the R_{ac} and thus the plasma concentrations at steady state. In vivo pharmacokinetic profiling of drugs based on their core parameters is a useful instrument in designing drug therapies. Although it is clear that refinements are needed for more than a rough classification, the estimates presented here provide important clues about tissue distribution, renal excretion, and biotransformation in the liver. They also allow predictions on possible drug interactions upon comedication, as well as on the plasma concentration–time curve to be expected upon multiple dosing.

13

Toxicokinetics

Toxicokinetics is the study of drug disposition in overdose. The biochemical processes that constitute the science of pharmacokinetics may be altered when drugs are administered in high concentrations. GI absorption may be altered in overdose due to delayed gastric emptying, changes in intestinal motility, and therapy with activated charcoal. Drugs such as morphine, ethanol, and barbiturates delay gastric emptying and as a consequence slow drug movement into the small intestine. In addition, morphine decreases intestinal motility, resulting in increased transit time through the intestine and increased absorption. Little is known about changes in drug distribution throughout the body after overdose. Several mechanisms may be at work in overdose to cause changes in drug disposition. For example, the bioavailability of a drug with a high first pass metabolism may be increased when the hepatic metabolizing enzymes become saturated. In a similar manner, the concentration of free drug in the plasma may be increased when protein binding becomes saturated. This may result in significant toxicity for those drugs that are highly plasma protein bound. Also, changes in peripheral blood flow due to the cardiac effects of some drugs may result in prolonged drug distribution and higher blood drug concentrations.

Drug metabolism may be altered in overdose when those enzymes responsible for metabolism become saturated. In this event, clearance is decreased, half-life is prolonged, and therefore high drug concentrations exist for a longer time. If multiple drugs are co-ingested, competitive inhibition of metabolism may occur. In addition, if hepatic blood flow is decreased, due to impaired liver function or cardiovascular drug effects, biotransformation of xenobiotics may be decreased.

Renal excretion may or may not be altered in drug overdose. Alteration of renal drug clearance may be utilized therapeutically to enhance drug elimination. Urinary pH is adjusted to increase the clearance of acidic and basic drugs. For example, administration of sodium bicarbonate will raise the urine pH above 7.5, concentrating the ionized form in the renal tubule and, therefore, enhancing elimination of salicylate. Conversely, acidification of the urine may be utilized to enhance renal excretion of basic drugs. However, with some drugs, such as phencyclidine, there is controversy about the role of urinary acidification in enhanced excretion and whether this procedure improves clinical outcome. Acidification is contraindicated with myoglobinuria and may also increase the risk of metabolic complications.

Factors Affecting Pharmacokinetic Parameters

Toxicokinetics is utilized to describe the changes in pharmacokinetic processes as a result of drug overdose. Other factors may contribute to changes in pharmacokinetic parameters when nontoxic doses are therapeutically or illicitly administered. Besides species differences in the variability in drug response, which are not discussed here, other factors that contribute to changes in parameters include drug formulation and route of administration, gender differences, age, weight or body composition, disease, genetic abnormalities, and drug interactions.

Genetic Factors

When a distinguishable difference between individuals is under genetic control, it is known as genetic polymorphism. Some drug responses have been found to be genetically determined. For example, the activity of the liver enzyme *N*-acetyltransferase differs between individuals such that the population may be divided into slow and fast acetylators. Approximately 60% of the U.S. population are slow acetylators and may show toxicity unless doses of drugs requiring acetylation for metabolism are reduced. Other inherited variations in pharmacokinetics include deficiency of one or more hepatic cytochrome-P450 isozymes or plasma cholinesterase.

Sex Differences

Examples of sex differences in drug pharmacokinetics have also been identified. These differences may be due to variations in body composition, hepatic metabolism, renal elimination, protein binding, or absorption. Differences in weight may influence muscle mass, organ blood flow, body water spaces, and hence affect the pharmacokinetic parameters of many drugs. In addition, women tend to have a higher percentage of body fat than men, which will affect the volume of distribution of lipophilic drugs. The clinical significance of differences in body composition is unclear but there are some important examples: women have a lower volume of distribution (V) of ethanol and a higher V for diazepam than men.

A number of studies have examined the effect of gender on hepatic metabolism and drug elimination. Greenblatt et al. found that young women have a significantly higher CL for diazepam than young men. In contrast, clearances of oxazepam and chlordiazepoxide are higher in men than in women and no sex difference has been observed in the metabolism of nitrazepam or lorazepam. Differences can be explained by differences in metabolic pathways because oxazepam is metabolized primarily through conjugation, nitrazepam is metabolized by reduction of the nitro group, and most of the other benzodiazepines are metabolized by various cytochrome P450 isozymes. It has been found that the isozyme cytochrome 3A4, responsible for the metabolism of many drugs, is approximately 1.4 times more active in women than men. The isozymes P2D6 and P2C19 display genetic polymorphism that is not influenced by gender. The isozyme P1A2 may be influenced by sex although the data are inconclusive. The work of Relling et al. suggests that the activity of this isozyme is lower in women than men. As mentioned above, gender differences have been demonstrated in the elimination of drugs that are metabolized solely by conjugation. The male:female clearance ratio for oxazepam is approximately 1.5:1.

When considering renal elimination, the glomerular filtration rate (GFR) is on average higher in men than women, but this may be a weight rather than a gender effect as GFR is directly proportional to weight. The effects of gender on tubular secretion and reabsorption have not been well characterized. The influence of gender on plasma protein binding appears to be minimal. Albumin levels are not altered by gender in contrast to the protein á1-acid glycoprotein, which is reduced by estrogen. Other plasma constituents whose levels are influenced by gender include corticosteroid binding globulin and various lipoproteins. Gender differences in the binding of diazepam and chlordiazepoxide have been demonstrated. Some studies have suggested that gender influences gastric emptying rate and intestinal transit time. Women empty solids from the stomach more slowly than men and the activity of a stomach enzyme, alcohol dehydrogenase, may be much lower in women. The GI tract also contains large concentrations of the isozyme cytochrome P3A4, so gender differences in the activity of this enzyme could affect the bioavailability of certain drugs. Gender differences observed after intramuscular drug administration may be due to differences in blood flow or incorrect injection into fat in women. Drug absorption in the lung may differ according to gender. Knight et al. found significantly less deposition of an aerosolized drug in women than men, which the authors attributed to differences in breathing characteristics. It should be noted that female-specific issues may have significant effects on drug distribution and metabolism. For example, pregnancy may increase the elimination of certain drugs, reducing their efficacy. In addition, oral contraceptive use can affect the metabolism of drugs. The effects of menopause, menstruation, and hormone replacement on the pharmacokinetics of drugs are largely unknown.

Age

Changes in the rate but not the extent of drug absorption are usually observed with age. Factors that affect drug absorption, such as gastric pH and emptying, intestinal motility, and blood flow, change with age. Gastric acid secretion does not approach adult levels until the age of 3 and gastric emptying and peristalsis is slow during the first few months of life. Because skeletal muscle mass is limited, muscle contractions, which aid blood flow, are minimal, and therefore will limit the distribution of intramuscularly administered drug. Higher gastric pH, delayed gastric emptying, and decreased intestinal motility and blood flow are observed in elderly individuals.

Drug and Disease Interactions

The pharmacokinetics of several drugs have been shown to be influenced by concurrent disease processes. The clearance of many drugs decreases in those individuals with chronic hepatic disease such as cirrhosis. In contrast, in acute reversible liver conditions, such as acute viral hepatitis, the clearance of some drugs is decreased or the half-life increased, and for others no change is detected. The volumes of distribution of some drugs are unaltered in hepatic disease while an increase is observed for other drugs, especially those bound to albumin in individuals with cirrhosis. This phenomenon is due to the decreased synthesis of albumin and other proteins. The influence of liver disease on drug absorption is unclear. It is probable, however, that the oral bioavailability of drugs highly extracted from the liver is increased in cirrhosis. The reasons are decreased first pass hepatic metabolism and the development of portal bypass in which blood enters the superior vena cava directly via esophageal varices. Renal diseases such as uremia may result in decreased renal clearance of certain drugs. Gastrointestinal diseases, such as Crohn's disease, result in increased plasma protein binding of several drugs due to increased levels of binding proteins. Further, respiratory diseases such as cystic fibrosis increase the renal clearance of some drugs.

Patients commonly receive two or more drugs concurrently and most individuals who abuse drugs are polydrug users. Multiple drug use may result in drug interactions. This occurs when the pharmacokinetics or pharmacodynamics of one drug is altered by another. This concept is important to consider because interaction may result in decreased therapeutic efficacy or an increased risk of toxicity. The degree of drug interaction depends on the relative concentrations and therefore dose and time. Changes in absorption rate, competition for binding sites on plasma proteins, oral bioavailability, volume of distribution, and hepatic and renal clearance have been demonstrated for therapeutic drugs. Few studies have systematically documented pharmacokinetic interactions between illicit drugs.

14

Antitumor Agents

Regional chemotherapy provides a treatment approach designed to improve the selectivity of chemotherapy, by increasing drug concentrations at tumor sites and lowering systemic drug exposure. Isolated lung perfusion (ILP) provides an alternative to achieve high concentration of anticancer drugs in tumor tissue. The main attractiveness of regional chemotherapy such as ILP is that high drug concentrations would target the tumor site, thus making the drug more efficacious. It is true that the therapy permits delivery of high drug levels over a relatively short period of time and this, in theory, results in considerably high tissue exposure. On the other hand, increased dose may not enhance the efficacy, but may induce toxicity when the maximum drug effect is reached. Therefore, it is important to keep in mind that regional drug therapy requires the knowledge of pharmacokinetics, such as the feasibility of reaching expected high concentrations in tumor tissue and the concentration–response relationship.

Evaluating the pharmacokinetics of anticancer agents via ILP is particularly important. It provides a quantitative perspective regarding the pharmacologic advantage of the anticancer drugs using ILP, and helps us to decide if clinical effort is necessary for a particular drug. Finally, pharmacodynamic factors must also be considered for the overall assessment of regional delivery.

Lung Anatomy and Physiology and Drug Pharmacokinetics

The lung is a complex and heterogeneous organ. There is considerable cellular heterogeneity, with approx 40 different cell types within the lung. Two classes of enzymes exist in the lungs that have direct implications for the disposition of drugs. The first class is the enzymes responsible for the active uptake of catecholamines and related drugs into the lung. These transport enzymes can be saturated and inhibited competitively. The other class is the enzymes that are required for drug metabolism in the lungs. The lung, generally, has low activities of many metabolic enzymes found in the liver. In humans, the enzyme activity in the lung varies from $< 1\%$ up to 34% of the liver enzyme activity for a range of drugs studied. Drug uptake into the lung is principally by diffusion, as well as active transportation. The lung has the smallest diffusion distances of all of the body organs; thus, the diffusion of drugs is very fast. The lung is also characterized by large surface areas in contact with blood and respiratory gases. The characteristics of lung anatomy and physiology have an influence on drug distribution and metabolism. The evidence suggests that the kinetics of drugs in the lung is highly variable with respect to both drug distribution and metabolism. These can have a significant impact on pharmacokinetic studies. The lung kinetics of many drugs has not been extensively examined in animals and in humans. Regional chemotherapy using ILP provides an opportunity to evaluate the pharmacokinetic behavior of many drugs in the lung.

Preclinical Pharmacokinetic Studies of ILP with Anticancer Agents

Many animal studies have been performed using ILP with different anticancer agents. Different animal models of ILP have been developed in different laboratories. Pharmacokinetic advantages of ILP using different anticancer agents have been evaluated, together with the evaluation of pharmacodynamics.

Cisplatin

ILP with cisplatin was reported by several investigators. Li et al. evaluated ILP with cisplatin in a rat lung tumor model. The results demonstrated that a significantly higher platinum concentration in the tumor was observed in the ILP treated rats with 0.1 mg/mL of cisplatin than in the rats treated with a 1-mg intravenous injection (6.7 ± 1.6 vs 2.5 ± 0.6 μg/g of tissue [$p < 0.05$]). In accordance with the findings of Wang et al., a lower cisplatin level was observed in the tumor nodule than in the lung tissue in the ILP rats, but almost the same levels were seen in the animals treated with intravenous cisplatin in this study. These results suggest that the pharmacokinetics for ILP and intravenous injection could be different. The study showed that ILP with cisplatin was pharmacokinetically superior to intravenous injection.

In another study, Li et al. investigated the pharmacokinetic differences of cisplatin in rat tumor and lung tissues after ILP, using different perfusion times and perfusate drug concentration. Isolated lungs were perfused over various times with perfusate cisplatin concentration of 25, 50, or 100 μg/mL. The total cisplatin concentration in the lung tissue increased significantly with perfusion time and increasing cisplatin perfusate concentration. The cisplatin concentrations in the lung tissue after a 60-min perfusion ranged from approx 4 to 21 μg/g of tissue. However, the total cisplatin concentrations in the perfused tumor tissues (tumor nodules developed were approx 4 mm in diameter) did not change significantly with the perfusion time or perfusate cisplatin concentration, ranging from 4.17 ± 0.82 to 4.95 ± 0.80 μg/g of tissue in all the perfusion groups. It was also observed that the cisplatin concentration in tumor tissue was inversely related to the weight of tumor nodules after IPL with cisplatin. The results indicate that different pharmacokinetics in the tumor and lung tissues exist following ILP with cisplatin in the rat sarcoma model. Further studies are required to raise cisplatin concentration to the tumor tissue.

2′-Deoxy-5-Fluorouridine

Port et al. studied the pharmacokinetics and effectiveness of ILP with 2'-deoxy-5- fluorouridine (FUDR) in a rat model. FUDR is well tolerated at 21 mg/mL at a rate of 0.5 mL/min for 20 min, which is above the rat lethal dose of intravenous bolus injection. The pharmacokinetics of FUDR via ILP was compared with intravenous administration. Isolated lung perfusion with FUDR at 21 mg/mL maximally elevated total lung FUDR and 5-fluorouracil (5-FU) levels (508.5 ± 96.4 μg/g) in comparison to the intravenous group (7.5 ± 4.1 μg/g). It is believed that the lung is an inefficient extractor of FUDR and is unable to catabolize FUDR beyond 5-FU. Less than 1% of FUDR extracted in this study supports the inefficient uptake by the lung. The pharmacokinetic advantage of high pulmonary FUDR levels, the lung's inefficient FUDR extraction, as well as the lung's inability to detoxify FUDR may be advantages for the treatment of pulmonary colorectal metastases with ILP.

Doxorubicin

Minchin and Boyd evaluated doxorubicin pharmacokinetics of ILP using an ex vivo rat model. The results demonstrated that doxorubicin concentration in the lung increased linearly with perfusion time and with increasing doxorubicin perfusate concentration. In another study, dog lungs were perfused with doxorubicin at concentrations ranging from 0.5 to 118.2 nmol/mL (0.27 to 64.1 μg/mL). Doxorubicin uptake in the lung increased with time but was saturable at perfusate concentrations above

20 nmol/mL (10.9 μg/mL) after 50 min. Doxorubicin lung uptake ranged from 1.3 to 65.1 μg/g tissue. Tumor levels of doxorubicin were always lower than in the pulmonary tissue surrounding the tumors. Random sampling of lung tissue from the upper, middle, and lower lobes showed that the drug was distributed uniformly throughout the tissue.

Baciewicz et al. studied the pharmacokinetics of ILP with doxorubicin in dog. Perfusate concentrations ranged from 1.95 μg/mL to 7.61 μg/mL and the lung concentration of doxorubicin ranged from 3.9 μg/g to 20.6 μg/g. A plateau of doxorubicin concentration in lung tissue appeared to be reached at a perfusate concentration of 5.79 μg/mL. The observed plateau in tissue doxorubicin levels could be explained by the lung tissue uptake of doxorubicin, perhaps by means of a carrier-mediated mechanism. Another explanation of the plateau is that perfusate concentration of 7.6 μg/mL caused a significant histologic injury of the lung, and once the lung is injured, increased uptake might not be expected.

Weksler et al. evaluated doxorubicin pharmacokinetics of ILP and intravenous injection in rats. Lung doxorubicin concentrations after ILP were 107.8–663.8 μg/mL and were significantly higher than those after intravenous doxorubicin (19.9–25.5 μg/mL). Lung doxorubicin concentration reached a plateau at a perfusate concentration of 255.2 ± 12.8 μg/mL of doxorubicin. Extraction ratio, the percent of doxorubicin extracted by the lung from the perfusate, appeared to be related to perfusate concentration, ranging from 38% to 58%. The optimal perfusate and other pharmacokinetic factors for ILP using doxorubicin were also investigated in rats. The mean lung concentrations of doxorubicin were < 100 and < 300 μg/g, respectively, for perfusate concentrations of 80 μg/mL and 320 μg/mL. Extraction ratios were 5.5 and 4.3, respectively, which were lower than those reported. The study also suggested that the dose per kilogram or per square meter of body surface area, the total infused dose of doxorubicin, and the rate of infusion were not important in the final lung concentration of doxorubicin. The results indicated that the doxorubicin perfusate concentration and the duration of perfusion are the only factors determining the final lung concentration of doxorubicin. An equation to predict final lung concentration of doxorubicin in rats was proposed: $\log(FLC) = 1.9 + 0.0071P + 0.186T$, where FLC is final lung concentration, P is measured perfusate doxorubicin concentration, and T is perfusion time in minutes ($r^2 = 0.91$).

Furrer et al. performed a study of ILP with doxorubicin in pigs by two different systems. Doxorubicin lung tissue concentrations were 17.5 μg/g to 21.9 μg/g at a dose of 50 mg/ m2 and were approximately six- to sevenfold higher than after intravenous administration at a dose of 10 mg/kg (3 μg/g).

Melphalan

Hendriks et al. studied ILP with melphalan and tumor necrosis factor for metastatic pulmonary adenocarcinoma in rats. Pharmacokinetic results demonstrated that ILP with melphalan was superior to intravenous injection. Lung melphalan levels in ILP groups were 30–50 times higher than in the intravenous groups, for both 0.5 and 1.0 mg of melphalan. No significant elevation of melphalan tissue levels could be detected when the dose was doubled from 0.5 mg to 1.0 mg. The concentration–time profiles were nearly identical and the decrease in metastatic nodules was similar between the two groups. The results may suggest that lower doses of melphalan may be used.

Paclitaxel

Pharmacokinetics of paclitaxel administered by ILP was first evaluated by Schrump et al. Nine adult sheep underwent ILP and one sheep received paclitaxel by 1-h intravenous infusion. Paclitaxel concentrations in lung tissues increased nonlinearly with escalating doses ranging from 2 to 800 mg and peaked between 60 and 90 min. Drug tissue levels rapidly declined during washout. In this study, lung tissue samples were collected at different time intervals for pharmacokinetic analysis. Paclitaxel peak concentration (C_{max}) and area under the concentration–time curve (AUC) in lung tissue increased with dose, gradually approaching a plateau. The average C_{max} in lung tissues following ILP at 200 mg was approximately twofold higher than that observed after systemic infusion of the same dose of paclitaxel over 1 h. Tissue AUCs under these conditions were relatively comparable. Higher C_{max} and AUC were achieved with increased dose (800 mg), and were higher than those with 1-h intravenous infusion (200 mg) (C_{max}: 90 vs 25.4 μg/g; AUC: 184 vs 73 $\mu g \cdot mg^{-1} \cdot h^{-1}$). The continued increase of C_{max} and AUC without reaching a plateau indicates that the transport of paclitaxel into lung tissue was not fully saturated. The results confirm the profound pharmacokinetic advantage for paclitaxel administered by ILP and provide a rationale for considering paclitaxel for ILP administration in clinical trials.

Clinical Pharmacokinetic Studies of ILP with Antitumor Agents

Pharmacokinetic studies of isolated lung perfusion with different antitumor agents have been evaluated in preclinical animal models. These animal studies have demonstrated that ILP with these drugs are superior pharmacokinetically to systemic administration, providing higher lung tissue (tumor) levels and lower systemic exposure. The results indicate a pharmacologic rationale for ILP in humans. Several clinical studies have been reported or are under evaluation. Some of the reported studies with pharmacokinetic results are discussed here.

Cisplatin

Johnston et al. reported ILP with cisplatin in patients with metastatic lung sarcoma or diffuse bronchioloalveolar carcinoma. Two patients received perfu sate with cisplatin at concentrations of 14 and 20 μg/mL. The drug concentrations in the tumor were about twofold higher than those in normal lung tissue. The drug was detectable in the mediastinal lymph nodes for one patient.

Ratto et al. reported administering cisplatin by ILP for the treatment of pulmonary metastases from soft tissue sarcoma in six patients. Cisplatin at a dose of 200 mg/m^2 was administered. The AUC (0–60 min) values in pulmonary plasma were about 43 times greater than those in systemic plasma (12.8 ± 5.6 vs 0.3 ± 0.2 $mg \cdot mL^{-1} \cdot min^{-1}$). Cisplatin concentration in mediastinal lymph nodes (the diameter < 1 cm) was 2.57 μg/g, and was similar to those achieved in normal lung tissue. In this study, cisplatin concentration in larger metastases was not investigated as they were removed during the operation.

In a clinical study of hyperthermic (41°C) ILP with cisplatin for the treatment of lung sarcoma metastasis, four patients were treated with high doses of cisplatin (70 mg/m^2). Initial cisplatin concentrations in the perfusate were higher than 100 μg/mL. At the end of the perfusion, a lung tissue sample was found to have a cisplatin concentration of 93.8 μg/g of tissue. This is the highest cisplatin lung concentration reported. However, cisplatin tumor concentrations were not reported in this study.

Doxorubicin

Minchin et al. first evaluated the pharmacokinetics of doxorubicin in isolated lung samples from humans and dogs. Three patients with sarcoma lung metastases were perfused at 25°C with doxorubicin perfusate concentration of 0.56–0.98 μg/mL. Drug concentrations in lung tissue increased steadily with time. Tumor concentrations of doxorubicin were consistently lower than in the lung tissue in all three patients, possibly owing to poor vascularity of the tumor tissue. Lung tissue doxorubicin concentrations in these patients were considerably lower than those seen in dogs treated with similar drug concentrations.

ILP with doxorubicin in patients with metastatic lung sarcoma or diffuse bronchiol-oalveolar carcinoma was reported by Johnston et al. Escalating doses of doxorubicin ranging from 1 to 10 μg/mL were administered in six patients. Although showing much variability, drug concentrations in tumor and lung tissue immediately after perfusion generally increased with higher doses. Doxorubicin concentration in tumor tissue appeared lower than in lung tissue, although there was no statistical difference.

Another Phase I trial of ILP with doxorubicin in patients with metastatic sarcoma was reported by Burt et al. Seven patients were treated with doxorubicin at a dose of 40 mg/m^2 or less, and one patient received 80 mg/m^2. The mean perfusate level of doxorubicin was 5.9 μg/mL in the group of patients receiving 40 mg/m^2 or less. The mean lung tissue level of doxorubicin in this group was 6.5 μg/g. Doxorubicin concentrations in lung and tumor appear to correlate with the amount of doxorubicin in the perfu sate. In general, tumors took up less drug than the healthy lung tissues. Thirteen percent of the drug (10 mg) was extracted during ILP.

Drug Penetration in Tumor Tissue and Isolated Lung Perfusion

Many solid tumors are rather resistant to chemotherapy. The mechanisms of genetically determined factors expressed in individual tumor cells includes the existence of drug efflux pumps (such as P-glycoprotein or multidrug resistance-associated proteins), changes in the expression of topoisomerase, alterations of drug metabolism, DNA repair, and apoptosis.Other areas of potential causes for drug resistance in solid tumors are those related to the solid tumor microenvironment and the problems relating to the drug delivery into the tumor cells.

With regional chemotherapy such as ILP, the maximum tolerated dose is given to achieve high concentrations at tumor site and kill all tumor cells. However, for the effective treatment of solid tumors, anticancer drugs must penetrate through the extravascular space to achieve a lethal concentration in all of the target cancer cells. The limited penetration of anticancer drugs through tumor tissue may be a very important cause of clinical resistance of solid tumors to chemotherapy, especially regional chemotherapy such as ILP.

Blood flow in tumors is often irregular. Blood vascular systems may be poorly formed, with variable rates of blood flow, and the intercapillary distance may be relatively large when compared with normal tissue. For drug to be effective, it must penetrate through multiple layers of solid tissue to reach all cells in a tumor. Thus, tissue penetration of anticancer drugs is likely more limited in tumors than in normal tissue. It is more difficult to predict pharmacokinetic behavior of the drugs. Many other factors would also affect drug distribution in tumors, such as drug delivery by the vascular system, the rate of diffusion through tissue, drug metabolism, and binding to tissue components. Tumor cell density, tumor blood supply, and the distance from tumor nodule surface all could have an impact on tumor tissue pharmacokinetic results. More variability of pharmacokinetic results could be expected with ILP.

The concentration of anticancer drugs in lung tissue and tumors has been compared in many preclinical and clinical ILP studies. Some studies show that high concentrations of anticancer drugs are achieved in normal tissue but not in tumors. Saeki et al. evaluated tumor size and weight with pharmacokinetic characteristics of ILP in tumor tissues. They found that the total platinum concentrations in tumor nodules were correlated inversely with the tumor weight (total platinum concentration in tumor = 1.167 × 1/tumor wt; $r^2 = 0.981$; $p < 0.001$). The results suggested that ILP may be more effective against small tumors than large ones. The results showed that large tumor legions may need to be debulked before utilizing ILP in patients with an unresectable lung tumor. To increase intracellular platinum concentration and enhance the antitumor effect of ILP with cisplatin, a combination study with cisplatin and digitonin, a detergent to increase cell permeability, was performed in rat. The rats underwent ILP with 100 μg/mL of cisplatin after 20 μmol/L of digitonin was injected. However, pharmacokinetic results showed that cisplatin concentration of tumor nodules in the rats treated with digitonin–cisplatin increased slightly, only 20% higher than in the cisplatin-only rats (5.48 ± 0.64 vs 4.5 ± 1.09 μg/g; $p = 0.067$), although the number of pulmonary nodules decreased significantly by digitonin use (1.3 ± 1.5 vs 9.7 ± 2). Preclinical and clinical studies indicate that ILP can deliver high concentrations of antitumor drugs to lung tissue with minimal systemic toxicity. High drug concentrations in lung and tumor tissue are achievable. The studies indicate there are pharmacokinetic differences in tumor and lung tissues following ILP with different anticancer agents. Perfusate concentration and perfusion time are important factors influencing drug pharmacokinetics in lung and tumor tissue. Other contributing factors may include tumor size, tumor types, poorly formed blood vascular system in tumor, site of biopsy, animal models, and so forth. Some of studies show that the drug concentrations are generally lower in tumor tissue than in normal lung tissue. The strategies to improve the penetration of anticancer drugs through poorly vascularized tumor tissue have considerable potential to improve the outcome of isolated lung perfusion for solid tumors.

Anticancer Drugs in Children

Several comprehensive reviews of the disposition of anticancer drugs in children with cancer have been published. However, recent advances in cellular and molecular biology techniques have led to the design and analysis of clinical pharmacology studies, which have increased our understanding of the age-related changes that govern drug disposition: absorption, distribution, metabolism, and elimination. Moreover, recent studies have characterized the disposition of new anticancer drugs in children, as well as contributed new insights into the use of currently available anticancer drugs. Thus, an update on pediatric pharmacokinetics of anticancer drugs in children is warranted.

In the past the US Food and Drug Administration (FDA) used data from adult clinical trials when making decisions about approval of a drug for pediatric use. However, in April 1999, the FDA instituted a rule mandating the conduct of clinical trials of new drugs or biologics intended for use in children. The rule also mandates studies of drugs or biologics already approved by the FDA and used in a substantial number of pediatric patients for which insufficient labeling could pose significant risks. In addition, the rule mandates studies in children if an approved drug would provide meaningful therapeutic benefit over existing treatments for children, and the absence of adequate labeling could pose significant risks to children. Before 1999, the FDA required studies of drugs in children only if information about pediatric use was included in the product labeling. However, clinical pharmacology studies are now performed in children on a more routine basis, and those data are used in the review and approval process. This change has occurred only after significant work by many individuals to clarify that it is critical to understand the relationship between drug disposition and drug effect in children. Furthermore, the relation between pharmacokinetics and pharmacodynamics of anticancer drugs in children cannot be extrapolated from what is known about the adult population for many reasons, including the different spectra of malignancies acquired by children and adults. Moreover, many age-related changes in drug disposition occur in children, which are the subject of this chapter.

In addition to age-related changes in physiology that contribute to the differences in pharmacokinetics between children and adults, wide interindividual variability has been well documented in the pharmacokinetics of many drugs in children. This interindividual variability that characterizes the pharmacokinetic parameters of many anticancer drugs in the pediatric population has significant clinical implications. For example, when standardized dosages are administered to children, some with relatively low levels of clearance will have increased systemic exposure, which can lead to toxicity. Conversely, those children with more rapid clearance may not have toxicity, but they may have unacceptable antitumor activity.

Differences in drug disposition among children can be attributed not only to developmental changes in physiology but also to variation in genetic composition of individuals. The genotype of drug metabolizing enzymes or drug transport proteins can often be correlated with a pharmacokinetic phenotype, further explaining a source of the variability in pharmacokinetics observed among individuals. Interindividual variation in disposition of anticancer drugs often results in interindividual variation in drug systemic exposure (i.e., uniform dosages can yield different systemic exposures in different children). Evaluation of the relationship between systemic exposure and drug effect (e.g., toxicity and efficacy) has become an important aspect of new drug development in children, as many clinical pharmacology studies have reported a relationship between systemic exposure and response. Understanding the pharmacokinetics of anticancer drugs in children is essential to develop new drugs and new combination regimens and to define rational dosing schedules for these drugs. The first section of this chapter reviews the basic principles of drug absorption, distribution, metabolism, and elimination in children and adolescents. Subsequent sections address the appropriate method to select drug dosages in children, practical issues associated with clinical pharmacokinetic studies in children with cancer, and the pharmacokinetics of specific anticancer drugs in children.

EFFECT OF MATURATION ON DETERMINANTS OF DRUG DISPOSITION

Influence of Age on Drug Absorption

Although many anticancer drugs are administered parenterally, several of the currently available drugs are administered orally, such as methotrexate, 6-mercaptopurine, etoposide, and temozolomide. Also, many agents that are administered intravenously are now being evaluated as the intravenous solution given orally. Knowledge of the age- related changes in factors associated with drug absorption will enhance the ability of the clinician to use oral anticancer drugs appropriately in children. Moreover, because many young children are unable to swallow whole tablets or capsules, a clinician must consider that crushing or dissolving tablets may alter oral absorption. Whether absorption will be increased or decreased depends on the physicochemical properties of the drug, and the clinician is advised to consult appropriate references prior to altering commercially manufactured dosage formulations.

Oral drug absorption is dependent on both physicochemical and physiological factors. Physicochemical factors, which can vary among individual agents and formulations, consist of molecular weight, size and shape, degree of ionization under physiologic conditions, and solubility at the site of absorption. Because these characteristics are drug specific they are not subject to maturational changes; however, they are relevant when one considers the practical implications of crushing or dissolving tablets for extemporaneous administration to children. Physiological factors can vary among individuals as well as with maturation. These factors include gastric emptying time, gastric pH, bile salt production, bacterial colonization of the gastrointestinal tract, gastrointestinal transit time, and pancreatic function.

Gastric emptying time is prolonged in children relative to adults, and this can reduce or delay the peak concentration of drugs administered orally. Moreover, the rate of gastric emptying is directly related to gestational and postnatal age and the type of feeding. Furthermore, meals with high caloric density can increase gastric emptying time further in premature infants. Gastric emptying time approaches values comparable to adults within the first 6–8 mo of life.

Gastrointestinal transit time, which can also affect the absorption of orally administered drugs, has been less extensively studied in children than gastric emptying time. Intestinal transit times of 3–13.1 h have been reported for full-term neonates aged 3–5 days. After 45 d, breast-fed infants had a longer transit time (> 10 h) than infants who were fed formula (< 10 h). In comparison to adults, who usually have an intestinal transit time of about 24 h, it is possible that infants could have reduced absorption of some agents. The frequency of defecation decreases with age, so that 85% of children 1–4 yr of age defecate once or twice daily. A proportionate decrease of high-amplitude propagating contractions occurs in toddlers compared to adults.

Gastric acid secretion and pH strongly influence gastrointestinal absorption. At birth gastric pH is neutral because of the presence of amniotic fluid in the stomach. However, within hours pH rapidly falls to 1.5–3.0. Acid secretion peaks during the first 10 d of life and decreases from 10 to 30 d after birth. Gastric pH usually reaches adult values by 2 yr of age. The volume of gastric acid secretions approaches adult values by 3 mo of age. The lack of acidity in the gut could decrease the absorption (and hence bioavailability) of anticancer drugs that are weak acids and increase the absorption of weak bases. For example, methotrexate absorption is reduced by coadministration with milk, which effectively reduces the acidity of the gut.

Both the rate of bile acid synthesis and the bile acid pool size are decreased in neonates compared to adults. These changes may alter the disposition of drugs that undergo enterohepatic recirculation, such as irinotecan. Also, the absorption of lipid soluble drugs may be decreased in neonates. However, within the first year of life bile acid synthesis and pool size increase to adult values.

Pancreatic enzyme activity is low at birth and is even lower in premature infants. Lipase activity is low in the neonate, and in combination with low bile acid production could reduce the gastrointestinal absorption of lipid soluble drugs. However, even with low pancreatic lipase, the neonate is able to absorb 90–95% of dietary fat through gastric and intestinal lipases. Lipase activity increases 20-fold during the first 9 mo of life to reach adult values. The secretion of both amylase and tryp sin remains low for the first year of life.

Colonization of the gastrointestinal tract by bacterial flora varies with respect to age, type of delivery, and type of feeding. Before birth, the gut lacks bacterial flora; thereafter, the gut acquires bacteria from the environment. For example, a vaginal birth would lead to colonization of the gut by the mother's vaginal and large intestinal flora. Owing to the presence of certain antibodies in the breast milk, an infant who is fed breast milk will acquire different types of bacteria compared to an infant who is fed formula. These age-related changes in bacterial colonization of the gastrointestinal tract have theoretical implications for drug absorption and metabolism, as discussed later in the section on irinotecan.

Influence of Age on Drug Distribution

The volume of distribution (V_d) is a pharmacokinetic parameter that relates the drug dosage to the plasma concentration. Although V_d is a pharmacokinetic parameter and a theoretical term, for many drugs the value is similar to physiological volumes. As such, clinicians often attach physiological relevance to this term, and similar to gastrointestinal absorption, drug distribution in children is dependent on physicochemical and physiological factors. As with physiochemical factors associated with gastrointestinal absorption of drugs, those associated with the volume of distribution remain relatively constant from patient to patient. However, the physiological factors that can change with age include body composition, extent of protein binding, tissue binding characteristics, and vascular perfusion.

Body composition, which can be expressed as the relative proportion of total body water, total extracellular water, and total body fat, varies widely from neonates to teenagers. Total body water (as a percentage of total body weight) falls from 85% and 77% in the premature and full-term neonate, respectively, to 73% at 3 mo, 59% at 1 yr, and to 55% by 12 yr of age. The clinical relevance of this observation is that relatively water-soluble drugs (e.g., topotecan) will have a larger volume of the central compartment in infants compared with adults, whereas lipid-soluble drugs (e.g., etoposide or SN-38, the active metabolite of irinotecan) will have a smaller volume of the central compartment. Similarly, extracellular water falls from 45% of total body weight in the full-term neonate to 33% at 3 mo, 28% at 1 yr, and 20% in the adult. Also, total body fat increases from infancy to about 10 yr of age. In boys during puberty, the percentage of total body weight that is fat begins to decrease at about age 17 to a mean of 12%. Conversely, in girls, the percentage of body weight that is fat rapidly increases during puberty to as much as 25%. These changes suggest that during adolescence, sex-related differences in volume of distribution play a more important role than they do in younger children or adults.

Drug distribution in children may also be affected by age-related changes in plasma proteins. Extent of protein binding depends on a variety of factors such as amount of plasma proteins and the presence of endogenous substances that may compete for binding (e.g., bilirubin). Protein binding is reduced in infants owing to the presence of fetal albumin and decreased albumin, γ-globulin, and α_1-acid glycoprotein. The concentrations of these proteins do not approach adult values until about 1 yr of life; thus, an infant given highly protein-bound drugs (e.g., etoposide or SN-38) will likely have decreased protein binding and an increased fraction unbound. This could lead to an increase in the systemic exposure to the unbound and putatively active drug. For anticancer drugs that have a very narrow therapeutic range, this could potentially be associated with toxicity. Theoretically, increases in the unbound fraction of a drug could also potentiate antitumor activity; therefore, the predicted changes in toxicity and efficacy resulting from changes in the unbound-drug fraction should be balanced when selecting appropriate dosages of highly protein-bound drugs in children. Even though protein concentrations are relatively stable from 2 yr to adulthood, other factors such as disease or malnutrition can decrease plasma protein concentrations and create similar circumstances potentiating both toxicity and efficacy of protein-bound drugs.

Tissue binding also affects drug distribution and changes with maturation. The absolute mass of tissue available for binding in each organ will increase with age. Therefore, younger children who have smaller organs have less tissue available for drugs to bind. This could lead to a greater amount of free drug in the plasma and a greater exposure to the drug. Each tissue has a different affinity for drug binding based on the physicochemical properties of the drug, and the maturational changes in the amount and composition of such tissues may significantly alter drug distribution.

To develop physiologically based pharmacokinetic (PB-PK) models that are age-specific, Haddad and colleagues performed a literature search to obtain previously published data on age-related changes in body weight and tissue weight. The authors were not comprehensive in their literature search and instead relied on two previously published databases to cover age groups between birth and 18 yr. Empirical relationships were then developed based on the body and tissue weight data found in these references, sometimes using one reference to develop equations for multiple organs and other times combining data from different sources to develop an equation for one organ/tissue. The authors suggest that the relationships/equations developed in this study can ultimately be used to estimate organ size in children when generating PB-PK models. Although the authors suggest that the equations may provide reasonable initial estimates for PB-PK models, one must be aware of the numerous limitations to this quasi-population analysis. For example, the demographics of the study population are not defined, the statistical analysis lacks sophistication, and the method for determination of body weight (i.e., lean body mass vs ideal body weight) was not specified. In the absence of these details the use of these equations cannot be recommended.

Influence of Age on Drug Metabolism

The cytochrome P450 enzyme system is a crucial pathway in the metabolism of xenobiotics, including many anticancer drugs. Furthermore, numerous medications used in the supportive care of the children with cancer are substrates, inducers, or inhibitors of CYP450 enzymes, which alter the metabolism, efficacy, and toxicity of anticancer agents that are metabolized via this pathway. Children exhibit higher clearance than adults for many drugs metabolized by the liver (e.g., busulfan and cyclophosphamide). This phenomenon has been ascribed, possibly falsely, to greater activity of the CYP450 enzyme system in children than adults; however, current data do not support this observation.

The literature regarding age-related changes in drug metabolism is rife with inconsistencies between activity of CYP450 enzymes, the level of expression of CYP450 protein or mRNA, and the clearance of CYP450 substrates. Consequently, it has not been possible to establish a link between the age-related changes in the CYP450 enzyme system and the age-related changes in drug metabolism. It has been demonstrated that antipyrine, which is a substrate of CYP450 3A4, 1A2, and 2C9, exhibits higher clearance in children than adults when normalized to body weight. However, no difference was observed in antipyrine clearance between children and adults on normalization to body surface area. Blanco and colleagues subsequently showed that in a panel of 52 normal human livers from individuals ranging in age from 0.5 to 93 yr, catalytic activity of CYP 1A2, 3A4/5, 2E1, 2C8, and 2C9 was not affected by age. Likewise, a panel of human livers from donors ranging in age from 9 to 89 yr demonstrated weak and insignificant correlation between age and total CYP450 content or activity of microsomes. Although a relationship has not been defined between CYP450 catalytic activity or content and the differences in clearance observed in children and adults, perhaps variation in oxygen tension or other currently unknown factors determine the maturational changes in drug metabolism responsible for the maturational changes in drug clearance.

de Wildt and colleagues reviewed the literature on the CYP3A family, which is the most abundant CYP450 subfamily in the liver. They noted the absence of a correlation between liver size and hepatic microsomal enzyme activity and hepatic CYP activity and microsomal protein amount. Therefore, plasma drug clearance may not be informative in determining the relationship between maturation and CYP3A activity. Furthermore, they cautioned against the use of corrections for body weight or body surface area to obtain a relationship between CYP3A substrate pharmacokinetics and age-related changes in metabolism of CYP3A substrates. Because a definitive relationship between development of drug-metabolizing enzymes and anticancer drug metabolism has not been established, the clinician who treats children with anticancer drugs must rely on the reports of metabolism of individual anticancer drugs in children of all ages rather than a paradigm of developmental physiology to predict the metabolism of an anticancer drug in a child of any given age.

Despite the controversy about the determination of age-related changes in CYP450 expression or catalytic activity, the use of isoform specific probes has allowed for the characterization of the ontogeny of CYP3A4 and 3A7. In the developing child, the catalytic activity of CYP3A7 reaches peak levels in the first week of life when CYP3A4 catalytic activity is very low. As CYP3A7 catalytic activity declines from 3 mo to 1 yr, there is a corresponding increase in that of CYP3A4. At approx 1 yr, CYP3A7 catalytic activity is negligible, and CYP3A4 has reached peak levels of catalytic activity.

In addition to the phase I oxidative metabolism reactions that are important in the disposition of drugs, phase II conjugation reactions are also important in the disposition of some drugs used in children with cancer. For example, the anticancer drug irinotecan, the opioid analgesic morphine, and the antipyretic/analgesic acetaminophen are all glucuronidated by uridine 5'-diphosphase glucuronosyltransferase (UGT). However, at least 10 different isoforms of UGT have been identified. Moreover, some UGT isoforms are polymorphic, which may affect the interindividual variability in the disposition of UGT substrates. Irinotecan and acetaminophen are metabolized by isoforms in the UGT1A family, which is subject to genetic polymorphism and undergoes maturational changes. UGT1A1 is virtually undetectable in the fetus, its activity increases immediately after birth, and adult levels are attained by 3–6 mo of life. The activity of UGT1A3 is approx 30% of adult levels in neonates. UGT1A6 (for which acetaminophen is a substrate) activity slowly increases after birth to 50% of adult levels at 6 mo and does not reach adult levels prior to 10 yr of age. The implications of these developmental changes in the expression and activity of the UGT1A for the metabolism of irinotecan in children are discussed later in this chapter.

UGT2B7, which catalyzes the metabolism of morphine to morphine-6-glucuronide (100 time more potent analgesic than morphine), has approx 10–20% of adult activity by 15–27 wk of fetal life. Adult levels of UGT2B7 activity are reached by 2–30 mo of life. However, the complete ontogeny of all of the UGT isoforms has not yet been determined, so the full impact of the development of UGT on drug metabolism, especially anticancer drugs, is unknown.

Influence of Age on Renal Excretion

In the treatment of children with cancer many of the anticancer drugs and their metabolites are excreted renally; thus, it is important to understand the effect of maturation on renal function. As with adults, anticancer drugs and supportive therapy (e.g., cisplatin, radiocontrast dye, aminoglycosides, or amphotericin B) can alter renal function. Also, the presence of disease (e.g., from high burden of leukemic blasts, renal obstruction) can impair renal function. Thus, the clinician must accurately measure renal function in the pediatric patient; however, accurate measurement of renal function in this population presents challenges.

At birth, the glomerular filtration rate (GFR) in full-term infants is 40 mL/min/1.73 m^2, and it reaches adult values (90–140 mL/min/1.73 m^2) by 3 yr of age. Miall and colleagues have demonstrated that plasma creatinine rises in preterm infants during the first 48 h after birth, and the greatest absolute increase and the longest time to the mean peak in plasma creatinine occurred in infants 23–26 wk compared to ≥27 wk gestational age. The elevated plasma creatinine observed in the preterm infant population for approx 2 d after birth could be attributed to reabsorption of creatinine by the renal tubule or a delay in the establishment of a normal GFR. In the preterm infant population studied, all of the patients had respiratory distress syndrome, which could have contributed to a decreased GFR. Furthermore, preterm infants are predisposed to a delay in the development of a normal GFR secondary to incomplete nephrogenesis, which reaches completion at approx 34 wk postconception. Although such young infants are rarely treated for cancer, the clinician must consider not only postnatal age but also postconceptional age to determine appropriate dosages of renally excreted anticancer drugs in light of the development of GFR.

Schwartz and colleagues have demonstrated that the mean GFR for neonates 5-7 d of age is 50.6 mL/min/1.73 m^2. During the first year of life, GFR increases exponentially to a mean of 87 mL/min/ 1.73 m^2. Because the growth of lean body mass increases more rapidly than GFR after 1 yr of life, serum creatinine gradually increases during childhood to reach the normal adult values of 1.0-1.5 mg/ dL during adolescence.

Despite its limitations (e.g., cost and radioactivity), ^{99m}Tc-DTPA clearance is the best method for assessing GFR in children with cancer. In an uncomplicated pediatric patient the clinician might depend on a paradigm of renal developmental physiology to predict the capacity to eliminate a renally excreted drug. However, in a child with altered renal function due to multiple factors (e.g., maturational changes, malignancy, anticancer drugs, supportive care drugs, sepsis), the clinician cannot rely solely on this paradigm and must measure renal function. Although it is recommended that ^{99m}Tc-DTPA clearance be determined, in those institutions not able to perform these studies the clinician must utilize the best available method to assess renal function when dosing renally excreted drugs in children with altered renal function.

Selecting the Appropriate Method to Dose Anticancer Drugs in Children

Several reviews have recently addressed the question of the selection of the appropriate method to dose anticancer drugs. Although many of the issues regarding dosing anticancer drugs in adults that were addressed in these reviews may be relevant in children, many of the issues are different. A potential source of variability in calculation of drug doses in children arises from the different methods used to calculate body surface area (BSA). Although the initial approaches to measuring BSA utilized direct measurement techniques, current practices rely instead on nomograms developed from early studies. In 1916, the DuBois formula for calculation of BSA was developed by measuring the BSA of nine subjects (one child) and conducting regression analysis of the known height and weight of subjects to yield BSA = $W^{0.425} \times H^{0.725} \times 71.84$. Height (or supine length) in centimeters and weight in kilograms are the major components of the most frequently used formulas for calculating BSA. Therefore, one of the primary determinants of accurate assessment of BSA is accurate measurement of height and weight, which can be difficult to obtain in children. Calculation of BSA from regression is limited further by the potential for either over- or underestimation of true BSA in a proportion of the population.

It is common practice to normalize drug doses to a measure of body size (e.g., total body weight, BSA) with the intention of reducing interindividual variability in drug systemic exposure and thus response (i.e., efficacy and toxicity). In 287 adults, Grochow and colleagues examined the correlation between the pharmacokinetic parameters of nine anticancer drugs and weight, BSA, or height. The clearance of only one drug, paclitaxel, was highly correlated with one measure of body size, height. Thus, normalizing doses of the studied drugs did not reduce interindividual variability in drug exposure, leading the authors to recommend the use of fixed doses. Since the letter by Grochow and colleagues, numerous drugs have been examined in adults for a correlation between dosage normalization and variability in pharmacokinetic parameters. Gurney and colleagues summarized these reports and found that only 4 drugs out of 20 had a possible correlation of BSA and a pharmacokinetic parameter. Sawyer and Ratain recently reviewed the question of whether BSA or body weight is more appropriate to determine the dose of anticancer drugs in adults. The use of BSA was originally introduced into clinical medicine to translate data from preclinical animal studies to starting dosages for first-time human clinical trials. As these authors correctly note, many discrepancies have been suggested among the formulas used to calculate BSA in adults. Also the authors noted that BSA was selected for its perceived correlation with organ function associated with drug elimination, which is not supported by the analysis of Grochow et al. or Gurney. Although liver volume measured by magnetic resonance imaging (MRI) in children with cancer correlated with BSA, owing to the inconsistencies in the results of studies of liver volume, body weight, BSA, and clearance of hepatically eliminated drugs, hepatic oxidative metabolism is unlikely to correlate with BSA. Moreover, creatinine clearance has not been shown to correlate with BSA. Lean body weight correlates more strongly than BSA with physiologic volumes. No correlation of BSA with the pharmacokinetics of epirubicin, carboplatin, and etoposide has been found. Sawyer and Ratain suggest that the use of BSA in the dosing of anticancer agents has not been sufficiently validated, and they recommend that BSA be evaluated prospectively along with age, renal and hepatic function, albumin, and other covariates in future pharmacokinetic studies of anticancer drugs to determine which covariate(s) most appropriately reduce the interpatient variability in response (e.g., efficacy, toxicity, systemic exposure). Although several experts in the pharmacokinetics of anticancer drugs in adults have recommended that the convention of calculating doses solely based on BSA be abandoned, the evidence to support completely abandoning this convention for children is still lacking. However, for selected drugs in some pediatric populations, dosing anticancer drugs based on body weight is more appropriate than dosing based on BSA.

Infants have proportionately higher BSA to weight than older children, so drug dosages based on BSA rather than weight may be too large for infants. Evans and colleagues have demonstrated a statistically significant difference in doxorubicin clearance when normalized to BSA between children < 2 yr old and children > 2 yr old; however, between these two groups a statistically significant difference was not observed in doxorubicin clearance normalized to weight. To minimize anthracycline-induced cardiotoxicity, it has been suggested to use either lower milligram per meter squared doses of doxorubicin in young children or to dose doxorubicin in young children in terms of milligram per kilogram, but no further studies have been published to validate this recommendation. Conversely, when comparing children < 1 yr ($n = 2$) and > 1 yr ($n = 23$), the same investigators demonstrated a statistically significant difference in etoposide systemic clearance between the age groups when normalized to body weight but not when normalized to BSA. Although this study contained a small number of subjects, a relationship between total body weight and clearance was defined. In addition, specific dosing recommendations based on body size are discussed for individual drugs later in this chapter.

Practical Issues Involved with Clinical Pharmacokinetic Studies in Children with Cancer

In addition to the effect of maturation leading to differences between children and adults in drug disposition, the clinician must also consider the practical aspects of pharmacokinetic studies conducted in children. Often children will have indwelling venous access for administration of anticancer drugs; however, this site is not practical for obtaining pharmacokinetic samples because of the need for repeated use of the line and infection concerns, excessive blood loss due to flushing of the line, and potential for drug adsorption, which might lead to falsely high plasma concentrations. Therefore, children enrolled in pharmacokinetic studies often need two separate lines, a central line from which blood is drawn and a peripheral line where the anticancer agent is administered. Another potential option for the patient with a double-lumen Hickman or Broviac central line is to use the same line for drug administration and sample acquisition; however, this must be done with appropriate attention to catheter care (e.g,. proper flushing and nursing care) and careful attention to the results of the pharmacokinetic study to determine if adsorption has occurred.

As noted previously, children have a smaller intravascular volume than adults, which places a practical limit on the volume of blood that can be safely collected from each subject for pharmacokinetic studies. Currently, no formal recommendation is available for the amount of blood that can be obtained from children for pharmacokinetic studies. However, the FDA has published guidelines for industry that state that the volume of blood withdrawn should be “minimized” in pediatric studies and institutional review boards/independent ethics committees should review and may define the maximum amount of blood (usually on a milliliters per kilogram or percentage of total blood volume basis) that may be used for pharmacokinetic studies. Some institutions use 5–7% of total blood volume in 24 h or 3–5 mL blood/kg over 8 wk as a guideline for the maximum amount of blood that can be withdrawn from a child for pharmacokinetic studies. Selection of the most informative sample times for pharmacokinetic studies in children is critical. However, even with appropriate selection of plasma sample times for pharmacokinetic studies the clinician should consider that for the individual child blood will be collected not only for pharmacokinetic studies but also for routine laboratory tests including serum chemistries, complete blood counts, bacterial cultures, and blood gases. In neonates and infants, even the discard volume from routine blood draws may be significant. Therefore, the clinician must coordinate pharmacokinetic studies with the clinical pharmacologist.

Population pharmacokinetic modeling and limited sampling models can help maximize the information obtained from pharmacokinetic studies in children with cancer. For example, for a given drug, data sets from a large population of patients can be analyzed to determine if any patient specific factors, such as age, weight, or renal function, correlate with the pharmacokinetic parameters (e.g., systemic clearance). These correlations between patient specific parameters and pharmacokinetic parameters can be useful to refine dosage selection as exemplified by carboplatin dosing based on a patient's renal function and desired carboplatin systemic exposure. Similarly, with analysis of concentration–time profiles collected from serial plasma samples, a limited sampling model can be derived that will minimize the number of plasma samples necessary for a pharmacokinetic study, yet maximize the information yielded from those samples. Thus, with the application of these techniques the clinician can derive much information from a child with cancer regarding the clinical pharmacology of a drug, while remaining attentive to the volume of blood taken from the patient.

Pharmacokinetics of Specific Anticancer Drugs in Children

Methotrexate

Methotrexate is a folate acid antagonist used as an antileukemic agent since the 1940s. Methotrexate competitively inhibits dihydrofolate reductase (DHFR), the enzyme responsible for converting folic acid to reduced folate cofactors, and interferes with several critical biosynthetic pathways including DNA and RNA synthesis. Methotrexate is FDA approved for use in the treatment of acute lymphocytic leukemia (ALL) and osteosarcoma in adults and children. Furthermore, methotrexate is used extensively in both adults and children for nonmalignant diseases such as rheumatoid arthritis. New regimens containing methotrexate are currently being evaluated in pediatric clinical trials for the treatment of ALL and osteosarcoma. Pharmacokinetic monitoring of patients receiving methotrexate has been shown to reduce morbidity and mortality associated with this drug.

The oral bioavailability of methotrexate is highly variable in adults and children, with reports ranging from 36–83% to 25–95%. Because some children who have received larger doses of oral methotrexate absorbed a smaller fraction of the dose, it is possible that the mechanism of methotrexate absorption may be saturable. Certainly, this trend can be seen when comparing studies with a range of dosages. Balis and colleagues observed a 30% higher methotrexate area under the concentration–time curve (AUC) in girls than boys after oral dosing and suggested that gender-related absorption mechanisms might be related. Also, it has been shown that when methotrexate is administered with milk a delay occurs in the time to peak methotrexate concentration as well as a decrease in the AUC. In addition, more recently Dupuis and colleagues have shown that time to peak methotrexate concentration was increased and bioavailability was decreased when it was administered orally after a meal.

The volume of distribution of methotrexate is approx 0.18 L/kg; however, its steady-state volume of distribution has been studied more recently and ranges from 0.4 to 0.8 L/kg. Methotrexate is approx 50% bound to albumin in plasma. Organs with the greatest distribution of methotrexate are kidney, gall bladder, bone marrow, small intestine, and liver. Methotrexate also distributes into pleural fluid and ascites, Even though concentrations in these "third spaces" reach only about 10% maximum serum concentrations, the movement of methotrexate from third spaces into the central compartment is slow, leading to a prolonged systemic clearance. Thus, the presence of ascites or pleural effusions should be documented so that a sufficient duration of leucovorin rescue can be provided.

Methotrexate cerebrospinal fluid (CSF) concentrations range about 1.5–2.5% of serum concentrations after a 24-h infusion. However, if higher dosages are used ($\geq$ 5 g/m^2 over 24 h), it is possible to achieve cytotoxic concentrations ($\geq$ 0.01 μmol/L) despite poor distribution into CSF. To attain putatively cytotoxic CSF concentrations methotrexate has been administered via the intrathecal route. Intrathecal dosage regimens based on body surface area underdose children < 8 yr old because they have larger CSF volumes relative to their body surface area. Because of these age-related changes in CSF volume, it has been suggested that intrathecal methotrexate dose should be based on age. However, Strother and colleagues did not find age to be significantly correlated with methotrexate dose in a group of patients treated with intra-Ommaya methotrexate.

The metabolism of methotrexate in children is primarily catalyzed by hepatic aldehyde oxidase, which yields the less active metabolite, 7-hydroxymethotrexate, which has been found in low concentrations (0.1–0.3 μM). However, the ontogeny of hepatic aldehyde oxidase has not been well characterized. Even though 7-hydroxymethotrexate is 40–200 times less active then methotrexate against DHFR it could still have clinical consequences. Because this metabolite is less soluble than methotrexate at physiologic pH, it may contribute to renal toxicity through precipitation in renal tubules. Bacteria in the gastrointestinal tract also metabolize both oral and enterohepatically recycled methotrexate to 4-

amino-4-deoxy-N^{10}-methylpteroic acid (DAMPA). This metabolite is rarely detectable in patients and is 200 times less active than methotrexate. Also in both adults and children, folyl polyglutamate synthetase metabolizes intracellular methotrexate to methotrexate-polyglutamates, which are more toxic to cells than methotrexate, because the polyglutamates are retained by cells for longer periods of time than methotrexate. Methotrexate-polyglutamates are at least as active as methotrexate, and therefore have a major role in the cytotoxicity of methotrexate.

Renal excretion of methotrexate is a primary route of methotrexate elimination, with approx 80% excreted unchanged in the urine in 24 h through renal tubular secretion and glomerular filtration. Less than 10% of a dose is excreted as the 7-hydroxymethotrexate metabolite in the urine; however, this has been shown to increase when methotrexate is administered as a prolonged infusion. Furthermore, methotrexate systemic clearance, which includes renal and nonrenal pathways, is higher in children than in adults and decreases with age. However, this can be due to a variety of factors that can alter the disposition of methotrexate such as renal function, pleural effusion, and gastrointestinal obstruction.

Hydration and urinary alkalinization can increase the renal clearance of methotrexate as shown in the study by Sand and Jacobsen. It is therefore recommended that patients are well hydrated with intravenous fluids and treated with sodium bicarbonate to alkalinize the urine prior to high dose methotrexate therapy (i.e., intravenous fluid [with 40 mEq $NaHCO_3$/L] administered at the rate of 200 mL/m^2/h for at least 2 h before the start of high-dose methotrexate). Urinary pH should also be monitored during infusion and additional sodium bicarbonate therapy be administered if the pH is $\leq$ 6.0. Acetazolamide may be used if systemic alkalosis limits the administration of bicarbonate for urinary alkalinization.

Murry and colleagues evaluated the effects of the variability in GFR on the pharmacokinetic variability of methotrexate clearance in children receiving remission-induction therapy for ALL. Because GFR accounted for only 37% of the variability in methotrexate clearance, the investigators concluded that tubular secretion and reabsorption, hydration, volume status, urinary alkalinization, and nonrenal clearance might also contribute significantly to methotrexate pharmacokinetic variability. In addition, they demonstrated that remission-induction therapy that included methotrexate, leucovorin rescue, prednisone, vincristine, daunorubicin, asparaginase, etoposide, and cytarabine was not associated with a significant reduction in GFR when compared to pretreatment values.

Methotrexate is also excreted into the bile, however, to a much smaller extent (approx 10%) than other routes of elimination. Although biliary excretion is not a major route of elimination, methotrexate can be reabsorbed from the gastrointestinal tract, which can prolong its terminal half-life.

Cyclophosphamide and Ifosfamide

The oxazophosphorine alkylating agents cyclophosphamide and ifosfamide are prodrugs that are activated by 4-hydroxylation via the CYP450 system to 4-hydroxycy-clophosphamide and 4-hydroxyifosfamide, respectively. Cyclophosphamide is approved for acute nonlymphocytic leukemia (ANLL), ALL, neuroblastoma, retinoblastoma, and Wilms' tumor. However, cyclophosphamide is also used in bone marrow transplantation, childhood germ cell tumors, Ewing's sarcoma, osteosarcoma, and rhabdomyosarcoma. Ifosfamide is used in Hodgkin's lymphoma, non-Hodgkin's lymphoma, Ewing's sarcoma, osteosarcoma, rhabdomyosarcoma, and Wilms' tumor.

Metabolic deactivation of ifosfamide to 2- and 3-dechloroethylifosfamide by CYP3A4 and 2B6 also yields an equimolar amount of chloroacetaldehyde, which has been implicated in the neurotoxicity associated with ifosfamide. Kerbusch and colleagues have demonstrated that coadministration of ketoconazole with ifosfamide can reduce the formation of the active metabolite 4-hydroxyifosfamide, which may lead to reduced antitumor efficacy. They also showed that coadministration of rifampin with ifosfamide increases the metabolism of ifosfamide to both the active metabolite and the two inactive metabolites 2- and 3- dechloroethylifosfamide, as well as the neurotoxic byproduct chloracetaldehyde. Thus, they concluded that administration of either the CYP inhibitor ketoconazole or the CYP inducer rifampin can reduce the therapeutic benefit of ifosfamide.

Yule and colleagues have evaluated the pharmacokinetics of cyclophosphamide in pediatric patients and reported a wide interpatient variability in drug disposition. The cyclophosphamide clearance varied from 1.2 to 10.6 L/h/m^2. The half-life varied from 1.1 to 16.8 h, and was significantly prolonged at high dosage levels. In a more recent study, Yule and colleagues have demonstrated that fluconazole inhibits the first step in the activation of cyclophosphamide in vitro. Moreover, in a group of 22 children ranging in age from 2 mo to 18 yr, they have demonstrated a statistically significant reduction in clearance and increase in half-life of cyclophosphamide when fluconazole is coadministered.

Because pharmacologically induced changes in the expression and/or activity of the cytochrome P450 system resulted in changes in the metabolism and clearance of cyclophosphamide and ifosfamide, similar variations could be observed in children of different ages treated with cyclophosphamide or ifosfamide owing to the maturational changes in the CYP450 system. Therefore, not only should the clinician be aware of specific CYP450 drug interactions (actual or potential) with cyclophosphamide and ifosfamide, but also the clinician should anticipate different patterns of metabolism of these drugs in children of various ages.

Vincristine

Vincristine is a naturally occurring alkaloid, which exerts its cytotoxic effects by binding to tubulin, thus stopping mitosis and leading to apoptosis. Vincristine has been approved by the FDA as part of a combination regimen to treat a variety of adult and pediatric malignancies, including, ALL, Hodgkin's disease, and Wilms' tumor. Because it lacks myelosuppression as a dose-limiting toxicity, vincristine is an attractive anticancer agent for use in combination with other myelo suppressive agents. In general, vincristine pharmacokinetics are associated with high intra- and interindividual variability in children; however, intraindividual variability is usually smaller than interindividual variability.

Vincristine is administered as an intravenous infusion or bolus dose due to poor oral absorption. Gidding and colleagues demonstrated that the vincristine volume of distribution at steady state is variable in children with acute lymphoblastic leukemia, non-Hodgkin's lymphoma, or Wilms' tumor (range: 56–1165 L/m^2). Within 15–30 min after intravenous administration vincristine is rapidly distributed, and $> 90\%$ distributes from the blood to the tissue where it is tightly (but not irreversibly) bound. Although CSF penetration of vincristine is poor, intrathecal administration is strictly contraindicated because of associated lethality.

Vincristine is metabolized by the CYP3A family into a variety of poorly characterized metabolites that are considered devoid of antitumor activity. Because coexpression of CYP3A4 and NADPH-P450 (hOR) in a Chinese hamster ovary (CHO) cell line decreased the cytotoxicity of vincristine compared to the parental CHO line, Yao and colleagues conclude that vincristine metabolism by the P450 system leads to inactivation. Furthermore, vincristine systemic clearance was significantly increased with a consequent significant decrease in the AUC in patients with brain tumors who were receiving the CYP3A4-inducing antiepileptic drugs carbamazepine or phenytoin compared to control patients who did not receive any CYP3A4 inducing agents. While it is unknown whether the induction of the clearance of the vinca alkaloids has a clinically significant consequence (i.e., reduction in efficacy or toxicity), inhibition of vincristine clearance has been shown to augment toxicity. Furthermore, age-related changes in the CYP3A system could contribute to the high interindividual variability in vincristine pharmacokinetics among children.

Conflicting reports about the similarities or differences in the pharmacokinetics of vincristine between pediatric and adult populations may reflect increased sophistication of assay methods with time. An early report of vincristine pharmacokinetics in children showed similar disposition in adults and children; however, this study was conducted in only four children using a radioimmunoas say rather than the more specific high-performance liquid chromatography (HPLC) method. Woods and colleagues demonstrated that a high incidence of neurotoxity in infants smaller than 0.5 m^2 and recommended that children with a BSA of < 1 m^2 receive dosages based on body weight. Delayed hepatic conjugation and clearance of vincristine and the large ratio of BSA to weight in infants could cause the observed increase in toxicity. A more recent study used a specific HPLC assay for vincristine and showed that the vincristine clearance in children with acute lymphoblastic leukemia was higher than in adults with lung cancer (431 vs 189 mL/min/m^2). This study, however, did not account for concomitant medications, such as steroids and antibiotics, which may have accounted for the increased vincristine clearance. Crom and colleagues used this same HPLC method, and in 54 children aged 2–18 yr reported a vincristine clearance similar to that reported by de Graaf (482 mL/min/m^2); however, in the Crom study only two patients received CYP450 inducers, so it is likely that children do have a higher vincristine clearance than adults.

Two recent reports discuss aspects of interindividual variability in vincristine pharmacokinetics in children. Gidding and colleagues showed that age had a weak positive correlation with vincristine clearance when normalized to body surface area, but a weak negative correlation when normalized to body weight. Their findings are consistent with the reports of Woods et al. and Crom et al., which also describe a significant relationship between weight and vincristine clearance. Drug–drug interactions also contribute to the interindividual variability seen with vincristine pharmacokinetics, as observed by Gidding and colleagues when they showed that children who received steroids, which induce CYP3A isoenzymes, had a significantly higher vincristine clearance ($p = 0.0092$). Groninger and colleagues administered vincristine as a single agent to children ages 1–16 yr and reported a clearance of 228 mL/min/m^2. This value, which is lower than that reported by other investigators, could be due to exclusion of very young children and the absence of enzyme-inducing drugs. However, they did find that $t_{1/2}\beta$ was significantly smaller and clearance was significantly higher in children who received cephalosporins, but did not offer any further pharmacological explanation (including details of cephalosporin therapy). The relationship between vincristine disposition and measures of biliary function have been investigated, as vincristine is eliminated mainly in the bile. Two authors found vincristine clearance to be inversely related to alkaline phosphatase and gamma-glutamyltransferase; however, these enzymes are not specific to biliary function. Other investigators have seen no correlation between vincristine clearance and total bilirubin, alkaline phosphatase, or albumin level.

Etoposide

Etoposide, a topoisomerase II inhibitor that can be administered orally or intravenously, is used in the treatment of children with ALL, AML, ANLL, Ewing's sarcoma, non-Hodgkin's lymphoma, neuroblastoma, retinoblastoma, rhabdomyo sarcoma, and Wilms' tumor. High-dose etoposide is also used in conditioning regimens for bone marrow transplantation.

Chen and colleagues determined that the mean (range) bioavailability of etoposide in 12 children with relapsed ALL is 60.6% (17.6–91.2%). By evaluating the disposition of oral etoposide in 16 patients ranging in age from 3 to 73 yr in comparison to intravenous etoposide in 18 different children ranging in age from 0.8 to 17 yr, Wurthwein and colleagues determined a similar mean apparent bioavailability of 59%.

In children with ALL, Relling and colleagues have studied the penetration of intravenous and oral etopo side into the CSF. Although only approx 0.3% of the concentrations of etoposide that are attained in plasma are reached in the CSF, it is thought that even these low levels of etopo side can be cytotoxic to leukemic blasts, depending on the inherent sensitivity of each individual child's disease to etoposide. The ratio of etoposide CSF and plasma concentrations in children with ALL are comparable to those observed in adults with brain tumors without tumor invasion of the ventricles or subarachnoid space (0.7%). Therefore, it is unlikely that age-related changes exist in the penetration of etoposide into the CSF; changes in CSF penetration are more likely due to the effects of specific disease (e.g., disruption of the blood–brain barrier).

Etoposide is extensively plasma protein bound (90–94%). In eight children ranging in age from 4.2 to 22 yr with refractory solid tumors, 45% of the parent drug was excreted unchanged in the urine. In children with refractory solid tumors investigators reported an inverse relationship between albumin concentration and etoposide renal clearance, which suggests that a changes in albumin concentration might influence the amount of free drug available for renal clearance.

In vitro, CYP3A4 catalyzes 3'-demethylation of etoposide, and CYP1A2 and 2E1 also have minor catalytic activity in this metabolic pathway. Ketoconazole, troleandomycin, verapamil, cyclosporin, vincristine, and prednisolone inhibited etoposide 3'-demethylation in human liver microsomes. CYP3A4 also catalyzes the *O*-demethylation of etoposide in vitro in human hepatic microsomes and heterologous expression systems, which can be inhibited by erythromycin, cyclosporin, dexamethasone, prednisone, midazolam, nifedipine, and troleandomycin. Furthermore, a high degree of variability was observed in the maximal microsomal activity among individual livers, which may account for some of the interindividual variation in the disposition of etoposide.

Wurthwein and colleagues have reported a population pharmacokinetic model of the disposition of high-dose etoposide in children ranging in age from 9.6 mo to 23.7 yr. The concentration–time data were best fit by a three-compartment model with a volume of distribution, clearance, AUC, and terminal half-life of 0.067 L/kg, 15.5 mL/min/m^2, 1175 mg/L·h, and 44.2 h, respectively. These values are similar to those reported by Evans and colleagues. High inter- and intraindividual variability in protein binding was observed in this study. Furthermore, they demonstrated a negative correlation between age and etoposide clearance normalized to body weight; however, they found no correlation between age and clearance normalized to BSA. However, Boos and colleagues demonstrated that etoposide clearance adjusted neither for weight or BSA was correlated with age. Thus, no relationship has been reported between etoposide clearance (normalized to weight) and age.

Topotecan

Topotecan, a water-soluble camptothecin analog, is a topoisomerase I inhibitor. Topotecan undergoes a reversible, pH-dependent conversion from the lactone form to carboxylate form at physiologic pH. Topotecan has been approved by the FDA as second-line treatment of small-cell lung cancer and ovarian cancer in adults; however, it has been shown to be effective in a variety of pediatric solid tumors and leukemias. Topotecan is currently being evaluated as a single agent or in combination in clinical trials in children to treat neuroblastoma, medulloblastoma, glioblastoma, ALL, and other childhood cancers.

The oral bioavailability of the intravenous solution of topotecan in children is approx 30%, which is similar to that reported in adults. After oral administration topotecan peak lactone plasma concentrations occurred from 0.75 to 2 h. The absorption half-life of topotecan lactone was 0.78 ± 0.54 h. Large interpatient variability was noted in oral topotecan pharmacokinetics, whereas intrapatient variability was relatively small.

The topotecan volume of distribution (V_{dss}) has shown high interindividual variability. In adults it is as large as 160 L; however, in children it has been reported to be 73 ± 27 L/m^2 and 13–458 L/m^2. A study in adults showed that topotecan also distributes into third spaces and pleural effusions without sequestration. Furthermore, these authors demonstrated that distribution into third spaces had no effect on topotecan disposition, but inadequate data were presented to evaluate fully the conclusion of the authors. Plasma protein binding of topotecan is 7–35% in adults and children, which is reasonably low. Alterations in plasma proteins in children, whether age-related or disease-related, will likely not alter topotecan disposition or pharmacologic effect.

Topotecan is metabolized by the CYP450 enzyme system to an active metabolite, *N*-desmethyl topotecan, and has also been found to exist as an *O*-glucuronide. However, topotecan primarily undergoes renal elimination, with 49–70% of a dose recovered in the urine as unchanged drug.

The renal excretion of topotecan includes both glomerular filtration and tubular secretion. A study of adults receiving topotecan demonstrated that patients with impaired glomerular filtration, as measured by creatinine clearance, had decreased topotecan renal clearance. Thus it is recommended that adult patients with creatinine clearance <39 mL/ min receive topotecan at reduced dosages. However, renal dysfunction in children receiving topotecan did not alter topotecan renal or systemic clearance. In a study of six children with unilateral nephrectomies due to Wilms' tumor, a topotecan clearance of 25.7 L/h/m^2 was reported. When compared with an age-, SrCR-, and BSA-matched cohort of patients the topotecan clearance was not statistically different ($p = 0.08$) although the Wilms' tumor patients had significantly reduced GFR ($p = 0.03$), as measured by ^{99m}Tc-DTPA clearance. It is likely that other mechanisms (i.e., increase in drug transporters, other unspecified metabolic pathways) may have compensated for the anticipated decrease in topotecan renal clearance. Based on these data, it is therefore not recommended that topotecan dosage be altered in children with decreased renal function as measured by ^{99m}Tc-DTPA clearance.

The disposition of topotecan in infants <2 yr has been evaluated and results have shown that clearance correlated with weight better than BSA. This finding supports the practice of dosing infants (<2 yr of age) by weight instead of BSA. Multiple studies of pharmacokinetically guided dosing to attain discrete target AUC have also been conducted. Thus far, we have been successful in adjusting individual patients' topotecan systemic exposure to reduce interindividual variability in drug exposure.

Irinotecan

Irinotecan also inhibits topoisomerase I and is a prodrug that must be activated by carboxylesterase to form SN-38, the active moiety of irinotecan. Similar to topotecan, irinotecan undergoes reversible pH-dependent hydrolysis from lactone to carboxylate at physiologic pH. The FDA has approved irinotecan for use in adults with colorectal cancer. Although irinotecan has not yet been approved for pediatric use, preclinical studies have shown that neuroblastoma is sensitive to both oral and intravenous irinotecan. Furthermore, in Phase I trials in children, irinotecan is active in a variety of solid tumors including neuroblastoma, hepatocellular carcinoma, pineoblastoma, glioblastoma, brainstem glioma, osteosarcoma, hepatoblastoma, rhabdomyosarcoma, and squamous cell carcinoma of the larynx.

Although irinotecan is only 8% bioavailable, in children (2–19 yr) with solid tumors, the relative extent of conversion of irinotecan to SN-38 is greater for oral administration (0.38 ± 0.31) than for intravenous administration (0.11 ± 0.06), suggesting that SN-38 is formed presystemically after oral irinotecan. Thus oral administration is a reasonable alternative to intravenous, and Phase I studies of oral irinotecan are ongoing.

The age-related changes in bacterial colonization of the gastrointestinal tract have theoretical implications for drug absorption and metabolism as exemplified by irinotecan. Irinotecan-associated diarrhea can be ameliorated in a rat model by administration of penicillin and streptomycin. These antibiotics can in effect inhibit the cleavage of SN-38 glucuronide to SN-38 in the gut by elimination of the β-glucuronidase-producing bacteria. In a follow-up study, the same group demonstrated that inhibition of β-glucuronidase increased the exposure of the large intestinal luminal tissue to SN-38 glucuronide and decreased the exposure of this tissue to SN-38. Furthermore, inhibition of β-glucuronidase did not alter the systemic pharmacokinetics or small intestinal luminal exposure of irinotecan, SN-38 glucuronide, or SN-38. These results have important implications for irinotecan-associated diarrhea. Because bacterial flora change with age, one should be aware of developmental stage when administering anticancer drugs for which the parent drug or the metabolite is a substrate of β-glucuronidase. In theory, very young children in whom gastrointestinal flora are not fully established would be less susceptible than adults or older children to irinotecan-induced diarrhea owing to a relative lack of β-glucuronidase, which increases the local exposure of the large intestine to the putative toxic moiety, SN-38.

SN-38 is highly protein bound. Children with serum albumin within normal limits (3.0–4.4 g/dL) exhibited approx 3.4% unbound SN-38 (range 0.7–6.5%). Thus, the clinician must be aware of possible interactions between irinotecan and other highly protein- bound drugs and pathophysiological changes that can alter a child's serum albumin. The clearance of irinotecan lactone in children is approx 55.5 L/h/m^2, which is similar to that observed in adults.

Irinotecan is extensively metabolized in the liver by carboxylesterase to form the active metabolite SN-38, which is subsequently metabolized by hepatic UDP-glucuronyltransferase (UGT) and CYP450. SN-38 is glucuronidated by the UGT1 family. Ciotti and colleagues have demonstrated that COS-1 cells transfected with UGT1A7 were 12- to 40-fold more active at pH 7.6 in the conjugation of SN-38 to glucuronide than nine other isoforms of the UGT1A family, including UGT1A1, which had been previously demonstrated to be the predominant isoform responsible for this reaction. In addition, Hanioka and colleagues have demonstrated that recombinant human UGT1A3, UGT1A6, and UGT1A9 expressed in microsomes of insect cells catalyze the glucuronidation of SN-38. Because the expression of the UGT1A family increases as a child matures and because this family of enzymes detoxifies SN-38, children may be subject to an increased risk of SN-38 toxicity compared to adults until the expression of UGT1A isoforms reaches adult levels. SN-38 is also metabolized by CYP3A to NPC and APC. NPC can be metabolized by carboxylesterase to SN-38; whereas APC is not converted to SN-38 in the presence of carboxylesterase. Although NPC appeared to induce topoisomerase I-mediated DNA cleavage, it is thought that this pharmacologic property is due to contamination with SN-38 rather than activity of NPC itself. Even though NPC is likely an inactive metabolite, it can be converted to the active SN-38; therefore, alterations in CYP3A metabolism through pharmacologic induction or inhibition, developmental stage, or genetic polymorphism could impact the pharmacokinetics of irinotecan and its metabolites and thus the clinical response to this anticancer drug.

Enzyme-inducing anticonvulsants (EIAs) have been shown to alter pharmacokinetics of irinotecan in children (age range 3–21 yr) with high grade glioma. Patients who received EIAs exhibited greater clearance of irinotecan lactone and lower SN-38 lactone AUCs than those who did not receive EIAs. Because those who received EIAs did not have a significantly greater median AUC of APC than those who did not receive EIAs, induction of CYP3A4 may not explain the alteration in the pharmacokinetics of irinotecan in the presence of EIAs. The mechanism for the increase in the systemic clearance of irinotecan without a consequent increase in the AUC of its metabolites has yet to be elucidated, but it is thought that EIAs may increase the biliary excretion of irinotecan through induction of MRP2 (ABCC2) and Pgp (ABCB1). When possible, EIAs should be avoided in children receiving irinotecan; if anticonvulsants are required, the newer non-enzyme-inducing anticonvulsants should be considered.

Temozolomide

Temozolomide is a methylating agent that is approved for treatment of refractory anaplastic astrocytoma in adults and is undergoing evaluation for use in pediatrics to treat high-grade gliomas and sarcomas. This highly bioavailable compound undergoes spontaneous base-catalyzed hydrolysis to form the methyl triazene, MTIC, which is the final active methylating species. MTIC is believed to exert its toxic effects through acid catalysis, forming the methyldiazonium ion, which ultimately leads to O^6-methylguanine formation in DNA plus the inactive metabolite, AIC.

Only one pediatric pharmacokinetic study has been published that evaluated temozolomide disposition. After oral administration temozolomide was rapidly absorbed, with maximal concentrations observed within 60 min. Based on the assumption of 0.98 oral bioavailability, the total body clearance of temozolomide was 100 mL/min/m^2 and the plasma elimination half-life was approx 100 min. The AUC seen with the 200 mg/m^2/dose was the same for a single dose or after repeated doses (d 1 vs d 5). Plasma elimination half-life and apparent total body clearance values were constant over the dose range of 100–260 mg/m^2.

Beale and colleagues showed that, although a theoretical possibility, increasing gastric pH by administration of an H_2-receptor antagonist did not alter the bioavailability of temozolomide. In the case of children who are unable or are too young to swallow temozolomide capsules, temozolomide capsules can be opened carefully and reconstituted in applesauce, apple juice, or orange juice. No clinically relevant difference has been observed in temozolomide pharmacokinetic parameters using this method of administration.

Recent advances in cellular and molecular biology techniques have led to an increased understanding of pediatric clinical pharmacology, and in many instances a more rational approach to dosing drugs in children. As described in this chapter, a stronger scientific basis for dosing drugs in children will be derived from an increased understanding of the effects of maturation on the physiological processes affecting drug disposition, concomitant drug therapy, and disease states. Moreover, a further evaluation of the most appropriate dosing approach (e.g., dose per weight, height, BSA, age) in the pediatric population is warranted. Because the importance of pharmacokinetic and pharmacodynamic studies in this age group has been highlighted, an improved understanding of the clinical pharmacology of many anticancer drugs in children has been gained. In addition, computer hardware and software has become readily available to enhance the conduct of pharmacokinetic studies. This improvement in technology has encouraged investigators to pursue additional aspects of clinical pharmacokinetic studies, including pharmacokinetically guided dosing, on a more routine basis in this age group. This approach is viewed as one method to reduce the wide interindividual variability that so often characterizes pediatric pharmacokinetic parameters. Finally, pharmacogenomic analysis in children with cancer will further explain the observed interindividual variability in pharmacokinetics, toxicity, and efficacy. Establishing phenotype–genotype correlations will improve the care of children with cancer.

15

PHARMACOKINETICS OF TOXICOLOGY

Monoclonal antibodies (MAbs) are presently being used to treat malignant and nonmalignant diseases. MAb therapy began several years after the development of hybridoma technology in 1975. Early clinical trials using murine MAbs showed that they were immunogenic and, with a few exceptions, had little benefit. Furthermore, they had a short half-life ($t_{1/2}$) in the circulation and poor Fc-mediated effector functions. The generation of human anti-murine IgG antibody (HAMA) usually precluded repeated administration because of rapid immune elimination and toxic side effects resulting from the formation of immune complexes. The therapeutic effect of murine MAbs was impaired not only by HAMA but also by their short $t_{1/2}$ before HAMA was elicited. The half-life of murine IgG in humans is 1 d, which is 20-fold shorter than that of human IgG. Conversely, in mice, both human and mouse IgG have $t_{1/2}$s of 5 d. The molecular basis of this behavior has recently been elucidated by analyzing the binding of IgG to mouse and human neonatal Fc receptor (FcRn). Data obtained using mice as a model for pharmacokinetics (PK) may therefore not always be relevant to humans.

To improve the efficacy of murine MAbs, several chemical and genetic approaches have been used to "arm" MAbs with toxic moieties (immunotoxins) (ITs). ITs consist of MAbs linked to toxin or toxin subunits from plants, bacteria, or fungi. ITs

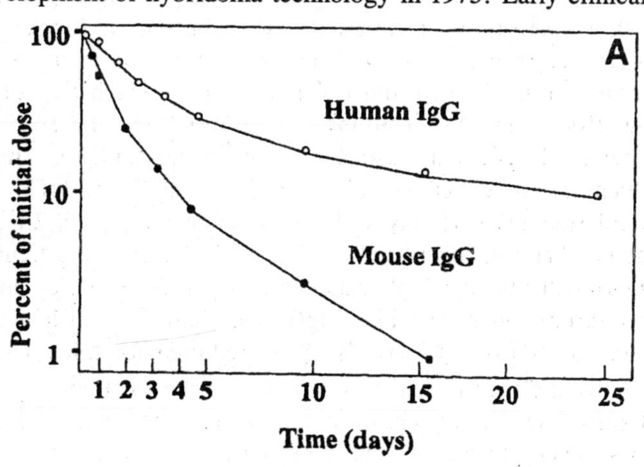

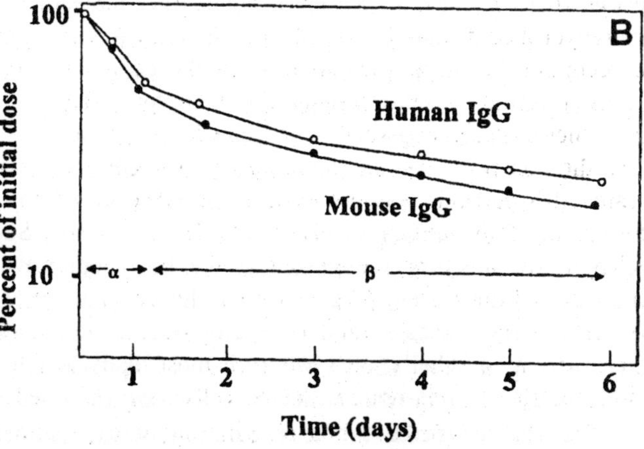

Fig. 15.1. Elimination curves of IgGs. A–Mouse and human IgGs in humans. B–Mouse and human IgGs in mouse.

are more cytotoxic to targeted cells than "naked" MAbs. In this case, the short persistence of the ITs in the circulation is not a drawback but an advantage because the body can rapidly eliminate the unbound cytotoxic IT. For the same reason, ITs constructed with fragments of murine IgG with short half-lives have been successfully used in some clinical trials. Murine MAbs radiolabeled with ^{131}I or ^{90}Y have been highly successful in the treatment of relapsed lymphoma despite their short half-lives and immunogenicity.

The development of chimerized (ch) and humanized (hu) MAbs has corrected two of the weaknesses owtmurine MAbs, that is, short $t_{1/2}$ and poor effector functions. The ch and hu MAbs have the same $t_{1/2}$ in the circulation as human IgG. The longer persistence of ch and hu MAbs results in increased penetration of tumors and better therapeutic activity. Their effector functions (recruiting FcR-bearing effector cells and complement components) are also excellent. The immunogenicity of ch and hu MAbs is considerably diminished, and they have few adverse effects. Clearly, the structure and PK of the MAbs and ITs have a major impact in their effectiveness in vivo. Therefore, understanding mechanisms that control their persistence in the circulation is of crucial importance.

Mechanisms Underlying the Persistence of IgG in the Circulation

Following infusion of an IgG antibody, its disappearance from the circulation can be divided into a short period of intravascular distribution, a longer phase of equilibration between intra- and extravascular compartments, and slow removal from the circulation by catabolism. IgG elimination curves can be divided into two phases from which the corresponding PK parameters can be calculated. The first is the fast equilibration α-phase and the second is the slow catabolic β-phase. However, some catabolism may also occur during the α-phase. The most documented parameter is the β-phase which is also called the biological $t_{1/2}$. The $t_{1/2}$ of IgG correlates directly with its persistence in the circulation and inversely with its catabolic rate ($= \ln 2/t_{1/2}$). Studies on the PK of IgG in humans have shown that catabolism is accelerated in myeloma patients who have increased levels of serum IgG (short half-life and high catabolic rate) and decreased in hypogammaglobulinemic patients who have low serum concentrations of IgG (long half-life and low catabolic rate). This catabolism–concentration effect of human IgG has also been reported for mice and other species.

To explain the relationship between the catabolic rate of IgG and its serum concentration in mice, Brambell et al. hypothesized that IgG is internalized into the cells involved in catabolism by fluid phase endocytosis and that a proportion of the antibody is then bound to intracellular receptors that recognize its Fc region. Receptor-bound IgG molecules are protected from lysosomal degradation and are recycled back into the circulation. In contrast, unbound molecules are degraded. Because the number of receptors is limited, an increase in the concentration of IgG in the circulation results in a shorter $t_{1/2}$ as a result of saturation of the receptors, that is, the proportion of internalized, unbound IgG molecules that are degraded is increased. Conversely a low concentration of IgG results in a longer $t_{1/2}$, as the receptors are not saturated and a smaller proportion of unbound molecules are destroyed. The Brambell hypothesis was proposed in the absence of any knowledge of the nature of the receptor(s) or the origin of the cell(s) involved in IgG catabolism. Subsequently, the receptor was identified as the FcRn. FcRn was first recognized as the Fc receptor which delivers maternal IgG across the neonatal intestine and the maternal–fetal barrier. Interestingly, FcRn is a heterodimer of an α-chain (homologous to MHC class I (chain) and β_2-microglobulin. Recent studies indicate that the FcRn is ubiquitously expressed in endothelial cells where it most likely acts to regulate levels of serum IgG. Further, studies using transfected and nontransfected cells have provided evidence that FcRn acts as an IgG transporter.

The role of FcRn in the regulation of the persistence of IgG in the circulation was clearly demonstrated by measuring the $t_{1/2}$ of mouse IgG_1 and IgG_1-derived recombinant Fc fragments in mice that do not express functional FcRn because of homozygous deletion of the gene encoding β_2-

microglobulin, a component of FcRn. The $t_{1/2}$s of IgG_1 and of the wild-type Fc fragment are considerably decreased in β_2-microglobulin knockout mice, and serum concentrations of IgG are 30 times lower as a result of the higher rate of IgG catabolism. In this case, the catabolism–concentration effect is absent because of the lack of FcRn. In contrast, IgA or a mutated Fc fragment of IgG, which are unable to bind to FcRn, have the same $t_{1/2}$ in both normal and FcRn-deficient mice.

Table 15.1. $t_{1/2}$s of IgG_1, Fc fragments, and IgA in normal and FcRn-deficient mice

Mice	*IgG_1*	*Half-life (h) of Fc*		*IgA*
		Recombinant	*Mutant*	
Normal	97.7	76.9	13.7	25.0
FcRn-deficient	17.6	12.6	14.8	24.0

The expression of FcRn in almost every tissue analyzed strengthened the hypothesis original proposed by Waldmann and Strober that the endothelial cells might be the site of IgG catabolism. Distribution studies of murine IgG_1 and anti-FcRn antibodies indicated that FcRn is expressed in the endothelium of small arterioles and capillaries of the skin and muscle and to a lesser extent in the liver and adipose tissue. Functional FcRn is present in both mouse and human endothelial cell lines.

Table 15.2. Affinity for FcRn and $t_{1/2}$s of recombinant mouse Fc fragments in mice

Fc fragment	*Relative affinity for mouse FcRn (%)*	*$t_{1/2}$ (h)*
Wild–type	100.0	119.1
Mutants:		
Ile253Ala	18.0	26.2
His310Ala	12.5	16.8
His433Ala	75.0	114.8
Asn434Ala	84.5	110.0
His435Ala	5.0	17.4
His436Ala	20.2	48.7

Delineation of the Amino Acid Residues Involved in the Catabolism of IgG

Mouse

The identification of the amino acid residues involved in regulating the persistence of IgG was facilitated by the observation that mouse IgG complexed with staphylococcal protein A (SpA) or its 7-kDa fragment B was rapidly eliminated from the circulation. Fragment B of SpA binds to the interface of the CH_2–CH_3 domains where the interaction site encompasses three regions comprising amino acid residues 252–254, 308–312, and 433–436. To test the hypothesis that the SpA-binding site overlaps the site of IgG involved in catabolism, amino acid residues from these three regions were altered by in vitro mutagenesis of recombinant Fc fragments. These mutants were tested for their PK in mice and for their binding affinity for recombinant mouse FcRn. Amino acids from both the CH_2 (Ile-253, His-310) and CH_3 (His-435, His-436) domains are essential for the regulation of IgG catabolism. Mutants with short $t_{1/2}$s bind to FcRn with lower affinity. The presence of highly conserved histidine residues at positions 310, 435, and, to a lesser extent, 436 provides an explanation for the strict pH dependence (binding at pH 6.0-6.5 and release at pH 7.0-7.5) of the FcRn–IgG (or Fc) interaction that was observed in binding studies. The pH dependence of the FcRn–IgG interaction explains how IgG salvage might take place in endothelial cells. Hence, it has been hypothesized that IgG molecules are ingested by fluid-phase pinocytosis, traffic into acidic intracellular vesicles (endosomes), and bind to FcRn. The IgG molecules bound to FcRn are recycled back to the membrane, where they are released into the circulation because of the slightly basic pH of the blood. Conversely, IgG molecules that do not bind to FcRn are destined for lysosomal degradation.

The crystal structure of Fc complexed with FcRn is consistent with the results obtained by site-directed mutagenesis, showing that Ile-253, His-310, His-435, and His-436 are involved in the FcRn–IgG interaction. In addition to these residues, amino acids at positions Thr-256, Pro-257, Pro-307, and Met-309 also play a role in building the FcRn interaction site of IgG in the mouse. The good correlation between serum persistence and affinity for FcRn of the Fc fragments (Pearson correlation coefficient = 0.78) suggested that an increase in the affinity of an Fc fragment or IgG would result in a longer $t_{1/2}$ in vivo. Subsequently, a mutated Fc fragment with a 3.5-fold higher affinity for FcRn was obtained from a phage display library. In this fragment, Thr-252, Thr-254, and Thr-256 were mutated to Leu, Ser, and Phe, respectively, and these mutations resulted in an increase in serum $t_{1/2}$ from 93 h to 153 h.

The IgG residues that are critical for FcRn binding are located on three spatially proximal loops that are noncontiguous in the primary sequence. This suggests that the relative positions of the residues might be dependent on the conformation of the β-strands that support them and also on the topology of the CH_2 and CH_3 domains relative to each other. Thus, the detrimental effect of mutating proline to alanine at position 257 on the serum half-life is most likely due to perturbation of the conformation of the loop encompassing Ile-253. The removal of the hinge region from the Fc fragment results in a shorter half-life, indicating that the hinge region determines the relative spatial orientation of the CH_2 and CH_3 domains and the configuration at their interface. In fact, replacement of the hinge sequence with a synthetic hinge containing a cysteine-cysteine bridge in the context of a different sequence generates an Fc fragment that has a $t_{1/2}$ similar to that of the wild-type fragment. The IgG molecule has two CH_2–CH_3 domain interfaces and both are necessary for its normal persistence in the circulation. This was demonstrated by using a hybrid recombinant mouse Fc fragment containing one functional and one mutagenized (and hence nonfunctional) FcRn interaction site.

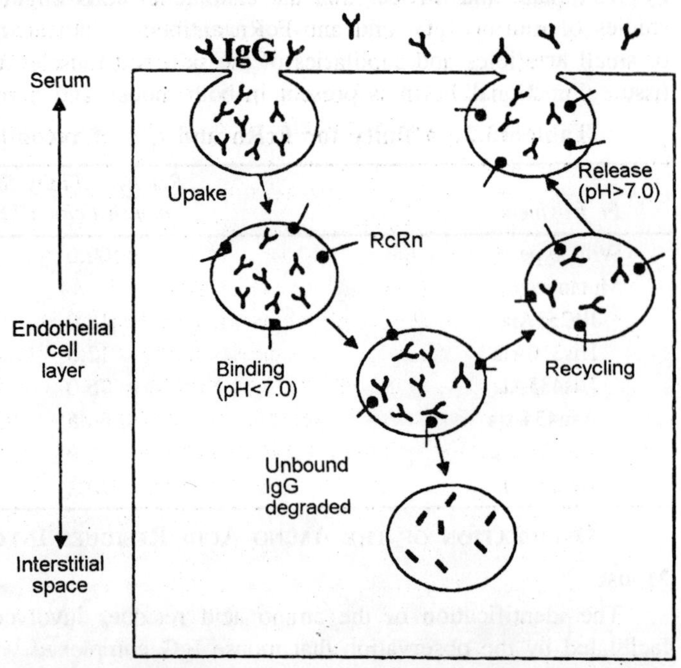

Fig. 15.2. The structure (a-carbon traces) of human Fc and rat FcRn with residues predicted to be involved in the interaction shown.

The $t_{1/2}$ of the hybrid was decreased by 50% as compared with the wild-type Fc fragment with two functional FcRn binding sites. This finding was in agreement with an earlier observation that a rabbit IgG complexed only with one of its CH_2–CH_3 domain interfaces to fragment B of SpA has only 20% of the persistence of the noncomplexed IgG in the circulation of rabbits. The same amino acid residues that are involved in the control of IgG catabolism are also involved in the control of the transfer of IgG from mother to offspring, a process also regulated by FcRn.

Human

For the genetic engineering of therapeutic ch and hu MAbs it is important to know whether the amino acid residues critical for FcRn binding in the mouse are equally important for the persistence of human IgG in humans. Ethical reasons precluded the use of humans for PK analyses, but mice provide a suitable model for the study of the catabolism of human IgGs. The $t_{1/2}$s and the affinities of mutated human Fc fragments for mouse FcRn have shown that Ile-253, His-3 10, and His-435 are also essential for regulating the $t_{1/2}$ of human IgG in mice. These results were confirmed by mapping the binding site for human FcRn on human IgG_1. In addition, it has been shown that other amino acid residues in human IgG_1 are important for its binding to human FcRn. These include Ser-254 and Lys-288 (both in the CH_2 domain), as well as Ser-415 and His-433 (both in the CH_3 domain). It has also been shown that a change in residue Asn- 434 to Ala yielded mutants with an increased affinity for FcRn. In the absence of PK, it is, however, difficult to evaluate how these mutants will be handled in vivo. The $t_{1/2}$s of ch IgG antibodies with shuffled constant regions have indicated that, as in the case for mouse IgGs, the conformation of the molecule also contributes to its persistence in the circulation. Thus, ch human-mouse IgG containing a γ_4 amino-terminus spliced to a γ_1 carboxy-terminus within the CH_2 domain had a half-life in SCID mice of 282 h, which was greater than either parental IgG (199 h for IgG1 and 77 h for IgG_4).

Mouse vs Human

Although the absence of carbohydrates on the Fc region of recombinant IgG has no impact on the persistence of mouse Fc, aglycosylated human recombinant Fc has a significantly shorter $t_{1/2}$ than its glycosylated counterpart. Thus, there appear to be differences in the requirements for glycosylation between the IgGs from these two species. A comparison of the X-ray crystallographic structures of human and mouse Fc regions has shown that the oligosaccharides attached to the CH_2 domain can form contacts (i.e., a bridge) between the two CH_2 domains in human IgG but not in mouse IgG. Thus, the contribution of CH_2 domain-linked carbohydrates to the conformation of CH_2 domains is species related.

The surprisingly short half-life of mouse IgG as compared with human IgG in humans has been explained previously by the assumption that some "natural" anti-galactose antibodies present in human serum can bind to the Galα_1-3Gal residues present *only* on mouse IgG (and IgGs from other mammals), thus shortening its $t_{1/2}$ in the circulation by immune elimination. However, therapeutic humanized MAbs produced in murine cells have been reported to have long $t_{1/2}$s, indicating that anti-Gal antibodies are not involved in the rapid removal of murine IgG. An alternative explanation for the decreased $t_{1/2}$ of mouse IgG in humans is based on the observation that the mouse IgG isotypes (with the exception of IgG_{2b}) fail to bind to human FcRn, whereas all human isotypes bind to homologous FcRn. As expected from PK analysis, both human and mouse IgG isotypes bind to mouse FcRn. These results provide a molecular explanation for the short half-lives of therapeutic mouse MAbs in patients as a consequence of their poor affinity for human FcRn.

The lack of an interaction between human FcRn and most mouse IgGs indicates that mice cannot be reliably used to extrapolate the $t_{1/2}$s of murine MAbs to humans. Even the PK of humanized MAbs in mice might be different from their PK in humans owing to differences in the fine specificity of FcRn across species. This is suggested by the discrepancy between the half-lives of human IgG isotypes in mice vs humans. For example, human IgG_3 has a significantly shorter $t_{1/2}$ than the other isotypes in both humans and mice (owing to the substitution of His by Arg in 435) but the $t_{1/2}$s of IgG_1, IgG_2, and IgG_4 differ considerably in both species. Although three isotypes have approximately the same $t_{1/2}$s in humans, in mice, IgG_2 has a much longer $t_{1/2}$ than IgG_1, and IgG_4. To predict the pharmacokinetics of a therapeutic MAb in humans, preclinical studies in mice should therefore be complemented by studies to measure the binding of the MAb to human FcRn. As in mice, FcRn also plays an essential role in the maternofetal transfer of IgG in humans. The same amino acid residues in human IgG that control the catabolism of IgG are involved in IgG transcytosis across the in vitro perfused placenta.

Localization of the Interaction Site for IgG on FcRn

Despite the homology of the α-chain of the FcRn with the major histocompatibility class (MHC) I molecule, the "peptide binding groove" of the FcRn is not occupied by peptide owing to close apposition of the α-helical segments that flank this groove. The genes encoding both the mouse and human FcRn α-chain have been isolated and characterized. These two proteins have a high degree of homology in the α_2-domain, which is involved in binding to the Fc region of IgG. The contact amino acid residues at the CH_2–CH_3 interface of IgG have been determined by both X-ray crystallography of the rat Fc–FcRn complexes and by site-directed mutagenesis. The residues in the α_2-domain that play a direct role in the interactions between IgG and FcRn are conserved in FcRn in both mice and humans with the exception of residues 132 and 137. The acidic nature of the four (or three for human) amino acid residues and the role of histidines in the binding of IgG to FcRn suggests that electrostatic forces may play a predominant role in mediating this interaction. Hydrophobic interactions between Trp-133 in FcRn and Ile-253 of IgGs are also involved. The amino-terminal residue of β_2-microglobulin (Ile), which is conserved in mice and humans, has also been implicated in the binding of IgG to residues Leu-309 and/or Glu-311, but to a lesser extent than the residues in the α_2-domain.

Differences between mouse and human FcRn occur at residue 132 (Asp in human, Glu in mouse) and 137 (Leu in human, Glu in mouse). Glu-137 (Asp in rat) forms a salt bridge with His-436 of IgG, and this interaction is precluded in the human FcRn owing to the replacement of Glu with Leu. Both human IgG and mouse IgG_{2b} have Tyr at position 436, a residue that may establish hydrophobic interactions with Leu-137 in human FcRn. This could explain the lack of binding of mouse IgG_1 and IgG_{2a}, the weak binding of mouse IgG_{2b}, and the strong interactions of human IgGs with human FcRn. However, neither sheep nor bovine IgGs can bind to human FcRn despite the fact that these proteins have Tyr at position 436. This suggests that other differences between human and mouse IgG and/or FcRn might also be responsible for the lack of interactions of some mouse IgG subclasses and human FcRn. Thus, in mouse, as compared with human FcRn, Trp-133 is more exposed to solvent. There is also a two-residue deletion in human FcRn that is located at the carboxy-terminal end of the α_1-domain, in the vicinity of the IgG-binding site. This shortens the α-helix of the α_1-domain and thereby creates a different conformation at the level of the α_1/α_2 platform of these two FcRns. This two-residue deletion also eliminates an Asn residue in human FcRn which is a potential site for glycosylation in mouse FcRn. It has also been suggested that to achieve maximal binding affinity for IgG, dimerization of FcRn is required. In the crystal structure of rat FcRn, dimerization is mediated by electrostatic interactions between the carbohydrate residues attached to Asn-225. There can be no such interactions in human FcRn because Asn-225 is replaced by Gln, as demonstrated by the propensity of rat FcRn (highly homologous with mouse) to form dimers in crystals, and by the lack of human dimers in such crystals.

PK of MAbs and ITs in Mice

Persistence of MAbs in Normal and Tumor-Bearing Mice

The preclinical testing of mouse or ch/hu MAbs in severe combined immunodeficiency (SCID) mice xenografted with various human tumors is usually followed by measuring tumor size (for subcutaneous tumors) or the survival of animals (for disseminated lymphomas and metastatic tumors). The persistence of murine MAbs in normal mice depends on the IgG isotype used. Both mouse and rat IgG_{2b} have a short $t_{1/2}$ as compared with the other isotypes. In the case of rat IgG_{2b}, the sequence difference at position 257 (Ala instead of Pro in the other isotypes) is most likely responsible for the short $t_{1/2}$ whereas for mouse IgG_{2b}, the short $t_{1/2}$ is probably due to the substitution of His-435 (in all other isotypes) with Tyr. The most frequently used mouse MAbs in clinical trials are of the IgG_1 isotype, which has one of the longest $t_{1/2}$s in mice.

In tumor-bearing mice the presence of the tumor acts as a sink for the injected MAb and decreases its $t_{1/2}$. However, if the tumor is saturated with the corresponding MAb, the $t_{1/2}$ is within its normal range. This behavior was demonstrated by using SCID mice xenografted with human Burkitt' s Daudi cells and injected with ^{125}I-labeled mouse RFB4 anti-human CD22 previously treated or not with an excess of unlabeled MAbs. The treatment of SCID/Daudi tumor mice with RFB4 prolonged the survival of mice from 30 d (untreated) to 46 d while the same amount of IT constructed with RFB4 and deglycosylated ricin A chain (dgRTA) was more efficient in extending the life of tumor-bearing animals to 73 d. Despite their small size and good tumor penetration, fragments of IgG antibody (Fab, Fv) have very short $t_{1/2}$s and therefore decreased tumor retention. To prolong their persistence in the circulation and increase their therapeutic potential, a site-specific chemical modification of human Fab fragments with polyethyleneglycol (PEG) was performed.

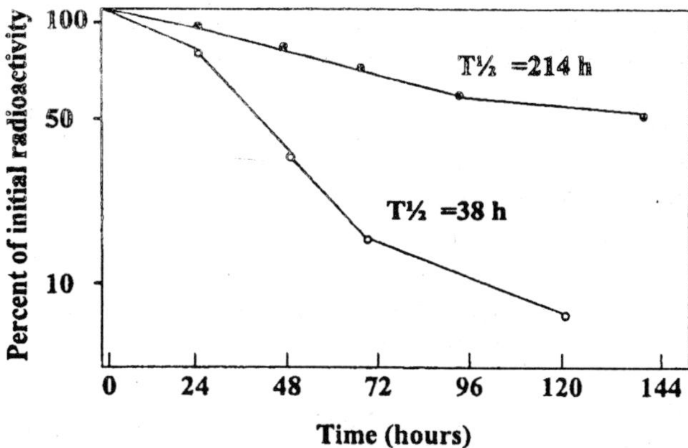

Fig. 15.3. Elimination curves of ^{125}I-RFB4 in SCID/Daudi mouse.

This conferred a longer $t_{1/2}$ and full retention of antigen-binding properties. Thus, the $t_{1/2}$ of a Fab–PEG conjugate in rats was prolonged from 0.3 h (nonconjugated Fab) to 4.9 h, which is close to the $t_{1/2}$ of 5.8 h for intact IgG. Similar results were obtained using cynomologus monkeys. It was noted that the majority of improvements in the PK were due to a large increase in the α-phase, indicating that less conjugate was lost from the circulation during the equilibration phase. However, the possible use of pegylated IgG fragments instead of the intact IgG in therapy may depend on the ability of such hydrophilic molecules to diffuse through the milieu of the interstitium.

Persistence of ITs in Normal and Tumor-Bearing Mice

The chemical attachment of toxins or their subunits to MAbs alters their PK. This is at least partially due to nonspecific interactions of the toxin with receptors on cells in a variety of tissues. The consequence of this interaction is the much shorter persistence in the circulation of IT vs the MAb used for its preparation. The decreased $t_{1/2}$ of ITs vs MAbs is not the result of the modification of the MAb molecule by the crosslinker used for the attachment of the toxin, as indicated by the same half-life of MAbs treated or not treated with *N*-succinimidyl 3-(2-pyridyldithiopropionate) (SPDP) or *N*-succinimidyloxycarbonyl-α-methyl (2-pyridyldithio)-toluene (SMPT) crosslinker. The MAb/IT ratios are inversely proportional to the number of mannose residues on the RTA molecule. Thus, following chemical deglycosylation, 5 of the 18 mannose residues in RTA remain. Recombinant RTA expressed in *E. coli* has none. The rapid clearance of the ITs is likely to be mediated through the recognition of mannose-rich oligosaccharides by hepatic Kupfer and sinusoidal endothelial cells which express mannose-binding receptors. The dose-limiting toxicity of ITs constructed with RTA and some other plant and bacterial toxins is vascular leak syndrome (VLS), which is characterized by an increase in vascular permeability resulting in interstitial edema, weight gain, and, in its most severe form, organ failure. The nonspecific cytotoxic effect of ITs is thought to be related to their ability to damage the integrity of the endothelial cells of the microvasculature. Because the predominant expression site of FcRn is the vascular endothelium, it is possible that treatment with ITs *per se* also alters their persistence in the circulation by altering the "salvaging" function of FcRn in the endothelium. This possibility is supported by results of studies designed to measure the persistence of ^{125}I-labeled mouse MAb in mice treated with an IT. The half-life of mouse MAb (RFB4) is considerably shortened after 3 d of consecutive treatment of mice with a dose of RFB4-dgRTA representing 40% of its LD_{50}. However, the effect of the IT was reversible, as shown by the elimination curves of RFB4, which are similar in normal mice and in mice used 2 wk after treatment with IT.

Recombinant ITs are molecules containing truncated toxins (e.g., *Pseudomonas exotoxin* [PE] or [PE40]) fused to a recombinant antigen-binding Fv fragment. The Fv fragment comprises the variable regions of the IgG heavy and light chains, which can be linked by either an engineered peptide linker (scFv) or an engineered disulfide bond (dsFv). These manipulations stabilize the association of VH and VL, which are normally noncovalently bound to each other. Compared to ITs containing intact IgG molecules, both types of recombinant ITs have improved intratumoral penetration in animals. However, the rapid blood clearance and monovalency of these small molecules result in significantly dęcreased tumor retention. Thus, the $t_{1/2}$ in mice of a dsFv IT containing a truncated PE was only 15–20 min. The very fast elimination is due to the rapid renal clearance of FvITs. This was demonstrated by biodistribution studies of FvIT in nephrectomized mice in which tumor retention of the FvIT was similar to that of IT containing intact. Therefore, to achieve antitumor effects in mice, these FvITs should be administered by continuous infusion using miniosmotic pumps. Improved $t_{1/2}$s and antitumor activity have been reported for an anti-EpCAM hu MAb fused at the carboxyl-terminal end of the heavy chain to interleukin-2 (IL-2). By introducing single amino acid changes in the junctional sequence between the MAb and IL-2, these fusion proteins showed reduced sensitivity to proteolysis and longer $t_{1/2}$s. This work demonstrated that, in addition to its interaction with FcRn, the persistence of these conjugates in the circulation was also dependent on their susceptibility to proteolysis. In support of the implication that the protease sensitivity of IgG affects its persistence in the circulation, human IgG_3, which is known to be more susceptible to papain/pepsin proteolysis than IgG_1, has the same affinity as IgG_1 for human FcRn. However, its $t_{1/2}$ in humans is three times shorter. In addition, the shorter $t_{1/2}$ of wild-type recombinant human Fc fragments as compared with Fc fragments generated by papain digestion is not due to a decreased affinity for FcRn, as both fragments bind equally well to FcRn-Sepharose. However, analysis of the sensitivities of these two human Fc fragments to pepsin-limited digestion demonstrated that the wild-type Fc fragment is digested about three times more rapidly than the Fc-papain fragment.

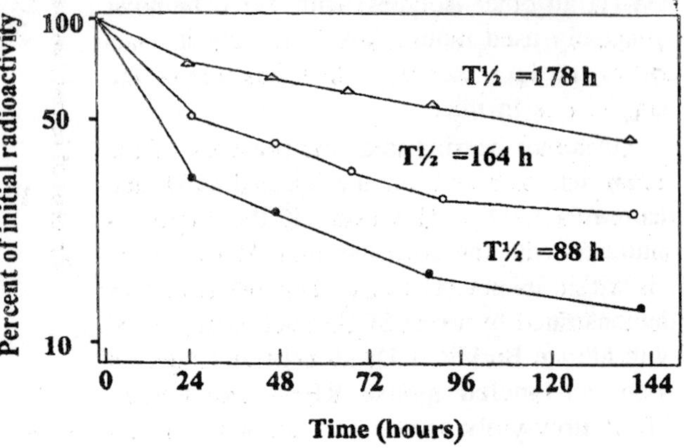

Fig. 15.4. The effect of IT treatment on the elimination curves of radiolabeled RFB4.

PK of MAbs and ITs in Cancer Patients

Persistence of MAbs in Cancer Patients

The $t_{1/2}$ of any heterologous or homologous IgG antibody infused into a normal recipient does not depend on the amount administered. However, this is not the case in tumor-bearing recipients in whom the tumor cells act as a sink. Therefore, it would be predicted that by increasing the dose, or by infusing repeated doses, the tumor will be saturated with the MAbs and the excess will be catabolized at a normal rate. Hence, in situations in which tumor cells are present, $t_{1/2}$s are dependent on the dose administered.

PK analyses of the anti-CD20 IgG_1 ch MAb (Rituxan) have demonstrated that its $t_{1/2}$ in patients with relapsed B-cell lymphoma is 445 ± 361 h, a value very close to 500 h for human IgG_1 in normal individuals. The half-life of another ch MAb directed against a high molecular weight mucin (TAG-72) expressed on colorectal tumors and constructed with an IgG_4 isotype was only 224 ± 62 h in patients with metastatic colon cancer. This value is considerably longer than that of its murine MAb counterpart (24–48 h) but shorter than that of Rituxan. The shorter half-life could be the result of the different type and burden of the two tumors and not on the isotype, as both IgG_1 and IgG_4 have similar $t_{1/2}$s in humans. The $t_{1/2}$ of the anti-TAG-72 ch MAb was considerably shorter (< 24 h) in patients who responded to treatment by eliciting HAMA, indicating that a process of immune elimination and not tumor capture took place.

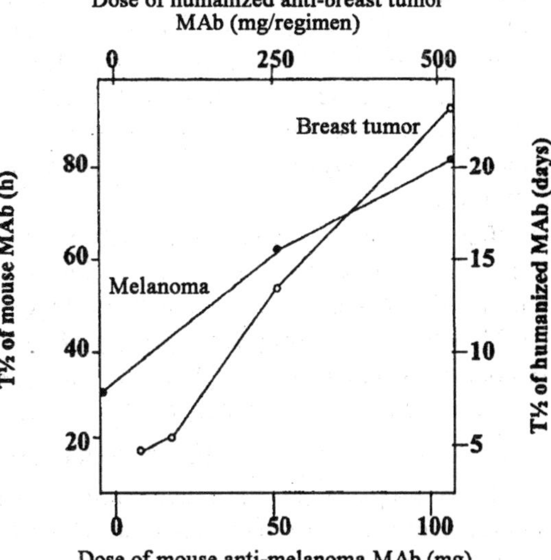

Fig. 15.5. Variations in pharmacokinetics of MAbs infused in increasing doses in melanoma and breast cancer patients.

Persistence of ITs in Cancer Patients

All ITs which have been used to date in clinical trials contain mouse MAbs. Hence, their persistence in the circulation and retention in the body is short irrespective of the toxin used. However, the size of the targeting antibody has an impact on the half life of the IT as shown in Phase I clinical trials using anti-CD22 (RFB4) IT constructed with dgRTA and intact IgG ($t_{1/2}$ = 7.8 h) vs its Fab' fragment ($t_{1/2}$ = 1.5 h). The ITs were administered intravenously in several bolus doses at 48-h intervals but therapeutic concentrations (~1 μg/mL) could be sustained only with ITs constructed with intact IgG. A high peak concentration of IT in serum and a longer $t_{1/2}$ correlated with both clinical response and toxicity. These results were consistent with those obtained in a murine lymphoma model where a longer $t_{1/2}$ resulted in a better antitumor response.

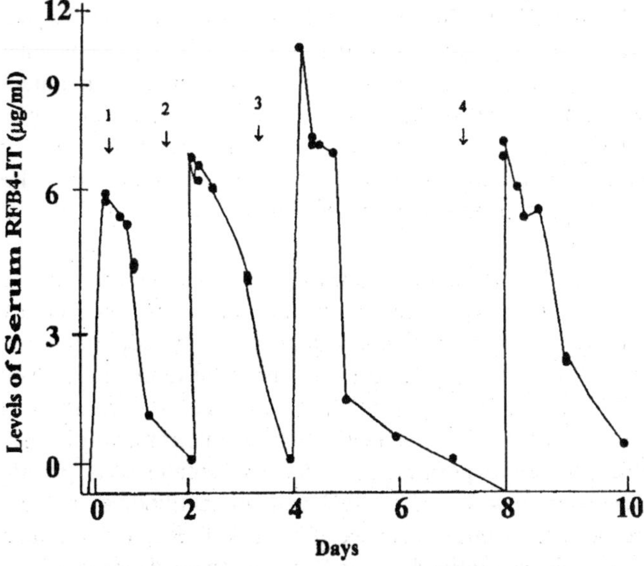

Fig. 15.6. Pharmacokinetics of RFB4-dgRTA IT.

To avoid toxic levels of ITs (> 1 μg/mL) in serum, and to maintain constant levels of IT in the blood, continuous infusion of anti-CD22 IT was evaluated. As compared to bolus infusion, a comparable $t_{1/2}$ (11.4 h), toxicity, immunogenicity, and clinical response were observed. Toxicity depended on the presence or absence of circulating tumor cells (CTCs) with less toxicity observed in patients with CTCs. The $t_{1/2}$ of the IT in patients with CTC was shorter (8.8 h) than in patients without CTCs (12.7 h), indicating that in these cases, the CTCs absorbed more IT and thereby reduced its $t_{1/2}$. However, this observation was not confirmed in subsequent clinical studies using combination therapy with a mixture of two ITs. In these studies, the $t_{1/2}$ of RFB4 IT was slightly longer for those patients with CTCs (32.1 h and 39.2 h for two dose levels) when compared to those without (24.4 h and 21.6 h for two dose levels). In contrast to the patients *lacking* these CTCs, patients with even small numbers of CTCs ($<50/mm^3$) tolerated even the highest dose of the combined ITs (30 $mg/m^2/192$ h). The PK of the anti-CD19 (HD37) IT in patients with B-cell lymphomas was similar to that of anti-CD22 IT. Thus, half-lives of 18.2 h and 22.8 h have been reported for anti-CD19 IT administered either by bolus or continuous infusions. In contrast, an anti-CD25 IT administered to patients with Hodgkin's lymphoma had a shorter $t_{1/2}$ (6.1 h), perhaps owing to the bioavailability of tumor cells.

Recombinant ITs constructed with mouse Fv fragments and truncated PE have a very short half-life (<1 h) in patients owing to the low retention of mouse Fv fragments in the circulation and the nonspecific uptake of PE by the liver. Despite unfavorable PK, a recombinant IT containing the anti-CD22 (RFB4) dsFv fragment fused to PE38 was efficacious in patients with hairy cell leukemia. Thus, in contrast to unconjugated MAbs, ITs may not require a long $t_{1/2}$ if the tumor cells are few in number and accessible to the circulation.

PK of Intravenous Immunoglobulin (IVIG)

IVIG preparations have been used to prevent infection in cancer patients and, in some cases, antitumor effects have been reported. Thus, as compared with untreated patients, mortality in the group of chronic lymphocytic leukemia patients treated with IVIG was lower. Similar observations were noted in a study in which regression of a Kaposi sarcoma occurred in human immunodeficiency (HIV) patients treated with IVIG. In a study using IVIG-treated SCID mice xenografted with human melanoma or sarcoma, fewer recurrences and prolongation of survival time was observed. This was confirmed in SCID mice xenografted with human lymphoma (Daudi) cells.

The PK of IVIG preparations were obtained by analyzing the plasma elimination curves after infusing IVIG into patients with immunodeficiencies. Alternatively, the elimination of some specific IgG antibodies present in the infused IVIG but not in the serum of the subject has been studied. The $t_{1/2}$ of various commercial IVIG preparations in patients with X-linked agammaglobulinemia or with various immunodeficiency syndromes ranged between 26 and 35 d. The dose of IVIG recommended for the treatment of patients with humoral immunodeficiencies is approx 0.4 mg/kg/mo, which is somewhat less than the amount of IgG in the intravascular pool of normal subjects but is sufficient to maintain levels above 5 g/L, which is considered to be a critical threshold. The $t_{1/2}$s of IgG_1, IgG_2, and IgG_4 isotypes were approx 30 d whereas the $t_{1/2}$ of IgG_3 was 20 d. This last value is higher than expected based on results from studies with radiolabeled IgG in normal subjects, suggesting that the IVIG preparation used in these studies might also contain a proportion of the IgG_3 allotype with His at position 435.

The effect of IVIG in the treatment of some autoimmune diseases may also be due to the concentration–catabolism effect in addition to the activation of inhibitory Fc receptors reported by Samuelsson et al. The increased catabolism of endogenous IgG (including autoantibody) by administration of high doses of IVIG (half-life decreased from 20 to 10 d) is the result of the saturation of FcRn in the patients which leads to the destruction of all IgG molecules present in excess. The contribution of enhanced IgG catabolism to the beneficial effect of IVIG in the treatment of some autoimmune diseases is also supported by the observation that the severity of experimental lupus erythematosus is greatly attenuated in β_2-microgloblin-deficient mice. The very low levels of IgG and autoantibodies in these mice are the cause of their protection from the disease. Hence, because they lack FcRn, they rapidly catabolize both their normal and their pathogenic IgG autoantibody. Furthermore these FcRn-deficient mice are protected against some other autoantibody-mediated diseases (e.g., bullous pemphigus), as the amount of IgG autoantibody reaching the epidermal target is greatly reduced because of its hypercatabolism.

Alterations in IgG PK in Non-Neoplastic Diseases

Alterations in the PK of IgG in individuals with hyper- and hypogammaglobulinemia has been explained by the concentration–catabolism effect inducing the accelerated or decreased catabolism of IgG in patients with high or low serum IgG concentrations, respectively. Hypercatabolism of IgG in diseases involving excessive loss of serum proteins through the kidney (nephrotic syndrome), gastrointestinal tract (protein-losing entheropathy), or skin (severe burns) can be explained by the irreversible loss of IgG in a new catabolic compartment. However, the hypercatabolism of IgG in unrelated diseases such as myotonic dystrophy, systemic lupus erythematosus, rheumatoid arthritis, Wiskott–Aldrich syndrome, and other diseases remains unexplained. In light of our present knowledge of the mechanism of IgG catabolism, the hypercatabolism of IgG in at least some of these diseases might be due to the lack of expression or malfunction of FcRn. With the exception of myotonic dystrophy this possibility has not yet been explored.

Myotonic Dystrophy (DM)

In an early study it was demonstrated that the mean survival time of IgG in individuals with DM was 11.4 vs 22.9 d in normal individuals, corresponding to a lower serum concentration (7.5 mg/mL) than in controls (12.1 mg/mL). The rate of IgG synthesis was normal (35.7 mg/kg/d) in patients with DM. Thus, the reduction in the concentration of serum IgG was due solely to the decreased $t_{1/2}$ of IgG. IgG isolated from normal individuals had a similar accelerated rate of catabolism in DM patients, suggesting that the defect is not in the IgG but in the patient's ability to catabolize it. Normal serum concentrations and catabolic rates were measured for albumin, IgM, and IgA, indicating that the alteration is restricted to a single class of serum proteins. One hypothesis to explain IgG hypercatabolism in DM patients is that the genetic alteration in DM suppresses FcRn expression, leading to decreased IgG protection and increased catabolism. The gene encoding the FcRn α-chain (*FCGRT*) is localized in the same chromosomal band as DM (19q13.3), 4.1 megabases away. This colocalization, however distant, may be compatible with a long range chromosomal effect induced by the DMCTG repeat. This hypothesis assumes that a potent *cis*-suppressive mechanism extends even to distant genes such as *FCGRT*inactivating the expression of functional FcRn. Because DM is caused by an expanded CTG repeat in the 3'-untranslated region of the DM protein kinase mRNA, this mRNA must be transcribed in the vascular endothelial cells where *FCGRT* itself is expressed and mediates IgG protection. The presence of DM protein kinase mRNA was confirmed in FcRn-positive human endothelial cells, suggesting that a long range effect of DMCTG expansion on *FCGRT* might explain the hypercatabolism of IgG in DM.

Systemic Lupus Erythematosus (SLE) and Rheumatoid Arthritis (RA)

In two studies published by different laboratories it was reported that patients with SLE have both higher serum IgG concentrations and higher catabolic rates of IgG than controls. There is excellent agreement between the data obtained in both laboratories indicating that IgG hypercatabolism is associated with an increased serum concentration. The increase in the concentration of serum IgG in SLE patients is a result of the increase in the synthetic rate, which surpasses the catabolic rate. Because the catabolic rates increase in patients with elevated serum IgG concentration (e.g., myeloma patients) a possible explanation is that hypercatabolism results from the higher concentrations of serum IgG in SLE patients. However, neither study found a correlation between the serum concentration and the fractional catabolic rate in these patients, indicating that the concentration–catabolism effect was not the cause of IgG hypercatabolism. The accelerated breakdown of IgG could not be explained by any of the factors known to alter IgG catabolism (e.g., loss of protein in urine or gastrointestinal tract) or the treatment with corticosteroids known to induce hypercatabolism of IgG. The nature of the phenomenon leading to the hypercatabolism of IgG in these SLE patients may correlate with alterations in the function of FcRn. This is supported by the results of experiments using MRL-lpr mice which develop SLE-like disease. As in its human counterpart, SLE in mice is characterized by the development of hypergammaglobulinemia and a severe autoimmune syndrome. β_2-Microglobulin-deficient mice that do not express FcRn are protected from hypergammaglobulinemia and show a reduction in the titers of autoantibody.

In agreement with these results, treatment of MLR-lpr mice developing SLE with a synthetic peptide that binds to IgG at its FcRn-binding site blocks the development of the disease in the majority of cases. These results indicate that modification of the function of FcRn in SLE may interfere with the catabolism of both endogenous IgG and autoantibody. If this is the case, mice with SLE should have an accelerated rate of catabolism of IgG. However, in disease-free, SLE-susceptible strains of mice, the $t_{1/2}$s of IgG were indistinguishable from those of resistant strains, suggesting that alterations in IgG catabolism take place only after the onset of the disease.

In a preliminary experiment using mice with lupus-like disease induced by treatment with pristane, the $t_{1/2}$ of mouse IgG_1 was considerably shortened from 208 ± 18 h to 76 ± 8 h 3 mo after treatment. However, the serum IgG concentrations in these treated mice was comparable to those of control mice. A possible link between the gene coding FcRn (*FCGRT*) and genes associated with SLE (*Sle3* and *Lrdm1*) was suggested. *FCGRT* has been proposed to be a suitable candidate for an SLE susceptibility locus.

Short $t_{1/2}$s have also been reported for patients with RA. In patients with SLE or RA, identical $t_{1/2}$s were reported whether the IgG was prepared from the patient or from a normal donor. This demonstrates that hypercatabolism of IgG in RA and SLE patients is a host defect. In RA patients the accelerated catabolism of IgG could be due to a defect in the function of FcRn, combined with the presence of rheumatoid factor (RF) which may bind to the administered radiolabeled IgG and remove it from the circulation as an immune complex. It is well known that immune complexes consisting of RF bound to IgG are commonly present in the serum and in the diseased joints. Because RFs bind to the FcRn-binding site on IgG, they may also accelerate the destruction of IgG by interfering with the protective function of FcRn.

Future Implications

The therapeutic efficacy of MAbs in vivo depends on characteristics such as affinity, FcR-and C-binding, serum persistence, and immunogenicity. It also depends on the nature of the disease being treated (primary vs metastatic tumor, early vs late stage).

The characteristics of the MAbs that have been most thoroughly studied are affinity and specificity for the targeted (tumor) antigen. Current technologies now enable us to prepare "custom-made" MAbs with restricted specificities and very high affinities. In contrast, although the amino acid residues involved in the various antigen-dependent effector functions of MAbs have been identified this knowledge has not yet been applied clinically. However, it is likely that a new generation of genetically engineered antibodies with improved effector functions will be available in the near future.

A major antigen-independent effector function that has an impact on the antitumor activity of MAbs is their ability to bind to FcRn and to persist in the circulation. A long $t_{1/2}$ results in a higher concentration gradient across cellular barriers with better penetration into the targeted tumor. It has been demonstrated in animals as well as in patients that the antitumor activity of MAbs is proportional to their concentration. The improved PK of ch and hu MAbs vs mouse MAbs is partially responsible for the therapeutic success of these MAbs. The persistence of ch and hu MAbs (which are already similar to "normal" human IgG) can be prolonged further by genetic engineering as suggested by recent experiments using mouse and human Fc fragments or IgG. To isolate ch and hu MAbs with increased serum $t_{1/2}$s, random mutagenesis and selection could be used to alter amino acid residues in the vicinity of those involved both in FcRn-binding and in modulating the flexibility of the interface angle between the CH_2–CH_3 domains. Mutants should be analyzed for their affinity for human FcRn, the pH dependence of binding, and their persistence in the circulation of mice. Only mutants with favorable features in all three areas should be developed for use in clinical trials. More attention to the PKs of MAbs in Phase I clinical trials should be given, for example, persistence in the circulation, correlations between doses, PKs, maximum tolerated doses (MTDs) and any biological effects.

A decrease in the size of antibody molecules is invariably associated with better tumor penetration. However, this effect is diminished by a much shorter $t_{1/2}$ and a decreased serum concentration due to rapid renal elimination from the circulation. Future goals would be to produce smaller MAbs with longer $t_{1/2}$s. This could be accomplished by attaching Fvs to CH_2-CH_3 domain interface-like peptides able to bind in a pH-dependent manner to FcRn. The demonstration that an Fc region-derived peptide encompassing residues 308–317 blocks the binding of streptococcal protein G to IgG suggests that peptides encompassing key FcRn-binding residues may be effective.

In contrast to MAbs, a decreased $t_{1/2}$ of ITs might be advantageous excess IT (not absorbed by the tumor) is quickly eliminated from the circulation, thus diminishing nonspecific side effects. Therefore the use of ch and hu MAbs instead of mouse MAbs for the construction of ITs would confer longer half-lives, a higher serum concentration, and a better tumor penetration but also an increased toxic side effect. If ch or hu MAbs are used, the portion of the toxin that induces side effects should be identified and altered.

Finally we must expand our knowledge of how FcRn functions in endothelial cells. This will allow us to control the persistence of MAbs in the circulation not only by altering the structure of MAbs, but also by modulating the function of FcRn. For this purpose, in vitro systems using cells originating from tissues involved in transcytosis of IgG have provided valuable information regarding the mechanisms of intracellular trafficking of IgG and FcRn. In the future we need to study endothelial cells originating from the vasculature of the tissues involved in IgG catabolism. This could answer the question of how expression of FcRn is regulated in endothelial cells and how fluctuations in the expression of FcRn influence the PKs of MAbs in vivo.

Pharmacokinetics of Biologicals

Present therapeutic approaches, including surgery, irradiation, and chemotherapy, will cure up to 50% of all patients with cancer, but many of the remainder will live with chronic disease for many years. There is therefore a need for new therapeutic agents, not only to achieve durable remissions, but also to increase quality of life for patients during and after treatment. This chapter describes the impact and pharmacokinetics of cytokines and monoclonal antibodies (MAbs) in cancer therapy when used as adjuvants to chemotherapy, as therapeutic support, and as anticancer agents in their own right. Such compounds often have a very complex mechanism of action, and multiple effects. The dose–response curve is bell shaped rather than linear, which makes it more difficult to estimate the optimal therapeutic dose (OTD), which is not usually the maximum tolerated dose (MTD) for these compounds. Pharmacokinetic studies provide important data; enabling clinicians to optimize therapeutic strategies.

Pharmacokinetics of Cytokines

Interferons

The potential of the interferons as antitumor and antiviral agents has been well established. The interferon (IFN) protein families, α (produced by leukocytes), β (by fibroblasts and macrophages), and γ (by T cells), all show rapid plasma clearance after intravenous administration. Serum concentrations are generally undetectable after 24 h. Terminal elimination half-lives range from 4 to 16 h (α), 1-2 h (β), and 25-35 min (γ). Intramuscular and subcutaneous administration of α and β IFNs results in protracted but reliable absorption: >80% for IFN-α and 30–70% for IFN-γ.

Interferon, in the vast majority of cases IFN-α is used clinically for cancer treatment. Meta-analysis evaluating IFN-α across 24 multiple myeloma (MM) trials involving 4012 patients showed that IFN-α improved progression-free survival by about 6 mo, but the overall survival benefit was small. A meta-analysis of treatment of MM and renal cell carcinoma (RCC) patients, with or without IFN-α, indicated that inclusion of IFN-α in the treatment of 1164 MM patients raised response rates from 17% to 24%; in the 525 RCC patients, IFN-α raised response rates from 8% to 14%.

IFN-α can be used in conjunction with IFN-γ and with other biologicals such as interleukin-2 (IL-2) for treatment of advanced RCC. When compared in a randomized trial, addition of IFN-γ to IFN-α increased the rate (from 12.5% to 20%) and duration of responses. IFN-γ may also be used alone, or in conjunction with IL-2 or IL-12.

The clinical utility of synthetic interferons has been hampered, however, by rapid clearance from the plasma and degradation by plasma and tissue enzymes. Various modifications have been carried out in an effort to overcome this. The degree and type of glycosylation, for example, has a profound effect on IFN pharmaco-kinetics: IFN-γ is a dimer containing four glycosylation sites that shows differential clearance due to glycosylation. High-mannose glycosylated recombinant IFN molecules expressed in insect cell cultures were taken up by the liver and so eliminated more rapidly from serum than unglycosylated recombinant forms, which in turn were eliminated faster than the natural form (low-mannose glycosylated). Clinical studies, in general, use forms of IFN grown in *Escherichia coli*. These are unglycosylated, which may explain why their clearance is faster than that of natural IFN. More recently, pegylation has been used to improve pharmaco-kinetics by addressing the problem of rapid clearance. Polyethylene glycol (PEG) moieties, inert long-chain amphiphilic molecules, are linked to any protein of interest, usually via amino groups of lysine residues or the target protein amino-terminus. This decreases antigenicity by steric hindrance of immune recognition, reduces renal clearance, and prolongs the maintenance of serum levels at or near the target dose. As a result, PEG compounds generally have longer serum half-lives and durations of bioactivity than their nonpegylated counterparts.

PEG-IFN-α-2a is currently approved for treatment of chronic hepatitis C infection, and pegylated forms of IFN-α and IFN-β are under investigation for use in other conditions. Pegylation has been shown to improve absorption, to increase the elimination half-life ($t_{1/2}\beta$) from 3–8 h to 65 hours, and to decrease systemic clearance (CL) 100-fold. There are no significant differences in subcutaneous bioavailability of pegylated forms of IFN.

Effective pegylation may be achieved by attaching a single, large PEG at a single site; a branched-chain PEG at a single site; or multiple small-chain PEGs at several attachment sites. PEGs of varying shapes and lengths (5000, 12,000, and 40,000 Da) have been attached to IFN-α-2a and to IFN-α-2b, and although they also extend half-life ($t_{1/2}$) to a similar degree, other pharmacokinetic parameters

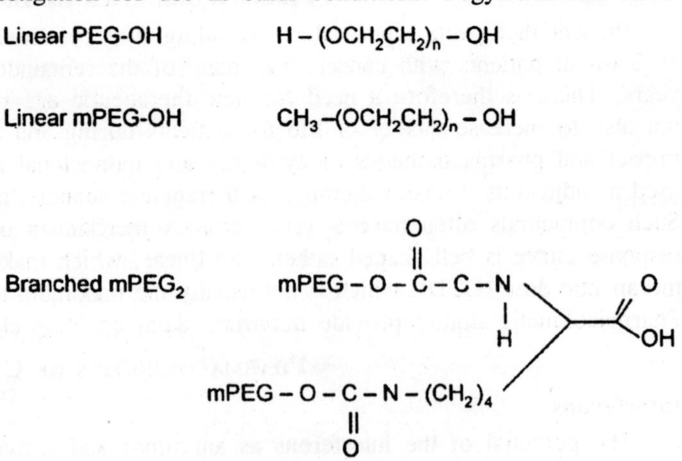

Linear PEG-OH $H-(OCH_2CH_2)_n-OH$

Linear mPEG-OH $CH_3-(OCH_2CH_2)_n-OH$

Branched $mPEG_2$ $mPEG-O-C(=O)-C-NH-$ … $-COOH$; $mPEG-O-C(=O)-N-(CH_2)_4$

Fig. 15.6. Structural formulae of poly(ethylene glycol) (PEG) molecules. mPEG and monomethoxypoly(ethylene glycol.)

are affected in a size-dependent manner, with the 5000-Da moiety behaving similarly to unmodified IFN in terms of volume of distribution (V_d) and absorption half-life ($t_{1/2abs}$). Only the 40,000-Da (branched-chain) moiety is associated with a highly decreased V_d and a much more sustained serum concentration. This provides for a much more convenient administration schedule, allowing the drug to be given once weekly. This schedule has safety and convenience advantages and can replace the frequently used three-times-weekly schedule or the daily schedule required for treatment of melanoma. Using the 40,000-Da PEG forms also allows for higher and more sustained virological responses than those achieved by standard therapy in patients with hepatitis C. Extensive randomized studies in patients with chronic hepatitis C infection have demonstrated the benefits of pegylated IFN.

An understanding about the distinct pharmacokinetic properties of PEG-IFNs when used as antiviral agents can also be applied to their use as antitumor agents. PEG-IFNs show the same advantages, allowing the intervals between treatments to be reduced from daily or three-times-weekly schedules. The 40,000-Da branched-chain PEG-IFN-α-2b derivative, administered subcutaneously on a weekly basis in RCC, demonstrated antitumor activity and established a dosage (450 μg/wk) suitable for further trials. A multicenter Phase II trial conducted in 40 previously untreated patients with advanced RCC using this schedule demonstrated a major response in five patients (four partial and one complete). Median time to progression was 4.8 mo, with 14 patients still under therapy. After 13 mo median follow- up, median survival has not yet been reached, but 72% of patients were alive at 1 yr. The toxicity profile was not appreciably different from that of standard IFN. Serum drug levels were studied in all patients. The mean peak serum concentration (C_{max}) at week 1 was 18 ng/mL, and levels were sustained at close to peak levels over 1 wk. With chronic dosing, drug concentration was increased two- to threefold, and steady state was achieved in about 5 wk. PEG-IFN is currently also under investigation in treatment of chronic myeloid leukemia.

These new schedules using PEG-IFNs offer equivalent efficacy and greater convenience and safety than nonpegylated IFNs.

Erythropoietin

The glycoprotein hormone erythropoietin (EPO) is the primary regulator of erythropoiesis. Recombinant forms of human EPO produced in Chinese hamster ovary (CHO) cells (rHuEpo) are used to combat chemotherapy- and cancer-related anemia, either replacing or supplementing red blood cell transfusion, and are highly effective in increasing quality of life. Two main recombinant forms of EPO are available, epoetin-α and epoetin-β. These differ slightly in glycosylation, with epoetin-α having more sialic acid residues than epoetin-β, and being more widely used.

A study comparing the pharmacokinetics of rHuEpo administered intravenously, intraperitoneally, or subcutaneously, showed that after intravenous infusion, serum rHuEpo levels decayed exponentially from a peak of 3959 mU/mL, with a half-life of 8.2 h. In patients on chronic hemodialysis treatment, bioavailability of ssubcutaneous rHuEpo (21.5%) was seven times greater than that of intraperitoneal rHuEpo. (2.9%). Further work showed bioavailabilities after subcutaneous injection of 31.7%, 36%, and 20–30%, with peak concentrations occurring about 18 h after injection of 5–10% of peak levels obtained after an intravenous dose.

Such studies have established the effectiveness, dosage, and optimal route of administration of rHuEpo and have indicated that the high levels reached immediately after intravenous doses are unnecessary either to induce or to sustain erythropoiesis. This encourages the use of subcutaneous administration. The constant presence of rHuEPO is critical to erythropoiesis, and although peak plasma values are achieved slowly after subcutaneous administration, rHuEpo levels are then maintained above the critical concentration required. The subcutaneous route sustains rHuEpo levels, prevents death of rHuEpo-dependent cells, and results in more efficient and more sustained erythropoiesis. Subcutaneous administration in 36 healthy adults allowed the pharmacokinetics of once-weekly injection and (fixed dose, 40,000 IU) three-times-weekly injections (weight adjusted 150 IU/kg) to be compared. This study showed that the peak serum concentrations (C_{max}) and the area under plasma concentration–time curve (AUC_{0-168}) for the once-weekly schedule were three times and six times higher than those achieved with the three-times-weekly schedule. Both groups showed similar changes in reticulocytes and red blood cells, and hemoglobin levels from baseline, indicating that these schedules can be considered clinically equivalent. The total weekly dose administered by single injection is greater than that required when three injections are administered.

To improve both pharmacokinetics and effectiveness, further modifications have been made to the glycosylation of rHuEpo. Human physiological EPO has a 40% carbohydrate content and studies have shown that there is a direct relationship between the sialic acid content and the serum half-life and biological activity in vivo. Although affinity for the EPO receptor diminishes with increasing sialic acid content, this does not translate to a decrease in activity. The recombinant rHuEpo (Epogen, epoetin-α) used in the majority of cases is a fraction containing molecules with 9–14 sialic acid residues. Isoform 9 has one third of the in vivo activity of isoform 14 owing to the difference in serum half-life.

Hyperglycosylated rHuEpo analogs have altered protein backbones that provide more glycosylation sites. The most active product, novel erythopoiesis stimulating protein (NESP), has five glycosylation sites and can contain up to 22 sialic acid residues. Comparative pharmacokinetic studies were performed in mice that showed that NESP was 3.6 times more potent than rHuEpo when administered three times weekly. Importantly, it also showed that NESP was 13–14 times more potent than rHuEpo when administered once weekly. Studies in dialysis patients and in pediatric renal disease patients also confirmed a longer serum half-life for NESP, and its ability to achieve suitable serum levels by subcutaneous administration in both pediatric and adult patients. Of these studies, the double- blind randomized trial in 11 dialysis patients compared the pharmacokinetics of a single dose of rHuEpo with an equivalent mass of NESP, both given by intravenous bolus; in a second comparative study, 47 patients were randomized to rHuEpo (three times weekly), NESP three times weekly, or NESP once weekly.

One NESP study of cancer patients used a single injection of NESP given as a single subcutaneous injection prior to the first cycle of chemotherapy, followed by further injections on day 1 of each cycle of subsequent chemotherapy. This study indicated that subcutaneous NESP is slowly absorbed, taking about 85 h to reach peak concentration, with a mean $t_{1/2}\beta$ of 32.6 h. Trough serum concentrations of NESP varied within chemotherapy cycles, most likely due to the impact of myelosuppression on pharmacokinetics: within a cycle, the lowest values were found in wk 1 (immediately prior to NESP and chemotherapy), whereas the wk 2 values (1 wk after chemotherapy) were the highest. This may indicate that bone marrow involvement may affect either the clearance or the distribution of NESP. For instance, reduction in erythroid precursors by chemotherapy would allow more NESP to remain in circulation. No antibodies to NESP were detected. These results demonstrate that the mean elimination half-life of NESP doubles when given sc because this value represents a balance between absorption from the injection site and elimination from the circulation. NESP terminal half-life also appears to be at least twice that achieved with sc rHUEpo.

Granulocyte Colony-Stimulating Factor (G-CSF)

The granulocyte colony-stimulating factor (G-CSF) is used to prevent febrile neutropenia, which is a frequent consequence of high-dose cancer chemotherapy and increases the risk of infectious complications. G-CSF may be given as primary prophylaxis or as support in response to neutropenia. It also has a role in allogeneic transplantation, as it is effective in mobilizing peripheral blood stem cells (PBSCs).

Like other recombinant cytokines, it can be produced in three ways: using bacterial (*E. coli*), yeast, or mammalian (usually CHO) cell lines. These recombinant products vary in the amount of posttranslational modification. Bacterial systems do not glycosylate the polypeptide backbone; yeast systems glycosylate to a limited extent; CHO cells glycosylate to a similar extent as the human physiological form of the cytokine.

Two main recombinant forms of G-CSF have been produced, the *E. coli* product, filgrastim, and the CHO product, lenograstim. In addition, an *E. coli* derived amino-terminal mutated form (nartograstim, rHuG-CSF-mutein, KW-2228), a pegylated version of nartograstim (Ro-25-83 15, PEG-rHuG-CSF-mutein), as well as a pegylated version of filgrastim (PEG-filgrastim, SD-01), are under investigation. Of these, filgrastim has been most extensively investigated in humans.

Filgrastim has consistent and predictable pharmacokinetics when given intravenously or subcutaneously. It is rapidly absorbed and peak serum concentrations are achieved 2–8 h after intravenous infusion. The elimination half-life after intravenous or subcutaneous dosing is 2–4 h. After discontinuation of dosing, concentrations decrease to physiological levels within 24 h. In cancer patients, dose-linear clearance can occur during severe neutropenia and after high-dose administration, presumably due to saturation of receptor-mediated clearance. It appears that, in cancer patients, administration of rHuG-CSF increases the number of G-CSF receptors per cell as well as circulating neutrophil counts, resulting in modulation of its own clearance. Conversely, dose-dependent clearance is seen after the administration of low doses prior to chemotherapy.

Pharmacodynamics and efficacy are directly related to pharmacokinetics, with dose- dependent increases in the numbers of neutrophils and metamyelocytes. Phase I/II trial results from 15 patients given doses ranging from 1 to 60 μg/kg/d demonstrated dose- dependent absolute neutrophil count (ANC) increases, achieving ANCs up to 80 × 10^9/L. Doses > 10 μg/kg/d can also produce dose-dependent increases in monocytes and small increases in lymphocytes.

Like filgrastim, lenograstim achieves higher maximum plasma concentrations after intravenous administration than after sub-cutaneous administration of the same dose. However, subcutaneous administration resulted in a longer elimination half-life, and a greater and more sustained neutrophil response. In controlled Phase II dose-ranging studies, which included 66 solid tumor and 121 bone marrow transplantation (BMT) patients, lenograstim doses from 2 μg/kg/d were shown to restore neutrophil counts, and a dose of 5 μg/kg/d was chosen for further clinical trials. Phase III double-blind randomized studies in a further 439 patients with solid tumors or post-BMT confirmed the clinical efficacy of the recommended therapeutic dose of lenograstim (150 μg/m^2/d) which is equivalent in efficacy to 5 μg/kg/d. Irrespective of route, the most common adverse events were headaches and back/spine pain, and at doses of up to 5 μg kg/d these were mild and generally well tolerated.

With regard to myelostimulation, low subcutaneous doses of lenograstim (1 μg/kg/d) in 72 healthy volunteers produced ANC increases that did not correlate to C_{max} or the plasma concentration–time curve. This upper limit to the rHuG-CSF transfer rate from subcutaneous tissue to blood may be dependent on the concentration of the G-CSF receptors.

Pharmacokinetics after sc administration of lenogastrim was studied in healthy subjects at doses of 2, 5, and 10 μg/kg/d, given for 5 d to mobilize PBSCs for allogeneic transplantation. In this study, peripheral neutrophils increased markedly by up to 13 times from baseline, peaking at about 40 × 109/L on d 5 for both the 5 and 10 μg/kg/d doses. Peak serum concentration (C_{max}) occurred 4 hours after administration and serum G-CSF then declined with time in a log-linear fashion. The C_{max} and 12-h AUC increased dose-dependently, but the minimum drug level increased up to d 2 and then decreased until d 5. Clearance decreased with increasing dosage at the first dose, and increased significantly at the last dose. There was a highly significant correlation between ANC and clearance for each dose. Adverse events most frequently occurred on d 6, with increases of alkaline phosphatase and lactate dehydrogenase, and onset of bone pain. Direct comparisons of the clinical effects of glycosylated and nonglycosylated forms on PBSCs showed that while differences in serum concentrations were observed, this did not influence their ability to mobilize progenitor cells when tested in monkeys, in healthy volunteers, or in humans with breast cancer.

Adverse events appear less frequent with filgrastim than lenograstim, although few comparative studies have been carried out. Nartograstim is a G-CSF mutant produced in *E. coli* in which five amino acids at the terminal region have been replaced. This compound has higher specific activity than the native protein owing to increased serum stability, although serum concentration–time profiles were found to be very similar to those of filgrastim in monkey studies. These pharmacokinetic studies comparing filgrastim, lenograstim, and nartograstim indicated that after intravenous injection, the serum concentration–time profiles of nartograstim were almost identical to those of filgrastim at either 1.5 or 5 μg/kg doses, but that the serum concentration decreased faster after lenograstim administration. After subcutaneous administration, no marked differences were observed between the three forms of rHuG-CSFs, although lenograstim showed lower serum concentrations than both filgrastim and nartograstim. The small differences in pharmacokinetics did not translate into any significant differences in pharmacodynamics, with all compounds having equivalent activity.

As with other cytokines, addition of PEG to G-CSF has great advantages, allowing active serum levels to be sustained over days rather than minutes. Pegylated forms of nartograstim and filgrastim are under investigation. The uninterrupted therapy possible using pegylated G-CSF may also prove more beneficial with regard to ANC recovery after transplant and with regard to efficient mobilization of PBSCs.

Addition of PEG to nartograstim produces a multi-PEG molecule (Ro-25-83 15, PEG-rHuG-CSF-mutein) that can further increase serum half-life compared with filgrastim, as first demonstrated in mice and monkeys, indicating that these compounds can maintain elevated neutrophil doses for extended periods, with the extent of pegylation directly proportional to the increase of in vivo activity. In monkeys receiving subcutaneous injections, peak neutrophil levels could be attained 6 d after a single dose of Ro-25-8315, while similar levels required six daily injections of PEG-rHuG-CSF.

In humans, Ro-25-83 15 has been compared with filgrastim in 52 healthy male volunteers. Part 1 of this study was a double-blind trial in which 40 adults were randomized to receive either placebo or a single subcutaneous dose of Ro-25-8315 at 10, 30, 60, 100, or 150 μg/kg, with eight patients assigned to each dose level in a dose-ascending manner. Part 2 of the trial assigned 12 adults to receive either 5 or 10 μg/kg of filgrastim (using the standard multiple dosing regimen). This consisted of a single subcutaneous dose of filgrastim given on d 1 and then, beginning on d 15, each adult received daily injections of filgrastim for 7 d.

Administration of Ro-25-8315 resulted in substantial increases in ANC, with both ANC_{max} and AUC_{ANC} increasing six- to eight-fold over placebo at the four highest doses tested. These increases were dose-dependent, although over 60 μg/kg the increases were modest. The time to reach maximum plasma concentration was also dose dependent, ranging from 30 h at 10 μg/kg to 104 h at 150 μg/kg. Effects on $CD34^+$ counts showed that mobilization peaked between day 4 and d 5 with Ro-25-8315, earlier than with filgrastim, and that the 60 μg/kg single injection achieved mobilization levels equivalent to daily administration of filgrastim for 1 wk.

Addition of a single chain (20,000 Da) of PEG to filgrastim produces PEG-filgrastim. Studies in rats of this pegylated protein suggest that it has an elimination half-life that is two to four times greater than that of filgrastim and comparative studies in humans have demonstrated its advantages. The first clinical study of PEG-filgrastim in humans was a randomized dose-escalation study carried out in 13 patients with small-cell lung cancer receiving carboplatin and paclitaxel chemotherapy. In this study, patients were randomized to receive either daily filgrastim (5 μg/kg/d) or a single injection of PEG-filgrastim at 30, 100, or 300 μg/kg per cycle. The maximum PEG-filgrastim serum concentration and AUC were dose dependent. In cycle 1, maximum values were similar to cycle 0. However, a prolonged plateau of serum concentrations began during cycle 1 and began to decline only with recovery of neutrophil counts. Prechemotherapy median ANCs in patients receiving PEG-filgrastim were increased in a dose dependent fashion, with the duration of this effect also being dose-dependent. After chemotherapy, median ANC nadirs were similar in the filgrastim cohort and the cohort receiving PEG-filgrastim 30 μg/kg; higher nadirs were seen in the cohorts receiving PEG-filgrastim at 100 or 300 μg/kg. No serious adverse events were attributed to G-CSF in any arm, with the most common adverse event in all arms being musculoskeletal pain lasting about 8 d during cycle 1. Mobilization of $CD34^+$ cells was also similar in all arms. Seroreactivity was seen in 4 of 19 samples collected, but no evidence of neutralizing antibodies was found. This work established PEG-filgrastim at 100 μg/kg as effective, with no excessive toxicity associated with prolonged pharmacokinetics.

Mobilization of stem cells by PEG-filgrastim has also been studied in detail in both mice and humans. The splenectomized mouse model confirmed that a single-bolus dose of filgrastim could not sustain elevated neutrophil counts beyond 24–48 h irrespective of dose, and that this duration could be extended only by giving multiple injections. A single dose of PEG-filgrastim, however, resulted in increased neutrophil levels for almost 5 d. In a neutropenic setting (induced in mice by chemotherapy with 5-fluorouracil) data indicated that PEG-filgrastim was superior to daily injection of filgrastim. Further, PEG-filgrastim mobilized stem cells in a pattern different from filgrastim. PBSC counts were three times greater after a single injection, and the peak was earlier than could be achieved with multiple-dose filgrastim.

These critical pharmacokinetic observations were confirmed in humans. Healthy subjects were randomized to receive either 30, 60, 100, or 300 μg/kg of PEG-filgrastim. Mobilized $CD34^+$ cells peaked at d 3. At the highest dose, values remained elevated until d 12 or 13, and at other doses, values returned to the normal range at d 9. The duration of this response was longer than that seen with mice. Although direct comparisons with filgastrim were not made, peak mobilization with PEG-filgastrim in humans appears to be earlier than the 5.3 d achieved with a 5-d daily regimen of filgrastim (10 μg/kg/d). Overall, results indicate that single-dose PEG-filgrastim is at least as effective as a five-dose schedule of filgrastim in subjects with normal white cell counts, and appears to have advantages in the neutropenic setting when given following myelosupressive therapy, and for mobilization of PBSCs.

One large multicenter trial compared pegylated G-CSF with nonpegylated G-CSF when used once monthly as part of a chemotherapy regimen in 310 breast cancer patients enrolled in 62 centers. A single ssubcutaneous injection of PEG-filgrastim (100 μg/kg per chemotherapy cycle, given on d 2, 24 h after chemotherapy) was demonstrated to be as safe and effective as daily sc injections of filgrastim (5 μg/kg/d, given until ANC recovery with an average of 11 injections per cycle). PEG-filgrastim was given to 154 patients and filgrastim to 156. Incidence of grade IV neutropenia and depth of the ANC nadir was similar in the two arms. In some parameters, such as the duration of grade IV neutropenia between cycles 2 and 4, and the incidence of febrile neutropenia, PEG-filgrastim performed better than filgrastim. Adverse events were similar in the two arms, and no adverse safety patterns or trends were seen with PEG-filgrastim. This work confirms earlier claims for a supportive role for PEG-filgrastim during cancer chemotherapy.

Granulocyte-Macrophage Colony-Stimulating Factor (GM-CSF)

Granulocyte-macrophage colony-stimulating factor (GM-CSF) is the most widely used hematopoietic growth factor used to augment immune responses, usually as an adjuvant to vaccination. This stimulation of immune effector functions aims to increase the potency of treatment and improve the outcome for patients with various disorders including hematopoeitic and nonhematopoietic malignancies.

Comparative pharmacokinetics studies of glycosylated (produced from CHO cells) and nonglycoslylated (produced from *E. coli*) recombinant GM-CSFs have explored the differences between these forms. Twelve patients were randomized to treatment with either bacterial or CHO rHuGM-CSF, first intravenously, then subcutaneously. Both GM-CSF types followed a two-compartment first-order pharmacokinetic model after intravenous administration. The bacterial form showed more rapid absorption, achieved higher peak serum concentrations, and was eliminated faster. The initial rate of clearance ($t_{1/2}\alpha$) of the bacterial form was also higher (7.8 min vs 20 min). After subcutaneous administration, clearance of the *E. coli* form was faster (reversion to pretreatment serum levels took 16–20 h vs > 48 h). However, the more rapid turnover of the bacterial form did not translate into a significantly different effect on neutrophil kinetics. While there was considerable variability between patients, both types of rHuGM-CSF induced an initial fall in ANC immediately after administration, then a sharp increase, passing baseline levels by about 3 h (intravenous) or 3–6 h (subcutaneous) and reaching maximum values after 4.5–9 h (intravenous) and 5–20 h (sub-cutaneous).

The effects of bacterial and mammalian rHuGM-CSFs on endogenous leukotriene biosynthesis have also been studied, in 21 healthy subjects, linking this marker to the frequency of adverse reactions. This study confirmed the more rapid kinetics of the *E. coli* form, linked to faster and larger increases in urinary leukotriene concentrations (2.1- to 44-fold vs 1.4- to 14-fold). Mammalian GM-CSF caused a number of skin reactions; other side effects (flulike symptoms, bone pain, gastrointestinal effects, and dyspnea) predominated in volunteers given bacterial GM-CSF.

Recombinant GM-CSF has potent augmentation effects. In addition to stimulating proliferation of myeloid cells, GM-CSF enhances phagocytosis and killing of invading pathogens and increases chemotaxis of neutrophils and macrophages. It also expands and activates antigen-presenting cells; activates eosinophils; and stimulates monocytes to increase production of IFN-γ, IL-12, and Il-15, so increasing natural killer (NK) cell functions. This has led to its investigation as an adjuvant, used to increase the immune response against tumor-specific antigens.

Tumor vaccines may consist of whole tumor cells, or cell lysates, or purified fractions of specific tumor antigens such as human carcinoembryonic antigen (CEA) or mucins (MUC-1). The cytokine adjuvant may be administered as soluble protein, as protein encapsulated in microsomes or by transfer of the cytokine DNA sequence into cells expressing the tumor protein(s) of interest. These vaccination protocols are of particular relevance to patients at risk of relapse after surgery has excised solid tumors, as in colorectal cancer (CRC), melanoma, and renal cell carcinoma.

Preclinical models established the importance of prolonged exposure to GM-CSF together with tumor cell proteins, showing that responses in mice were better with low doses of GM-CSF given for 4 d than for 1 d, and that good results could be obtained when GM-CSF was encapsulated in slow-release microspheres. These preclinical results supported the use of low doses of GM-CSF given for 4 d. Most CRC cells express CEA, and vaccination using this antigen alone can stimulate antibody production.

With the addition of GM-CSF these effects are greatly enhanced. This latter study treated 18 CRC patients without macroscopic disease, after surgical excision of primary tumor. Local administration of soluble GM-CSF was used, rather than generation of retrovirally GM-CSF-transduced cells. Nine patients received baculovirus-produced rHuCEA alone (100, 300, or 1000 μg), while nine received the same dose plus GM-CSF. All patients in the GM-CSF group developed a strong rHuCEA-dose-dependent IgG antibody response compared with the weak antibody response seen in only one third of the non-GM-CSF patients. All patients in the GM-CSF group also developed a strong rHCEA-specific proliferative T-cell response, and induced IFN-γ production in type 1 T cells. In addition, 45% of GM-CSF patients showed IL-4 production by type 2 T cells. Further studies are indicated to develop regimens that present the recombinant rHuCEA in such a way as to maximize production of antibodies that can recognize the native protein. After follow-up periods of at least 18 mo from the last vaccination, strong T-cell responses against rHuCEA remained in the GM-CSF group; in the non-GM-CSF group the original weak responses had disappeared.

This work has demonstrated that local administration of soluble GM-CSF is an inexpensive, simple, and reproducible therapeutic procedure for the successful induction of immunity. The majority of colorectal carcinomas also express the tumor antigen GA733 (CO 17-1A, KSA, EPCAM). In one study, responses were maintained for the whole observation period of 10 mo after only three injections of GM-CSF with rHuGA773. The responses observed include a strong type 1 T-cell response that seems to be major histocompatibility class (MHC) I as well as class II restricted.

The idiotypic immunoglobulins on the surface of myeloma cells can be treated as tumor- restricted antigens, and used in vaccination. The use of GM-CSF in such protocols appears to be mandatory for frequency and magnitude of the antigen response. In five myeloma patients vaccinated with purified M-protein plus low-dose (75 μg/d) GM-CSF at six intervals over a 14-wk period, a transient rise of B cells producing IgM antiidiotypic antibodies was seen in all patients. The T-cell response could be characterized as a type 1 response (IFN-γ production), which seemed preferentially to be MHC I restricted. Patients with a low tumor burden are expected to respond most favorably to this kind of therapeutic intervention. GM-CSF-transduced autologous melanoma cells may also be used to treat metastatic melanoma. This case history reported a temporary tumor response in a patient who had rapidly progressive disease at the time of vaccination.

RCC may also respond to vaccination strategies, as shown in a Phase I trial in which 16 such patients were treated. Patients were treated in a randomized, double-blind dose-escalation study with equivalent doses of autologous, irradiated RCC vaccine cells with or without ex vivo human GM-CSF gene transfer using a retroviral vector. Patients vaccinated with GM-CSF-transduced vaccines showed histology changes, such as an intense eosinophil infiltrate, while patients who received nontransduced vaccines did not. Treatment was well tolerated, with one patient achieving a partial response.

Mixed administration of GM-CSF with other cytokines is under increasing investigation for the treatment of RCC and melanoma. One combination of GM-CSF, IL-2, and IFN-α, resulted in considerable expansion and/or activation of various effector cells. In this study, of eight patients with progressive metastatic RCC after nephrectomy, three achieved a complete remission; one out of seven patients with metastatic melanoma achieved a partial remission. MAbs may also be added, such as anti-GA733-3 (anti-CO17A). The use of anti-GA733-3 with GM-CSF and recombinant human IL-2 in 20 CRC patients has produced mixed results. Although one patient obtained a partial remission and two patients achieved stable disease for 7 and 4 mo, respectively, the effect of the antibody was less than that anticipated from in vitro studies.

IL-2

Il-2 is an immune modifier able to activate cytotoxic T lymphocytes (CTL) and NK cells. It therefore has potential to treat cancers such as RCC and melanoma. In RCC, RHuIL-2 monotherapy can achieve overall response rates (ORR) of 20% (CR 5%), while in metastatic malignant melanoma, ORRs are about 13%. Early studies, reviewed in Anderson and Sorenson, indicated that effective treatment of cancer required repetitive long-term high-dose treatment to its very short half-life. Efforts to improve scheduling include pegylation—as for other cytokines that use the kidney as the main site of elimination, pegylation will sustain peak serum levels. Low-dose peritoneal administration also produces longer duration of action. Other approaches include administering rHuIL-2 in combination with an anti-IL-2

MAb to enhance targeting and distribution, or with other cytokines and MAbs to promote immune modulation.

L-12

Like Il-2, IL-12 can stimulate CTL and NK cells, and also has the unique property of promoting development of CD4 T cells, which have a critical role in cell-mediated immunity. This gives it a role as an antitumor agent also capable of restoring immune function.

Studies in rats and monkeys established that the terminal half-life of rHuIL-12 (produced in *E. coli*) was relatively long ($t_{1/2}\beta$ of up to 14 h) compared with other cytokines such as Il-2. This is likely to be a consequence of its larger molecular weight—Il-12 is a dimer composed of 35,000- and 40,000-Da subunits, compared with the more typical 15,500-Da molecular length of Il-2. It also has a low subcutaneous bioavailability (20-30%).99 Such pharmacokinetic data led to the adoption of once-weekly single subcutaneous injection for treatment of metastatic melanoma and RCC.

In a pilot study 10 patients with melanoma were given rHuIL- 12 (0.5 μg/kg) on d 1, 8, and 15, for two consecutive 28-d cycles. Peak serum levels were reached 8–12 h after the first injection, and became lower with subsequent injections, being undetectable at the end of the second cycle. This adaptive response may be due to greater removal of IL-12 from peripheral blood, inhibition of access of injected IL-12 to the bloodstream; or up-regulation of IL-12 receptors. Anti-IL-12 antibodies were not implicated, as assays for such antibodies proved negative. The attenuation in serum levels was reflected in attenuation of immuno-modulation such as stimulation of IFN-α.

A Phase I study in 51 RCC patients randomized them either to three fixed-dose rHuIL-2 injections (0.1, 0.5, and 1.0 μg/kg; $n = 24$) or to an up-titration scheme (lower levels in wk 1, increased to maintenance doses of 0.5, 0.75, 1.0, 1.25, and 1.5 μg/kg in wk 2; $n = 27$). With the up-titration scheme, the maximum tolerated dose was 1.5 μg/kg: at this level, serum IL-12 levels peaked at 706 μg/mL. Peak serum levels were achieved 8–24 h after the first injection, and decreased with a $t_{1/2}\beta$ of 7–21 h. Serum levels after the first maintenance dose in the up-titration scheme were lower than those seen with the equivalent fixed-dose scheme, although half-life and peak time were unchanged. Of the 50 patients evaluable for response, 34 had stable disease, 14 progressed, and 3 were lost to treatment.

In a multicenter Phase II trial, 46 patients with previously untreated advanced RCC were assigned (2:1) to either subcutaneous rHuIL-12 or IFN-α treatment. An escalating-dose schedule of rHuIL-12 was used: d 1, 0.1 μg/kg; d 8, 0.5 μg/kg; and d 14, 1.25 μg/kg. Subsequent doses were 1.25 μg/kg. IFN-α was given at 9×10^6 units, three times weekly. Pharmacokinetic studies were carried out in 10 patients. Peak serum concentrations occurred at about 12 h. In contrast to fixed-dose results, no adaptive response was seen, with C_{max} and AUC remaining constant after repeat dosing. Despite this, low disease responses to rHuIL-12 stopped accrual into this arm after an interim analysis. This modest clinical activity in RCC and melanoma suggests that the most promising use for IL-12 may be in combination with other cytokines, or as a vaccine adjuvant. One such vaccination study has reported on 48 patients with resected melanoma, vaccinated with two tumor antigen peptides ($gp100_{200-217}$, $tyrosinase_{368-376}$) with or without IL-12. IL-12 augmented cytokine release and enhanced the immune response to the tumor antigens. However, the time to relapse of the IL-12 group was identical to that of the non-IL-12 group (20 mo in the whole cohort). Tumor peptide-reactive CTLs did not increase to a plateau until at least six vaccinations had been given over 3 mo. This suggests that prolonged vaccination schedules may be required for melanoma.

Antigenicity of Cytokines

One drawback of using proteins of nonhuman origin for therapeutic purposes is an increase in antigenicity and the risk of triggering an immune response. Detection of such antibodies may predict clinical response and exact information on epitope recognition may also provide information of clinical relevance.

The different forms of recombinant interferon show different immunogenicities. Typical incidences of neutralizing antibodies are 17% after IFN-α-2b treatment, and up to 45% (plus 38% binding antibodies) after IFN-α-2a treatment. Neutralizing antibodies are associated with treatment failure. Conversely, patients, such as those with multiple myeloma, treated with natural leukocyte interferon do not produce antibodies. Changes in the polypeptide backbone in recombinant proteins can render the protein immunogenic, as has been seen in the case of EPO. Sporadic cases of anti-EPO development have been reported, in some cases causing red-cell aplasia. Neutralizing antibodies were identified and characterized in 13 patients with red-cell aplasia who had received rHuEpo-α (12 patients) or -β (1 patient) to treat chronic renal failure.

The antibodies did not target glycosylated moieties. They were shown to be reactive with epitopes specific for folded forms of the protein backbone, except in one case where antibody species reactive with both conformationally folded and linear epitopes were seen. Although, in theory, the additional alterations in the protein backbone of NESP might render this molecule more immunogenic, monitoring of patients treated with NESP has not shown the development of neutralizing antibodies. However, antibodies developed during treatment with rHuEpo-α showed cross-reactivity with other forms of recombinant EPO including NESP. NESP therefore is not likely to be able to rescue patients who have already developed red-cell aplasia as a consequence of EPO treatment and the development of neutralizing antibodies.

Binding or neutralizing antibodies have also been seen in response to GM-CSF. The purity of the recombinant product is one factor involved, with some preparations triggering antibodies to contaminant bacterial proteins. In a study of the significance of binding and neutralizing antibodies in 45 patients, binding antibodies were assayed using solid-phase indirect enzyme-linked immunosorbant assay (ELISA), using the same clinical-grade *E. coli*-derived recombinant human GM-CSF as was used for therapy. Neutralizing antibodies were assayed using the TF-1 cell line which proliferates in response to GM-CSF, using known quantities of GM-CSF used after pre- incubation with dilutions of patient serum. No patients had antibodies directed against GM-CSF at baseline. However, following therapy, while none of the four MM patients had developed reactivity, 15 of the 41 CRC patients had developed reactive antibodies (37.5%). The incidence was greatest in patients receiving high-dose therapy, and was related to cumulative dose. None of the reactive antibodies were capable of neutralizing GM-CSF activity, and no difference was observed in the stimulation of monocytes or other immune effector cells in patients with or without reactive antibodies.

These results were confirmed in a study of 64 CRC patients, in which it was found that only neutralizing antibodies (seen in 9 patients) impaired biological activity, while binding antibodies (seen in 47 patients) did not. These findings indicate that non-neutralizing antibodies to GM-CSF do not reduce an immune response. However, non-neutralizing antibodies to some biologicals may perturb pharmacokinetics by forming aggregates that remove the active molecule from circulation. The effect of binding antibodies has been clearly shown in studies of IL-2 pharmacokinetics in patients with and without anti-IL-2 antibodies. Of 19 CRC patients tested for the presence of IL-2 antibodies during therapy with rHuIL-2, rHuGM-CSF, and MAb17-1A, 10 developed antibodies (10 binding, 1 binding/neutralizing). Titers of anti-IL-2 antibodies increased with repeated treatment and reverted to undetectable levels 4–6 mo post-therapy. The presence of antibodies was shown to affect pharmacokinetics significantly, regardless of their neutralization potential. The reduction in serum IL-2 concentration and increased clearance by antibodies also reduced IL-2 impact on lymphocyte counts. These results indicate that non-neutralizing antibodies may be as important clinically as neutralizing antibodies.

Pharmacokinetics and Antigenicity of Therapeutic MAbs

Many clinically effective MAbs have now been generated, able to target specific cancers, including CRC, chronic lymphocytic leukemia (CLL), non-Hodgkin's lymphoma (NHL), melanoma, and breast cancer. MAbs directed against cell-surface tumor markers can kill their target cell by a variety of mechanisms including antibody-directed cellular cytotoxity (ADCC), complement-dependent cytotoxicity, (CDC) and apoptosis. The exact mechanism of killing varies among unconjugated antibodies: alemtuzumab appears to act primarily by ADCC and is less effective in bulky tumors which are poorly supplied with effector cells; rituximab cytotoxicity has strong apoptotic and complement-mediated components; and trastuzumab may act primarily by nonimmune effector mechanisms triggered by signal transduction. While all these MAbs are of largely similar molecular weight (about 145,000 Da), their pharmacokinetics vary greatly as a consequence of the different affinities for, and distribution of, the target antigen. However, increasing doses increased AUC, which augments the exposure of tumor cells to the MAb.

As with cytokines, the production of an anti-MAb response may limit efficacy after repeat administration. When rodent antibodies are shown to be immunogenic, this can be addressed by the production of chimeric MAbs, retaining only the rodent variable region, or humanized MAbs, retaining only short sequences of rodent hypervariable regions. Although some humanized MAbs show low immunogenicity after repeated dosing, others, such as MAb-A33, have triggered responses in a large numbers of patients (in 26 of 41, 63% in one study).

The antibodies produced to MAb-A33 included type 1 antibodies (49% of cases: early onset; declined with further treatment), which were associated with accelerated MAb clearance, and type 2 antibodies (17% of cases: late onset, increased with treatment), which were associated with infusion-related adverse reactions. The type 1 response appears to be unique to the A33 system. This persistent immunoreactivity is being addressed by using PEG-Mab-A33, which has shown slowed pharmacokinetics and decreased immunogenicity in xenograft models.

Major advances in producing stable and effective therapeutic biological agents have been made in the last decade. Antitumor vaccination programs have been boosted by the use of GM-CSF as an immunomodulator, and further progress is underway as the effects of additional cytokines such as IL-1 and IL-12 are elucidated, individually and in combination. The use of cytokines as chemotherapy support can achieve not only more effective therapy, allowing higher chemotherapy doses to be given, but also a better quality of life, even in patients who are not cured by therapy.

The introduction of more convenient dosing schedules of cytokines such as EPO and G-CSF, made possible by using PEG-cytokines, is also likely to have a beneficial effect on the quality of life of patients with cancer. In the case of EPO, tailoring glycosylation for maximum serum stability has also improved treatment schedules with regard to convenience and efficacy. Pegylation also has the advantage of reducing immunogenicity, which may prove to be of particular value when applied to MAbs with inherent immunogenicity, such as anti-A33.

The large scale production of clinical-grade MAbs achieved in recent years has paved the way to their successful therapeutic use in many conditions, now further enhanced by the synthesis of new humanized and/or pegylated molecules. Significant advances in the treatment of previously intractable forms of cancer have already been made, and these new generations of MAbs, in combination with chemotherapy, have great potential to achieve durable remissions in increasing numbers of patients.

16

FLUORESCENCE TECHNIQUE

A number of areas exist in pharmacogenomics research where it is desirable to determine the relative abundance of the two alleles of a gene or marker. For example, humans have a number of mast cell tryptase genes, and the number of copies of beta-tryptase is associated with asthma. Routine genotyping can only determine the presence or absence of the beta-tryptase gene but cannot determine the number of copies of beta-tryptase gene found in the genome. Another scenario concerns the duplication or deletion of genes in tumor cells caused by somatic mutation. Being able to determine whether a gene is duplicated or deleted is very helpful in studying cancer progression. An emerging area of research has to do with regulation of gene expression. Here, the relative abundance of alleles of a genetic marker in coding sequences can be used to monitor the expression differences between the allelic genes from the two chromosomes in the cell. In extreme cases, one can estimate the allele frequencies of genetic markers in pooled samples in genetic association studies.

Although a number of quantitative assays are available for allele frequency estimation, most are difficult and expensive to develop or implement. In this chapter, we describe the most versatile and least expensive assays for allele frequency estimation, namely, the template-directed dye-terminator incorporation assay with fluorescence quenching detection (the FQ-TDI assay). The FQ-TDI assay is a real-time homogeneous primer extension assay based on two principles, namely, that deoxyribonucleic acid (DNA) polymerase catalyzes the allele-specific incorporation of a dye-terminator at the polymorphic site and that the fluorescence intensities of a fluorescent dye decreases significantly when it is incorporated into primers.

The TDI assay procedure is quite simple. First, the DNA template containing a SNP site is amplified by polymerase chain reaction (PCR). After the excess PCR primers and deoxynucleotides (dNTPs) are degraded by exonuclease I and shrimp alkaline phosphatase, a SNP primer designed to hybridized one base upstream of SNP is allowed to anneal to the target DNA in the presence of DNA polymerase and dye-labeled acycloterminators. The SNP primer is extended one base by the acycloterminator complementary to the allele present on the target DNA. By determining which terminator is incorporated, one can infer the genotype of the target DNA sample. The primer extension has been used in various format for SNP genotyping and proven to be highly specific and sensitive.

If the TDI assay is monitored in real time, one can calculate the rate of incorporation, which is proportional to the amount of allelic target present. Therefore, one can estimate the allele frequency in the sample by determining the relative incorporation rate of the two terminators. A simple way to monitor the progress of the TDI assay is to take advantage of the physical phenomenon of fluorescence quenching. The fluorescence of some conjugated fluorescent dyes is sensitive to their local environment,

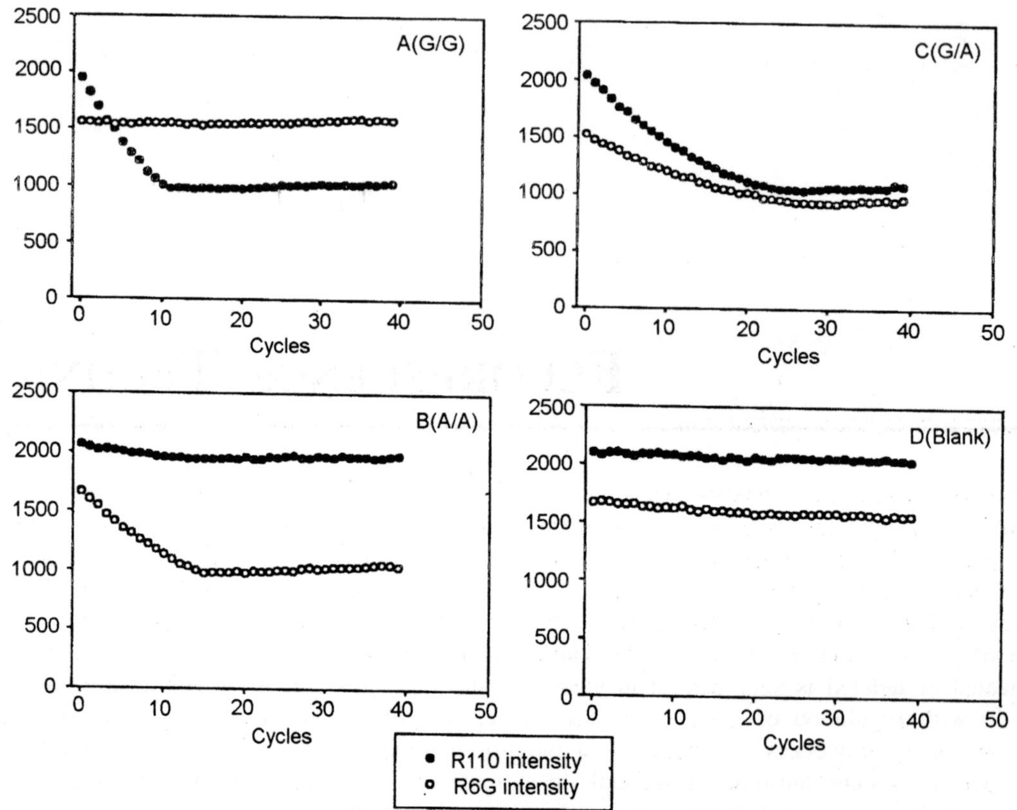

Fig. 16.1. The real-time fluorescence intensity profiles of four representative samples tested for SNP marker rs 154162 during thermal cycling of the primer extension step of the TDI assay.

such as the presence of DNA nearby. The fluorescence quenching caused by DNA–dye interactions has been reported for many different fluorescent dyes. We found that R110- and R6G-labeled acycloterminators were heavily quenched upon incorporation into oligonucleotides, especially those containing Gs within 10 bases of the incorporation site. Figure 16.1 shows the real-time fluorescence intensity profiles of four representative samples tested for SNP marker rs154162 during the primer extension step of the TDI assay. The fluorescence readings correspond to the emission maxima for R1 10-G (525 nm) and R6G-A (535 nm) acycloterminators are normalized by multicomponent analysis to account for the crosstalk between the two dyes. In Fig. 16.1A, the G/G homozygous sample directs the incorporation of R110-G (but not R6G-A) and the fluorescence reading shows a progressive drop in R110 fluorescence (filled circles) but no change in R6G fluorescence (open circles) as thermal cycling proceeds. The homozygous A/A sample in Fig. 16.1B shows that R6G-A is incorporated (but not R110-G) with a drop in R6G fluorescence but no change in R110 fluorescence. The heterozygous G/A sample in Fig. 16.1C shows that both R1 10-G and R6G-A are incorporated, with both R110 and R6G fluorescence dropping as the reaction proceeds, albeit at a slower rated than those observed in homozygous samples. In contrast, the fluorescence intensity profile of a negative control sample shows no change for both dyes because neither is incorporated.

The rate of change of the R1 10 and R6G fluorescence intensities is proportional to the amounts of the allelic target present in the reaction, with the initial slope of change for the heterozygote being approximately half of that for the homozygote.

Because the amounts of dye terminators used in the primer extension reaction are fixed by the manufacturer, the larger the number of target DNA molecules containing a particular allele that is present, the faster the dye terminators are used. The initial rate of change in fluorescence intensity (the steepness of the slope) of a dye-terminator is therefore a reflection of the amount of DNA molecule

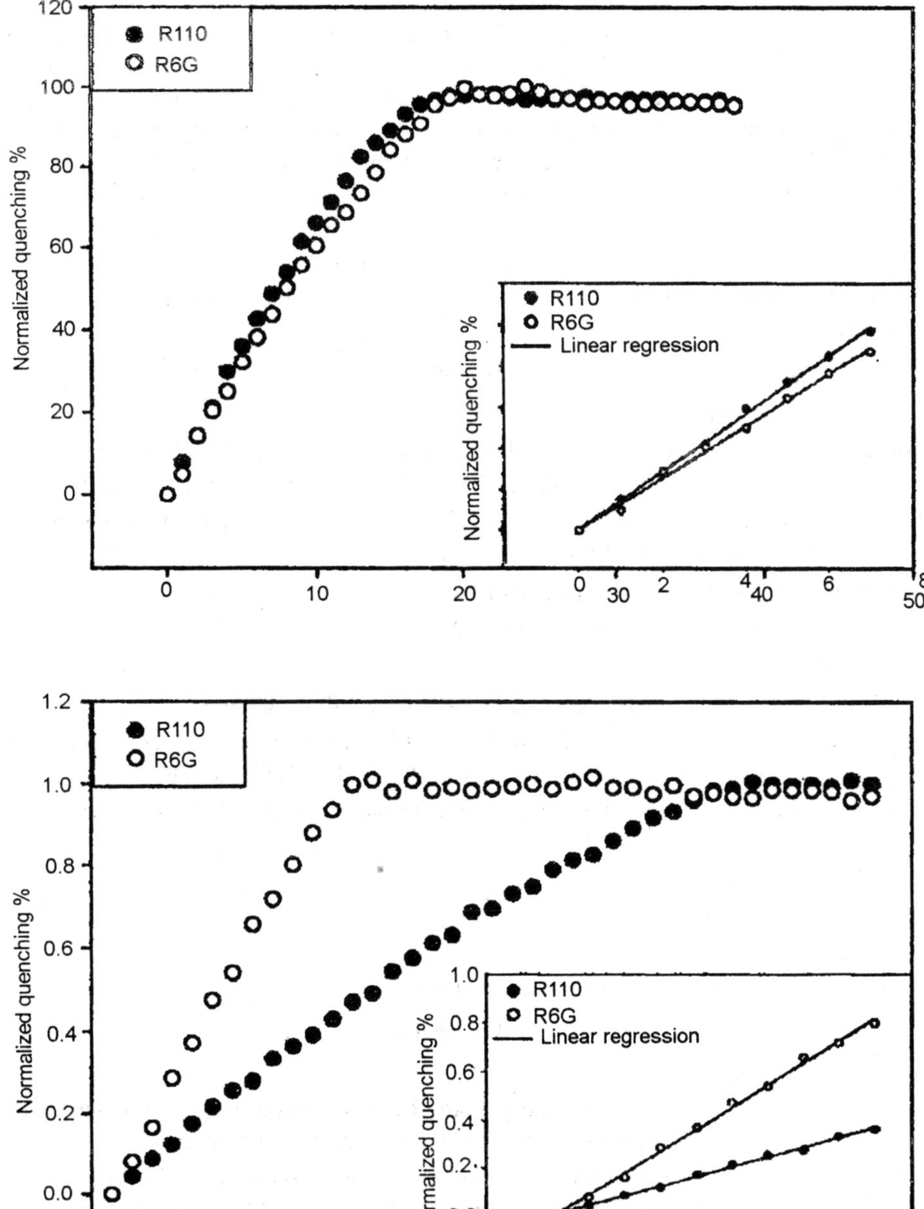

Fig. 16.2. The basis of determining allele frequency for pooled DNA samples.

containing the allele corresponding to the dye-terminator incorporated. By monitoring the fluorescence profile during the primer extension reaction, one can calculate the initial rate of change of fluorescence intensity. Comparing the initial rate of change of fluorescence intensity between a test sample and a heterozygous reference sample allows one to infer the relative amounts of the alleles found in the test sample. The top panel is a normalized real-time quenching curve for a heterozygous sample of rs922365. The linear regressions of the first eight cycles are shown in the inset, and the ratio of the two slopes is calculated as 0.93 (allele 2 [R6G]/allele 1 [R110]), which indicates that the AcycloPol enzyme incorporates R110-G slightly faster than R6G-A. The ratio of two slopes (S_2/S_1) of the pooled sample reflects the relative amount of allele present in the pooled sample. The higher the value of the slope, the more copies of this particular allele are present in the pooled sample. To calculate the absolute allele frequencies, one needs to correct differential incorporation efficiency of two dye-acyloterminators by the polymerase using a heterozygous sample $C = (V_1/V_2)$ as indicated in Eq. 1.

$$p_1 = 1/[1 + C(S_2/S_1)] \qquad \ldots(1)$$

where p_1 is the frequency of allele 1 and V_1/V_2 is the ratio of the slopes for alleles 1 and 2 of the heterozygous reference sample.

MATERIALS

Polymerase Chain Reaction

1. PlatinumTaq DNA polymerase with 10X PCR buffer and 50 m*M* $MgCl_2$ solution.
2. dNTP mixture: 2.5 m*M* dATP, 2.5 m*M* dCTP, 2.5 m*M* dGTP, and 2.5 m*M* dTTP.
3. PCR primers were designed using modified Primer 3. Working solutions of the PCR primers (P_1 and P_2) are prepared at concentration of 2.5 μM.

Degradation of Excess PCR Primers and dNTPs

1. Exo-Sap (Exonuclease I and shrimp alkaline phosphatase).

Primer Extension

1. SNP detection kit, including 10X reaction buffer, AcycloPol enzyme.
2. R110-acycloterminators (aATP, aCTP, aGTP, aTTP) and R6G-acycloterminators (aATP, aCTP, aGTP, aTTP). Unlabeled acycloterminators (aATP, aCTP, aGTP, aTTP).
3. SNP-specific primers were designed with a custom made program. The SNP primer stock solution is prepared at 10 μM concentration.

Instrument

1. 96-well or 384 well optic plates.
2. Thermocycler.
3. Applied Biosystems 7700 or 7900 Sequence Detector.

METHODS

Pool DNA Sample Preparation

1. DNA concentration is quantified by using both the absorbance at 260 nm and a DNA specific fluorescence dye, PicoGreen according to the manufacturer's instructions.
2. Construct the population pool samples by adding equal amounts of DNA from each of the 32 individuals to yield a pooled sample containing a final DNA concentration of 10 ng/μL.

PCR Amplification

1. Amplify genomic DNA (10 ng) in 5 μL reaction mixtures containing 0.5 μL of PCR primers, 0.25 μL of $MgCl_2$, 0.5 μL of 10X PCR buffer, 0.2 U of Platinum Taq polymerase, and 0.2 μL of dNTP mix.

2. The thermal cycling sequence is as follows: the reaction mixture is held at 95°C for 2 min (to activate the Taq polymerase and to denature the genomic DNA) followed by 40 cycles of 92°C for 10 s, 58°C for 30 s, and 68°C for 30 s. After the final extension step of incubating the reaction mixtures at 68°C for 10 min, they are cooled down and held at 4°C until further use.

Degradation of Excess PCR Primers and dNTPs

1. Dilute Exo-Sap solution with water in 1:1 ratio.
2. Add 2 μL of the diluted Exo-Sap solution to the PCR product from above.
3. Incubated the mixture at 37°C for 45 min to degrade the excess PCR primers and excess dNTP. Heat inactivate the enzymes were at 80°C for 15 min before the single-base extension reaction.

Single-Base Extension

1. Make 1 μM stock solution of acycloterminator mix with each of four acycloterminators according to the SNP alleles. For example, prepare a terminator mix containing R110-G, R6G-A, unlabeled acycloterminator C, and T for a G/A SNP.
2. Prepare the TDI cocktail (13 μL) with 1 μL of terminator mix, 0.05 μL of acycloPol polymerase, and 2 μL of 10X TDI buffer.
3. Add the TDI cocktail (13 μL) to the reaction mixtures (7 μL) from the previous step.
4. Add the standard R110 and R6G emission spectra were added to ABI 7700 or 7900 according manufacturer's instructions.
5. Set up the protocol in ABI 7700 or 7900 sequence detector using R1 10 as reporter and R6G as Quencher.
6. The thermal cycling sequence is as follows: incubate the reaction mixture at 95°C for 2 min followed by 40 cycles of 95°C for 10 s, 57°C for 30 s.
7. Collect data at 57°C of each cycle.
8. At the end of the reaction, the mixture is held at 4°C on an ABI 7900 sequence detector.

Data Analysis

1. Analyze data using the ABI multicomponent option.
2. The results of the multicomponent analysis data can be visualized with ABI software and can then be exported into a text file.
3. The results in text file format can then be imported into any graphing program, such as Excel, SigmaPlot.
4. The original file can be plotted. The quenching is calculated using the intensity of the first cycle minus the intensities of subsequent cycles. The inset is the linear regression of first 8 cycles used to calculate the slope of allele 1 (S_1) and the slope of allele 2 (S_2).
5. The allele frequency of allele 1 is determined as $p = 1/[1 + C(S_2/S_1)]$. C is the correcting factor, which is slope ratio (V_1/V_2) using a heterozygous sample.

Notes

1. The amount of templates from PCR is critical for the FQ-TDI assay; 0.1 pmol PCR templates should be adequate.
2. Because higher quenching will give better results, one can select the sense or antisense primers based on which primer has a G base closer to the 3' end and which primer has more G bases within 10 bases next to 3' end.
3. If R110 and R6G standard emission spectra cannot be added to the ABI software, the standard emission spectra of Fam and Joe can be used for R110 and R6G instead.

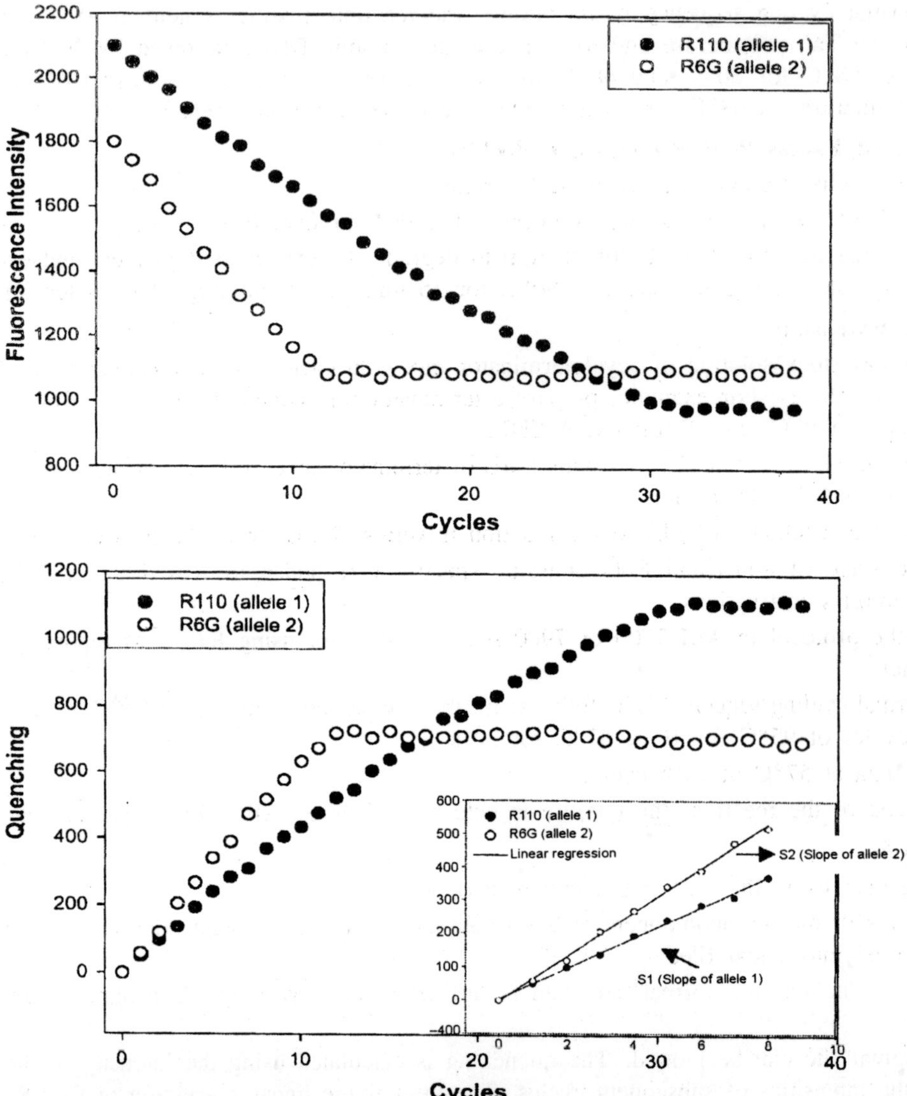

Fig. 16.3. Data analysis. The top panel is the original data plotted as intensity vs cycles. The bottom panel is the quenching plot, determined as the intensity of first cycle minus the intensity of subsequent cycles.

4. Although both R110 and R6G are reporters in this assay, the ABI 7700 or 7900 software requires the user to enter a "reporter" and a "quencher" to run the program for data acquisition during thermal cycling. Entering R110 as reporter and R6G as quencher fulfills this requirement and allows the data acquisition to proceed during the primer extension reaction.
5. FQ-TDI works well for SNPs with minor allele frequency between 0.05 and 0.5, and it generates more accurate results for the SNPs with minor alleie frequency closer to 0.5. It generally does not work for the SNPs with minor allele frequency less than 0.05, as the slopes of linear regression vary greatly for these SNPs.

17

PHARMACOKINETICS OF SPECIFIC DRUGS

The term *amphetamine* refers to the group of stimulants that includes amphetamine, methamphetamine, methylenedioxyamphetamine, and methylenedioxymethamphetamine. These low-molecular-weight basic drugs are sympathomimetic phenethylamine derivatives possessing central and peripheral stimulant activity. Amphetamines suppress appetite and produce CNS and cardiovascular stimulation. These effects are mediated by increasing synaptic concentrations of norepinephrine and dopamine either by stimulating neurotransmitter release or inhibiting uptake, or both. Clinical uses of amphetamine and methamphetamine include chronic administration for the treatment of narcolepsy in adults and attention-deficit/hyperactivity disorder in children.

AMPHETAMINE

These drugs are abused for their stimulant effect. The effects are usually longer lasting than those of cocaine and may prevent fatigue. The latter factor has led to their study in athletes and in military field situations. It is postulated that the disturbances in perception and psychotic behavior, which may occur at high doses, may be due to dopamine release from dopaminergic neurons and also serotonin release from tryptaminergic neurons located in the mesolimbic area of the brain.

Amphetamine and methamphetamine occur as structural isomers and stereoisomers. Structural isomers are compounds with the same empirical formula but a different atomic arrangement, e.g., methamphetamine and phentermine. Stereoisomers differ in the three-dimensional arrangement of the atoms attached to at least one asymmetric carbon and are nonsuperimposable mirror images. Therefore, amphetamine and methamphetamine occur as both D- and L-isomeric forms. The two isomers together form a racemic mixture. The D-amphetamine form has significant stimulant activity, and possesses approximately three to four times the central activity of the L-form. It is also important to note that the D- and L-enantiomers may have not only different pharmacological activity but also varying pharmacokinetic characteristics.

When indicated for therapeutic use, 5 to 60 mg or 5 to 20 mg of amphetamine or methamphetamine, respectively, are administered orally. An oral dose of amphetamine typically results in a peak plasma concentration of 110 ng/ml. When abused, amphetamines may be self-administered by the oral, intravenous, or smoked route. The last route of administration is common for methamphetamine. With heavy use, addicts may ingest up to 2000 mg per day.

Absorption

Limited data are available on the GI absorption of amphetamine in humans. Beckett and Rowland reported serum concentrations of amphetamine in two healthy volunteers after a 15-mg oral dose of the D-isomer. Peak serum concentrations of 48 and 40 ng/ml were achieved at 1.25 h when the volunteers' urine was acidified. Slightly higher serum concentrations were observed (52 and 47 ng/ml) if the urine pH conditions were not controlled. Rowland observed a peak blood concentration of 35 ng/ml, 2 h after a 10-mg oral dose of D-amphetamine to a healthy 66-kg adult. The half-life for the D-isomer was 11 to 13 h compared with a 39% longer half-life for the L-isomer. If the urine were acidified, excretion was enhanced and the half-lives of both isomers were reduced to approximately 7 h. Amphetamine demonstrates a linear one-compartment open model over the dose range 20 to 200 mg.

Distribution

The plasma protein binding of amphetamine in humans is approximately 16 to 20% and is similar in drug-dependent and naive subjects. Research by Rowland and Franksson and Anggard indicated that there was a difference in the volume of distribution between non-users (3.5 to 4.6 L/kg) and drug-dependent individuals (6.1 L/kg). It has been suggested that the larger V_d observed in drug-dependent subjects may be due to a higher tissue affinity for amphetamine in these individuals. Evidence to support this suggestion is found in studies with amphetamine-dependent animals in which higher tissue concentrations of amphetamine were found.

Metabolism and Excretion

Amphetamine is metabolized by deamination, oxidation, and hydroxylation. Deamination produces an inactive metabolite, phenylacetone, which is further oxidized to benzoic acid and then excreted in urine as hippuric acid and glucuronide conjugates. In addition, amphetamine is also converted to norephedrine by oxidation and then this metabolite and the parent compound are *p*-hydroxylated. Several metabolites, including norephedrine, its hydroxy metabolite, and hydroxyamphetamine, are pharmacologically active. The excretion of amphetamine depends on urinary pH. In healthy men who were administered 5 mg of isotopically labeled D,L-amphetamine, approximately 90% of the dose was excreted in the urine within 3 to 4 days. Approximately 70% of the dose was excreted in the 24-h

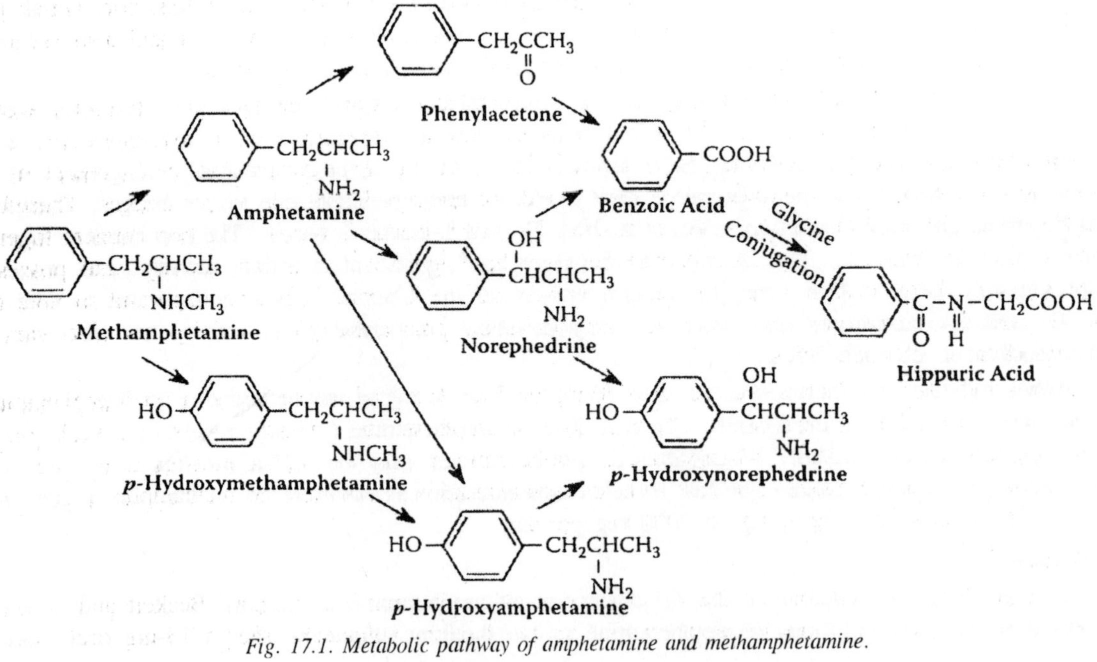

Fig. 17.1. Metabolic pathway of amphetamine and methamphetamine.

urine with 30% as unchanged drug. This was increased to 74% under acidic conditions and reduced to 1% in alkaline urine. Under normal conditions, <1% is excreted as phenylacetone, 16 to 28% as hippuric acid, 4% as benzoylglucuronide, 2% as norephedrine, <0.5% as *p*-hydroxynorephedrine, and 2 to 4% as *p-hydroxyamphetamine*. L-Amphetamine is not as extensively metabolized as the D-isomer. When volunteers were orally administered 5 to 15 mg of D- or L-amphetamine, the mean excretion of unchanged D-amphetamine was 33% of the dose and that of the L-isomer was 49% of the dose.

The metabolism of amphetamine has been studied in those presenting with amphetamine psychosis. In the presence of acidified urine, the renal elimination of amphetamine increased significantly. The intensity of the psychosis was found to correlate with the amount of basic polar metabolites excreted in the urine, such as norephedrine and *p*-hydroxyamphetamine, and not with the plasma amphetamine concentration. This suggests that these metabolites may play an important role in the development of paranoid psychosis in chronic amphetamine users.

Methamphetamine

D-Methamphetamine, the *N*-methyl derivative of amphetamine, was first synthesized in 1919. Methamphetamine is available in the D- and L-forms. The D-form has reportedly greater central stimulant activity than the L-isomer, which has greater peripheral sympathomimetic activity. The D-form is the commonly abused form while the L-isomer is typically found in nonprescription inhalers as a decongestant. Although initially available as an injectable solution for the treatment of obesity, D-methamphetamine hydrochloride is currently available as conventional and prolonged release tablets. Illicit methamphetamine is synthesized from the precursors phenylacetone and *N*-methylformamide (DL mixture) or alternatively from ephedrine or pseudoephedrine by red phosphorus/acid reduction.

Absorption

Doses of 5 to 10 mg methamphetamine typically result in blood concentrations between 20 and 60 ng/ml. In one study, six healthy adults were orally administered a single dose of 0.125 mg/kg methamphetamine. Peak plasma concentrations were achieved at 3.6 h with a mean concentration of 20 ng/ml. In a second study, Lebish et al. observed a peak blood concentration of 30 ng/ml, 1 h after a single oral dose of 10 mg methamphetamine to one subject. In a study by Schepers et al., eight subjects were administered four oral doses of 10 mg methamphetamine hydrochloride as sustained release tablets within 7 days. Three weeks later five subjects received four oral 20-mg doses. After the first dose, methamphetamine was detected in plasma between 0.25 and 2 h; the c_{max} was 14.5 to 33.8 ng/ml (10-mg dose) and 26.2 to 44.3 ng/ml (20-mg) and occurred within 2 to 12 h. Methamphetamine was first detected in oral fluid in this study 0.08 to 2 h post dose, with a c_{max} of 24.7 to 312.2 and 75.3 to 321.7 ng/ml after the 10- and 20-mg doses, respectively. Peak methamphetamine concentrations in oral fluid occurred at 2 to 12 h and the median oral fluid- plasma concentration ratio was 2.0 for 24 h. In general, the detection window for drug in oral fluid exceeded that in plasma.

Metabolism and Excretion

In humans, both the D- and L-forms undergo hydroxylation and *N*-demethylation to their respective *p*-hydroxymethamphetamine and amphetamine metabolites. Amphetamine is the major active metabolite of methamphetamine. Under normal conditions, up to 43% of a D-methamphetamine dose is excreted unchanged in the urine in the first 24 h and 4 to 7% will be present as amphetamine. In acidic urine, up to 76% is present as parent drug compared with 2% under alkaline conditions. Approximately 15% of the dose was present as *p*-hydroxymethamphetamine and the remaining minor metabolites were similar to those found after amphetamine administration. Urine concentrations of methamphetamine are typically 0.5 to 4 mg/L after an oral dose of 10 mg. However, methamphetamine and amphetamine urine concentrations vary widely among abusers. Lebish et al. reported urine methamphetamine concentrations of 24 to 333 mg/L and amphetamine concentrations of 1 to 90 mg/L in the urine of methamphetamine abusers.

L-Methamphetamine is biotransformed in a similar manner to the D-isomer but at a slower rate. Following a 13.7-mg oral dose, the 24-h urine contained an average of 34% of the dose as L-methamphetamine and 1.7% of the dose as L-amphetamine. Oyler et al. described the appearance of methamphetamine and amphetamine in urine after volunteers ($n = 8$) ingested 4×10-mg doses of methamphetamine hydrochloride daily for 7 days followed by 4×20 mg daily several weeks later. Parent and metabolite were generally detected in the first or second void post dose in a concentration range of 82 to 1827 and 12 to 180 ng/ml, respectively. Peak methamphetamine urine concentrations (1871 to 6004 ng/ml) occurred within 1.5 to 60 h after a single dose.

D-Methamphetamine is commonly self-administered by the smoked route. Both the free-base and hydrochloride salt of methamphetamine are volatile and >90% of parent drug can be recovered intact when heated to temperatures of 3 00°C. When cigarettes containing tobacco mixed with methamphetamine were pyrolyzed, amphetamine, phenylacetone, dimethylamphetamine, and *N*-cyanomethyl methamphetamine were the major resulting products. Cook conducted a study in which six volunteers were administered 30 mg D-methamphetamine from a pipe that was heated to approximately 300°C. Blood samples and physiological and subjective measures were collected after drug administration. Plasma methamphetamine concentrations rose rapidly after the start of smoking. However, concentrations plateaued (40 to 44 ng/ml) after 1 h with a slight increase in concentration over the next 1 h. Thereafter, concentrations in plasma declined slowly, reaching the same concentration at 8 h on the downward side of the curve as reached at 30 min on the upward side. The authors used a noncompartmental model to determine an average elimination half-life of 11.7 h with a range of 8 to 17 h. These authors also administered methamphetamine (0.250 mg/kg) orally and the resulting plasma data were fit to a one-compartment model with first-order elimination and a lag time. A maximum plasma concentration of 35 to 38 ng/ml was achieved at 3.1 h with a terminal elimination half-life of 10 h. Although the plasma concentration time curves for smoked and oral methamphetamine appeared similar, the subjective effects were markedly different, with a greater "high" being reported after smoked methamphetamine. This indicates that it may be the rate of change of plasma drug concentrations that is a significant factor in determining subjective effects. Other investigators have reported the bioavailability of methamphetamine after intranasal and smoked drug to be 79 and 67% (of estimated delivered dose), respectively. Maximum blood concentrations of parent drug occurred at 2.7 and 2.5 h after intranasal and smoked doses ($n = 8$).

3,4-Methylenedioxyamphetamine

3,4-Methylenedioxyamphetamine (MDA) is a potent psychotropic amphetamine derivative first synthesized in 1910. It has no accepted medical use but is self-administered orally or intravenously in doses of 50 to 250 mg for illicit use. Blood concentrations following normal use have not been reported and, to date, there are no reported clinical studies delineating the pharmacokinetic or pharmacodynamic characteristics of this drug. Blood concentrations in humans have been reported following overdose. The average blood concentration in 12 fatal cases was 9.3 mg/L (range 1.8 to 26). The metabolism of MDA in humans has not been studied, but in other animals MDA is metabolized by *O*-dealkylation, deamination, and conjugation.

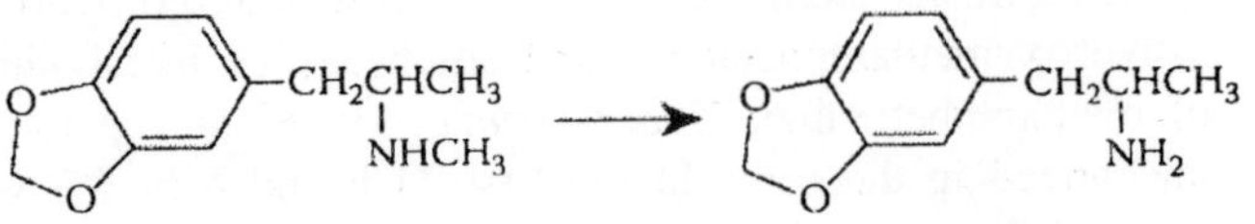

MDMA (3,4-Methylenedioxy-methamphetamine) → **MDA (3,4-Methylenedioxy-amphetamine)**

Fig. 17.2. Structures of MDA and MDMA.

Polymorphically expressed CYP2D6 is the major isozyme catalyzing the metabolic steps in the metabolism of MDA and MDMA.

3,4-Methylenedioxymethamphetamine

3,4-Methylenedioxymethamphetamine (MDMA) is a ring-substituted derivative of methamphetamine that has widespread use as a recreational drug. Self-administration is typically by the oral route in doses of 100 to 150 mg. Helmlin et al. reported a mean peak plasma MDMA concentration of 300 ng/ml at 2.3 h after an oral dose of 1.5 mg/kg to adult subjects; de la Torre et al. studied eight healthy volunteers and reported a peak MDMA concentration of 180 ng/m occurring 1.8 h after a 75-mg oral dose, with an MDA peak of 78 ng/ml 5 h after administration. MDMA presents nonlinear pharmacokinetics. In a randomized double-blind crossover placebo-controlled study with nine healthy male subjects, Farre et al. reported increased plasma MDMA concentrations after a second dose of 100 mg, 24 h after the initial dose, were greater than expected by accumulation. The authors suspected the reason to be due to metabolic inhibition. Parameters such as blood pressure, heart rate, and subjective effects were higher after the second dose than after the first.

MDMA is metabolized to MDA with 65% of the dose excreted as parent drug within 3 days. Both MDMA and MDA are hydroxylated to mono- and di-hydroxy derivatives and subsequently conjugated before elimination. The plasma half-life has been reported to be 7.6 h.

If MDMA is co-administered with ethanol, as 100 mg plus 0.8 g/kg ethanol, plasma concentrations of the former demonstrate a 13% increase compared with MDMA administered alone. Plasma concentrations of ethanol decreased 9 to 15% after MDMA administration ($n = 9$).

MDMA has also been reported in alternative biological specimens. After a single oral dose of 75 mg in human volunteers, MDMA concentrations in oral fluid exceeded those in plasma with a mean peak concentration of 1215 ng/ml ($n = 12$) and a range of 50 to 6982 ng/ml compared with an average peak plasma concentration of 178 ng/ml (range 21 to 295 ng/ml). In sweat the average concentration was 25 ng/wipe when measured 4 to 5 h after ingestion of a similar dose. When MDMA and MDA concentrations measured in ante-mortem samples have been compared, consistent and significant increases in the postmortem concentrations have been observed.

Barbiturates

Barbituric acid, 2,4,6-trioxohexahydropyrimidine, was first synthesized in 1864. In 1903 it was marketed for use as an antianxiety and sedative hypnotic medication. Barbituric acid is without CNS depressant activity but by substituting an aryl or alkyl group on C-5, anxiolytic and sedative properties may be conferred. Substitution of sulfur on C-2 produces the thiobarbituates, which have characteristically greater lipophilicity. Generally, structural changes that increase lipophilicity result in decreased duration of action, decreased latency to onset of action, increased biotransformation, and increased hypnotic potency. Although the use of barbiturates as sedative-hypnotic agents has largely been replaced by the benzodiazepines, the barbiturates maintain an important role as anticonvulsant and anesthetic drugs.

Pharmacology

As a class of drugs, barbiturates exert hypnotic, sedative, anxiolytic, anticonvulsant, and anesthetic properties. The clinical use of these drugs is based on their shared properties and also unique properties of individual drugs within this class. As CNS depressants, barbiturates exert effects on excitatory and inhibitory synaptic neurotransmission. Barbiturates are known to decrease excitatory amino acid release and post-synaptic response in experimental animals by blocking the excitatory glutamate response. This may be due to a direct effect on the glutamate-sensitive channel, or an indirect effect on calcium channels. The ultrashort-acting barbiturates used for anesthesia, such as thiopental, depress excitatory neuronal transmission to a greater extent than the anticonvulsant barbiturates.

Barbiturates also exert an effect on gamma-amino butyric acid (GABA) neurotransmission. Barbiturates, such as pentobarbital, enhance the binding of GABA to $GABA_A$ receptors. This effect occurs both in the CNS and the spinal cord. The enhanced action of GABA depresses both normal physiological processes, such as post-synaptic potential evocation, and pathophysiological processes such as seizures. Barbiturates also enlarge GABA-induced chloride currents by extending the time for chloride channel opening. It is important to note that some barbiturates such as 5-(1,3-dimethylbutyl)-5-ethyl barbituric acid (DMBB) promote convulsions by directly depolarizing the neuronal membrane and increasing transmitter release.

Absorption

When utilized as sedative hypnotics, barbiturates are administered orally. They are rapidly and completely absorbed by this route with nearly 100% bioavailability and an onset of action ranging from 10 to 60 min. Sodium salts are more rapidly absorbed than free acids. Intramuscular injections of sodium salts should be made deep into the muscle to prevent pain and tissue damage. Some barbiturates are also administered rectally; barbiturates utilized for the induction and maintenance of anesthesia (thiopental) or for treating status epilepticus (phenobarbital) are administered intravenously.

Pentobarbital is a short-acting barbiturate available for oral, intramuscular, rectal, and intravenous administration. After a single oral dose of 100 mg, peak serum concentrations of 1.2 to 3.1 mg/L were achieved at 0.5 to 2.0 h. These concentrations diminished slowly to an average of 0.3 mg/L at 48 h. When administered intravenously, in a 5-min continuous infusion of 50 mg, plasma concentrations averaged 1.18 mg/L ($n = 5$) at 0.08 h, declining to 0.54 mg/L after 1 h and reaching 0.27 mg/L after 24 h. Repeated intravenous doses of pentobarbital, typically 100 to 200 mg every 30 to 60 min, are administered to reduce intracranial pressure and decrease cerebral oxygen demand in patients with severe head trauma or anoxic brain damage. Doses are adjusted to maintain plasma concentrations between 25 to 40 mg/L.

Amobarbital is a barbituric acid derivative of intermediate duration of action. It is administered orally in doses of 15 to 200 mg as a sedative hypnotic and in ampoules of 65 to 500 mg for intravenous and intramuscular injection for the seizure control. Following a single oral dose of 120 mg, peak serum concentrations averaged 1.8 mg/L after 2 h. After an oral dose of 600 mg distributed over a 3-h period, the peak blood concentration was achieved after 30 min, averaging 8.7 mg/L, with a decline to 4.1 mg/L by 18 h. Phenobarbital is utilized as a daytime sedative and anticonvulsant. It also induces several cytochrome P450 isozymes. Compared to other barbiturates, phenobarbital has a low oil/water partition coefficient, which results in slow distribution into the brain. It is available for oral, intravenous, or intramuscular administration. Doses for epileptic patients range from 60 to 200 mg per day. After a single oral dose of 30 mg, peak serum concentrations averaged 0.7 mg/L ($n = 3$). Repeated doses over a period of 7 days resulted in an average peak concentration of 8.1 mg/L. Chronic administration of 200 mg per day as anticonvulsant medication resulted in an average blood concentration of 29 mg/L (range = 16 to 48 mg/L).

Distribution

Barbiturates are generally widely distributed throughout the body. The highly lipophilic barbiturates, especially those used to induce anesthesia, undergo redistribution when administered intravenously. Barbiturates enter less vascular tissues over time, such as muscle and adipose tissue, and this redistribution decreases concentrations in the blood and brain. With drugs such as thiopental, this redistribution results in patients waking up within 5 to 15 min after injection of a anesthetic dose.

Pentobarbital is 65% plasma protein bound with a volume of distribution of 0.5 to 1.0 L/kg. After intravenous administration, estimates of the plasma half-life have averaged between 20 and 30 h.

Amobarbital is similar to pentobarbital in the degree of plasma protein binding (59%) with a slightly larger volume of distribution (0.9 to 1.4 L/kg). The plasma half-life, however, is dose dependent, with a range of 15 to 40 h. Phenobarbital is approximately 50% plasma protein bound with a volume of distribution of 0.5 to 0.6 L/kg. The plasma half-life averages 4 days with a range of 2 to 6 days.

Metabolism and Elimination

Generally, barbiturates are metabolized by oxidation and conjugation in the liver prior to renal excretion. The oxidation of substituents at the C-5 position is the most important factor in terminating pharmacological activity. Oxidation of barbiturates results in the formation of alcohols, phenols, ketones, or carboxylic acids with subsequent conjugation with glucuronic acid. Other metabolic transformations include *N*-hydroxylation, desulfuration of thiobarbiturates to oxybarbiturates, opening of the barbituric acid ring, and *N*-dealkylation of *N*-alkylbarbiturates to active metabolites, e.g., mephobarbital to phenobarbital. Pentobarbital is biotransformed by oxidation of the penultimate carbon of the methyl butyl side-chain to produce a mixture of alcohols, and by *N*-hydroxylation. The alcoholic metabolites of pentobarbital are pharmacologically inactive. Approximately 86% of a radioactive dose is excreted in the urine in 6 days, about 1% as unchanged drug and up to 73% as the L- and D-diastereoisomers of 3′-hydroxypentobarbital in a 5.4:1 ratio, and up to 15% as *N-hydroxypentobarbital.* None of these metabolites is eliminated as a conjugate.

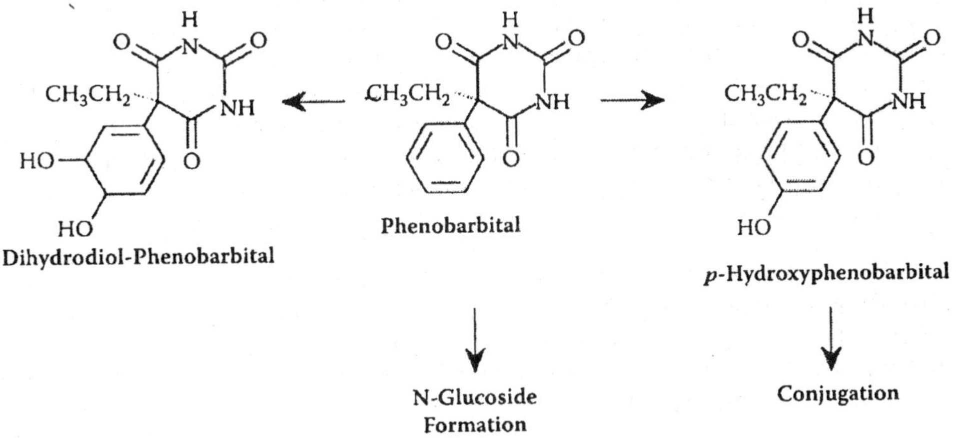

Dihydrodiol-Phenobarbital ← Phenobarbital → *p*-Hydroxyphenobarbital

Phenobarbital ↓ N-Glucoside Formation

p-Hydroxyphenobarbital ↓ Conjugation

Fig. 17.3. Metabolic pathway of phenobarbital.

Amobarbital is extensively metabolized to polar metabolites in a process that is saturable and best described by zero-order kinetics at therapeutic doses. Two major metabolites are produced by hydroxylation and *N*-glycosylation. 3′-Hydroxyamobarbital possesses pharmacological activity. Approximately 92% of a single dose is excreted in the urine with 5% excreted in the feces over a 6-day period. Approximately 2% is excreted unchanged in the urine, 30 to 40% is excreted as free 3′-hydroxyamobarbital, 29% as *N*-glycosylamobarbital, and 5% as the minor metabolite, 3′-carboxy-amobarbital.

Phenobarbital is primarily metabolized via *N*-glycosylation and by oxidation to form *p*-hydroxyphenobarbital followed by conjugation with glucuronic acid. A dihydrohydroxy metabolite has been identified in minor amounts, thought to arise from an epoxide intermediate. Approximately 80% of a single labeled dose is excreted in the urine within 16 days. Unchanged drug accounts for 25 to 33% of the dose, *N*-glucosyl-phenobarbital for 24 to 30%, and free or conjugated *p*-hydroxyphenobarbital for 18 to 19%.[12] When administered chronically, approximately 25% of the dose is excreted unchanged in the 24-h urine with 8% free and 9% conjugated *p*-hydroxyphenobarbital.

BENZODIAZEPINES

The benzodiazepines are among the most commonly encountered prescribed drugs in forensic analysis. It has been estimated that between 10 and 20% of the adult population in the Western world has ingested these drugs within any year. They are prescribed for the treatment of anxiety or panic disorder, and as a sleeping aid, anticonvulsant, or muscle relaxant. Abuse of this family of drugs is observed primarily in two forms: persistent therapeutic use, i.e., use longer than generally recommended; and illicit use, in which the drug is self-administered without physician approval or supervision. The former type of abuse is common and typically involves use at low doses compared to the rarely encountered illicit use that may involve high doses and clear indications of acute intoxication and impairment.

Pharmacology

Benzodiazepines exert central depressant effects on spinal reflexes, in part mediated by the brainstem reticular system. For example, chlordiazepoxide depresses the duration of electrical after-discharge in the limbic system. Most benzodiazepines elevate the seizure threshold and therefore may be used as anticonvulsant medications. Diazepam, clonazepam, and clorazepate may be prescribed for this therapeutic purpose. Benzodiazepines potentiate the inhibitory effects of GABA and neurophysiological studies have identified specific benzodiazepine binding sites in the cerebellum, cerebral cortex, and limbic system. These sites are located in a complex protein macromolecule that includes $GABA_A$ receptors and a chloride channel. Binding of benzodiazepines is modulated by both GABA and chloride. Several benzodiazepine antagonists, such as flumazenil, and inverse agonists (compounds with opposite physiological effects to benzodiazepines), such as ethyl-β-carboline-3-carboxylate, competitively inhibit the binding of benzodiazepines. Benzodiazepines are used as hypnotics because they have the ability to increase total sleep time. They demonstrate minimal cardiovascular effects, but do have the ability to increase heart rate and decrease cardiac output. Most CNS depressants, including the benzodiazepines, exhibit the ability to relax skeletal muscles. Clozapine, a dibenzodiazepine, is used in the treatment of schizophrenia. It has both sedative and antipsychotic actions, and is the only FDA-approved medication indicated for treatment-resistant schizophrenia, and for reducing the risk of suicidal behavior in patients with schizophrenia. This drug can have potentially life-threatening side effects, but appears to have no abuse potential and will not be considered further.

Absorption

The benzodiazepines comprise a large family of lipophilic acids (diazepam pKa = 3.4) with high octanol/water coefficients. They demonstrate a wide range of absorption rates when orally administered. Diazepam is absorbed rapidly, with peak concentrations occurring in 1 h in adults and as rapidly as 15 to 30 min in children. Following a single oral dose of 10 mg, peak blood diazepam concentrations averaged 148 ng/ml at 1 h, declining to 37 ng/ml by 24 h. Bioavailability is dependent on drug formulation and route of administration, with approximately 100% bioavailability of diazepam when administered orally as tablets or in suspension, decreasing to 50 to 60% when administered intramuscularly or as suppositories. The rapid rate of absorption may be explained in part by the lipophilicity of diazepam. In contrast, less lipophilic benzodiazepines, such as lorazepam, exhibit slower rates of absorption, with an average time to peak blood concentration of 2 h. Prazepam and clorazepate act as prodrugs and are decarboxylated in the stomach to nordiazepam. Consequently, absorption is slowed and a delay occurs to the onset of action of these drugs.

Distribution

The benzodiazepines exhibit a two-compartment pharmacokinetic model. Central compartment distribution is rapid and a slower distribution occurs into less perfused tissues, such as adipose. One-compartment pharmacokinetic models have been described for some benzodiazepines, such as lorazepam. It is obvious that the more lipophilic benzodiazepines distribute more rapidly than less lipophilic drugs. Therefore, after a single dose, diazepam, a highly lipophilic drug, will have a shorter duration of action than lorazepam because it will be rapidly redistributed throughout the body. This may not be easily understood when considering the half-life because diazepam has a longer half-life (approximately 30 h) than lorazepam (12 to 15 h). Therefore, a long elimination half-life does not necessarily imply long duration of action after a single dose. The majority of benzodiazepines are highly bound to plasma proteins (85 to 95%) with apparent volumes of distribution ranging from 1 to 3 L/kg due to rapid removal from plasma to brain, lungs, and adipose tissue.

Metabolism and Elimination

The benzodiazepines are extensively metabolized producing multiple metabolites, many of which share common pathways. Metabolic processes include hydroxylation, demethylation, and glucuronidation. Diazepam undergoes *N*-demethylation to an active metabolite, nordiazepam. Both of these compounds are then hydroxylated to temazepam and oxazepam, respectively. These metabolites are also active, but are usually rapidly excreted and do not accumulate in plasma. Only small amounts of diazepam and nordiazepam are detected in urine, with 33% of a dose excreted as oxazepam glucuronide and another 20% excreted as various conjugates. Oxazepam, the 3-hydroxy metabolite of nordiazepam, is rapidly conjugated with glucuronic acid to form an inactive metabolite. This conjugate accounts for

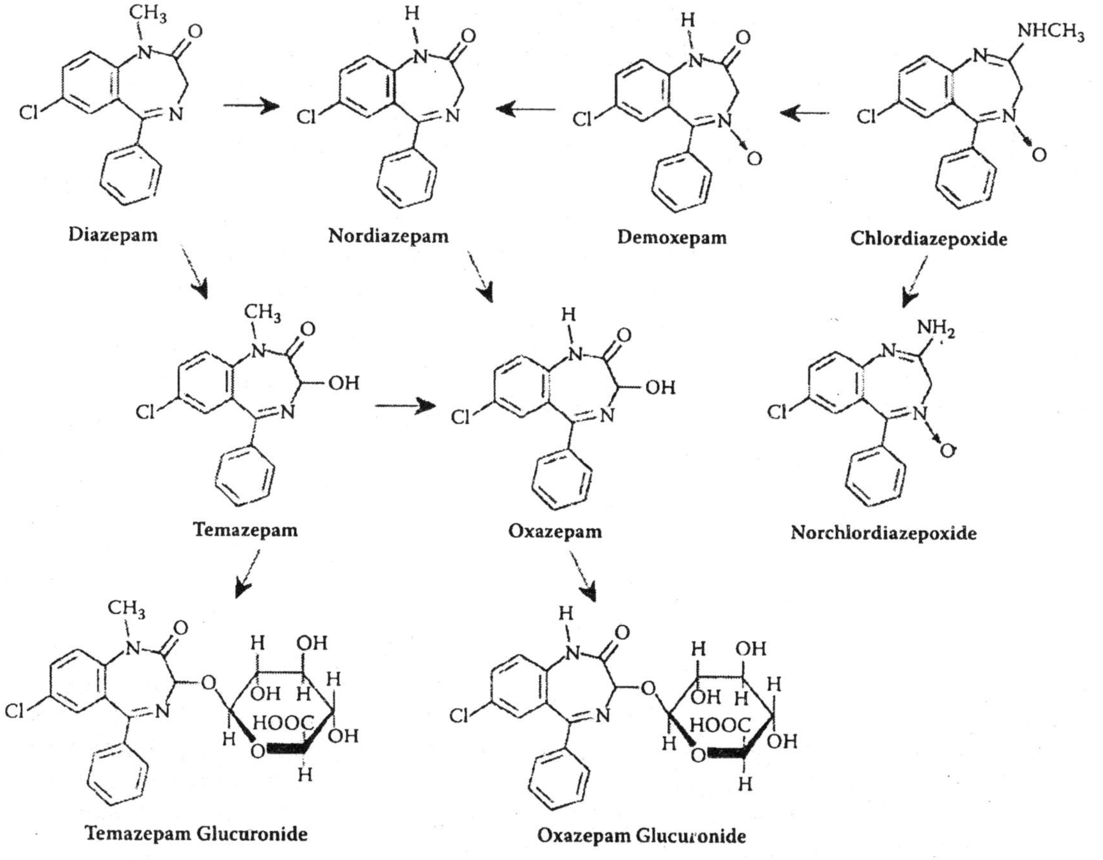

Fig. 17.4. Metabolic pathway of the benzodiazepines.

61% of an oral dose in the 48-h urine. Trace amounts of free drug are detected in the urine and other hydroxylation products account for less than 5% of a dose. Lorazepam is also rapidly conjugated, forming the inactive product, lorazepam glucuronide. This conjugate is not rapidly excreted but may achieve plasma concentrations exceeding the parent drug, with an elimination half-life of approximately 16 h. Approximately 75% of a dose is eliminated in the urine as the conjugate over 5 days. Minor metabolites, such as ring hydroxylation products and quinazoline derivatives, constitute another 14% of the dose. Trace amounts of free drug are found in urine.

Chlordiazepoxide is metabolized to four active metabolites. The drug is *N*-demethylated to norchlordiazepoxide, then deaminated to form demoxepam. These metabolites demonstrate pharmacological activity similar to the parent drug. Demoxepam is reduced to form nordiazepam, which accumulates in plasma with multiple dosing. Nordiazepam is then hydroxylated to produce oxazepam. Less than 1% of the dose is excreted unchanged in the urine with approximately 6% excreted as demoxepam and the rest as glucuronide conjugates. Temazepam undergoes *N*-demethylation to form the active metabolite oxazepam. Both parent and metabolite are subsequently conjugated. An average of 82% of a dose is excreted in urine and 12% in the feces.

Alprazolam, a triazolobenzodiazepine, is also extensively metabolized by oxidation and conjugation. Metabolites include a-hydroxyalprazolam, 4-hydroxyalprazolam, and a,4-dihydroxyalprazolam. The first two metabolites possess approximately 66 and 19% of the pharmacological activity of the parent, respectively. 3-Hydroxy-5-methyltriazolyl, an analogue of chlorobenzophenone, is also formed. Approximately 94% of a dose is excreted within 72 h with 80% excreted in the urine. Flunitrazepam, the *N*-methyl-2′-fluoro analogue of nitrazepam, undergoes biotransformation via *N*-demethylation, 3-hydroxylation, and glucuronidation. In addition, the nitro group is reduced to an amine and is subsequently acetylated. Approximately 84% of a labeled dose is excreted in the urine over 1 week, and 11% is excreted in the feces. Less than 0.5% is excreted unchanged. Norflunitrazepam and 7-aminoflunitrazepam may be detected in plasma for 1 day after a single dose of 2 mg. Triazolam is extensively metabolized by hydroxylation and subsequent conjugation. The major metabolite, 1-hydroxymethyltriazolam, possesses pharmacological activity. Only trace amounts of unchanged drug are excreted in the urine, with approximately 80% of a dose appearing in the urine in 72 h, mainly as glucuronide conjugates.

Since benzodiazepines are metabolized by the cytochrome P450 family of isozymes, potential inhibitors of these may produce significant increases in blood concentrations of benzodiazepines. An example of this inhibition is the drug midazolam, administered as a presurgical anesthetic. Lam et al. reported a mean increase in the area under the curve of midazolam by ketoconazole (772%) and nefazodone (444%) in a group of 40 healthy human subjects administered 200 mg ketoconazole per day and 400 mg nefazodone per day. The authors concluded that caution should be exercised when use of midazolam is warranted with potent CYP3A4 inhibitors.

COCAINE

Cocaine is a naturally occurring alkaloid obtained from the plant *Erythroxylon coca* L. This plant grows in the Andes region of South America, ideally at elevations between 1500 and 5000 ft. A second closely related species has been identified, *Erythroxylon novogranatense* H., and each species has one variety known as *E. coca* var. *ipadu* Plowman and *E. coca novogranatense* var. *truxillense*, respectively. Cocaine may also be chemically synthesized with cold aqueous succinaldehyde and cold aqueous methylamine, methylamine hydrochloride, and the potassium salt of acetone-dicarboxylic acid monomethyl ester. Cocaine is used medically by otorhinolaryngologists and plastic surgeons as an epinephrine cocaine mixture. Solutions for topical application are typically less than 4% cocaine hydrochloride. In the U.S. cocaine is a scheduled drug under the federal Controlled Substances Act of

1970. Refined cocaine, in the form of the base or hydrochloride salt, is self-administered by many routes, including snorting, smoking, genital application, and by injection.

Pharmacology

Cocaine inhibits the presynaptic reuptake of the neurotransmitters norepinehrine, serotonin, and dopamine at synaptic junctions. This results in increased concentrations in the synaptic cleft. Since norepinephrine acts within the sympathetic nervous system, increased sympathetic stimulation is produced. Physiological effects of this stimulation include tachycardia, vasoconstriction, mydriasis, and hyperthermia. CNS stimulation results in increased alertness, diminished appetite, and increased energy. The euphoria or psychological stimulation produced by cocaine is thought to be related to the inhibition of serotonin and dopamine reuptake. Cocaine also acts as a local anesthetic due to its ability to block sodium channels in neuronal cells.

Absorption

Cocaine is rapidly absorbed from mucous membranes and the pulmonary vasculature. However, the rate at which cocaine appears in the blood is dependent on the route of administration. Coca leaves have been chewed by native South Americans for more than 3000 years. Recent studies of the oral route of administration found that chewing powdered coca leaves containing between 17 and 48 mg of cocaine produced peak plasma concentrations of 11 to 149 ng/ml ($n = 6$) at 0.4 to 2 h after administration. In another study, healthy male volunteers were administered cocaine hydrochloride (2 mg/kg) in gelatin capsules. Peak plasma concentrations of 104 to 424 ng/ml were achieved at 50 to 90 min. One of the most common routes of self-administration of cocaine in North America is the intranasal route. Wilkinson et al. found that peak plasma concentrations of cocaine were reached 35 to 90 min after "snorting," but another study using equivalent doses found that peak plasma concentrations were achieved between 120 and 160 min. Intravenous administration of 32-mg cocaine hydrochloride resulted in an average peak plasma concentration of 308 ng/ml at 5 min.

Cocaine may also be self-administered by the smoked route in the form of cocaine base, commonly called "crack," or by a process known as "free-basing" in which powdered cocaine hydrochloride is converted into its base form. In a study of six subjects who each smoked 50 mg of cocaine, the average peak plasma cocaine concentration of 203 ng/ml was achieved at 5 min. The bioavailability of cocaine after smoking depends on several factors including the temperature of volatilization and drug loss in main- and sidestream smoke.

Perez-Reyes et al. estimated that only 32% of a dose of cocaine base placed in a pipe is actually inhaled by the smoker. Cone compared the pharmacokinetics and pharmacodynamics of cocaine by the intravenous, intranasal, and smoked routes of administration in the same subjects. Venous plasma cocaine concentrations peaked within 5 min by the intravenous and smoked routes. Estimated peak cocaine concentrations ranged from 98 to 349 ng/ml and 154 to 345 ng/ml after intravenous administration of 25-mg cocaine hydrochloride and 42-mg cocaine base by the smoked route, respectively. After dosing by the intranasal route (32 mg cocaine hydrochloride) estimated peak plasma cocaine concentrations ranged from 40 to 88 ng/ml after 0.39 to 0.85 h. In this study, the average bioavailability of cocaine was 70.1% by the smoked route and 93.7% by the intranasal route. Jenkins et al. described the correlation between pharmacological effects and plasma cocaine concentrations in seven volunteers after they had smoked 10 to 40 mg cocaine. The mean plasma cocaine concentration 2 min after smoking 40 mg cocaine was 153 ± 107.5 ng/ml. Peak concentrations ranged from 160.8 ± 99.1 ng/ml. Increases in pupil diameter, systolic and diastolic blood pressure, heart rate, and subjective measures of drug effect occurred early after drug administration, with maximum effects observed at 2 min (first measure) for blood pressure and subjective measures, or after a brief delay (at 5 to 10 min post dose) for others, notably heart rate and pupil diameter.

Distribution

After an intravenous dose of radiolabeled cocaine to rats, the highest concentrations were found in the brain, spleen, kidney, and lung after 15 min, with the lowest concentrations in the blood, heart, and muscle. Plasma protein binding in humans is approximately 91% at low concentrations. Cocaine binds to the plasma protein, albumin, and also to α1-acid glycoprotein. The steady- state volume of distribution is large (1.6 to 2.7 L/kg), reflecting extensive extravascular distribution. In 1991 Ambre et al. studied the pharmacokinetics of benzoylecgonine in nine human volunteers. The metabolite is much more polar than the parent and liphophobic, explaining why the measured mean V_d was only 0.71. A two-compartment open linear model has been described for the pharmacokinetic profile of cocaine after intravenous administration. The distribution phase after cocaine administration is rapid and the elimination half-life estimated as 31 to 82 min. Cone fitted data to a two-compartment model with bolus input and first-order elimination for the intravenous and smoked routes. For the intranasal route, data were fitted to a two-compartment model with first-order absorption and first-order elimination. The average elimination half-life ($t_1/2\beta$) was 244 min after intravenous administration, 272 min after smoked administration, and 299 min after intranasal administration.

The disposition of cocaine in nontraditional testing matrices has been described. For example, Lester et al. measured cocaine and benzoylecgonine (BE) concentrations in skin, interstitial fluid (IF), sebum, and stratum corneum in five volunteers after the intravenous 1-h infusion of 1 mg/kg cocaine d5. Peak cocaine concentrations in the skin were achieved at 1.5 h and were undetectable after 6 h. No BE was measured in the skin. Peak cocaine concentrations were achieved at 5 h after administration in the IF and were nondetectable by 24 h. BE was found in the IF. In the sebum peak cocaine concentrations occurred between 3 to 24 h but in the stratum corneum cocaine was detected in only one subject.

Metabolism

In humans, the principal route of metabolism of cocaine is by hydrolysis of the ester linkages. Pseudocholinesterase and liver esterases produce the inactive metabolite, ecgonine methyl ester (EME). The second major metabolite, BE, is formed spontaneously at physiological pH. In addition, there is evidence that BE may be formed enzymatically from cocaine by liver carboxylesterases. *N*-Demethylation of BE produces benzoylnorecgonine. Further metabolism of EME and BE produces ecgonine. Further hydrolysis of cocaine and BE produces minor metabolites, meta- and para-hydroxy-cocaine and -BE. The proportion of each metabolite produced and the activity of the individual metabolites have yet to be completely determined.

Cocaine may be *N*-demethylated by the cytochrome P450 system to produce an active metabolite, norcocaine. Further breakdown produces *N*-hydroxynorcocaine and norcocaine nitroxide. Further metabolism produces a highly reactive free radical that is thought to be responsible for the hepatotoxicity observed in cocaine users.

When cocaine is coadministered with ethanol, cocaethylene (CE) is formed in the liver by transesterification by liver methylesterase. CE may also be formed by fatty acid ethyl synthase. This lipophilic compound crosses the blood–brain barrier and is known to contribute to the psychological effects produced by cocaine. Harris et al. administered deuterium-labeled cocaine (0.3 to 1.2 mg/kg) intravenously 1 h after an oral dose of ethanol (1 g/kg) to ten volunteers. When co-administered with ethanol, 17 ± 6% (mean ± S.D.) of the cocaine was converted to cocaethylene. Ethanol ingestion prior to cocaine administration decreased urine BE levels by 48%. When cocaine is smoked, a pyrolysis product, anhydroecgonine methyl ester (AEME), is formed. Therefore, the presence of this compound indicates exposure to smoked cocaine. The pharmacological and toxicological properties of this compound have not been studied.

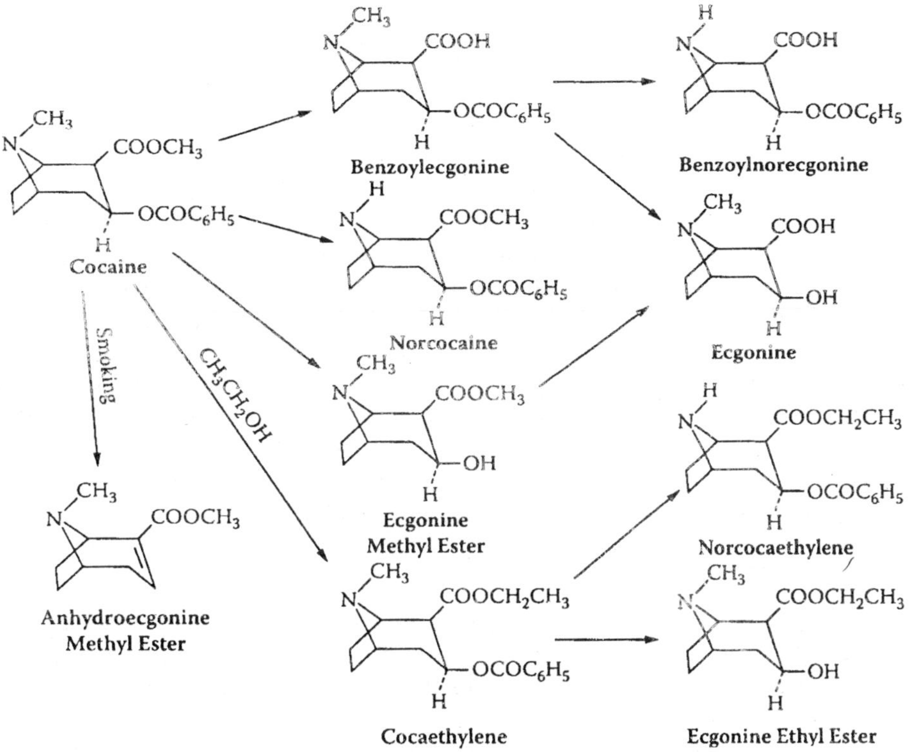

Fig. 17.5. Metabolic pathway of cocaine.

Elimination

Approximately 85 to 90% of a cocaine dose is recovered in the 24-h urine. Unchanged drug accounts for 1 to 9% of the dose depending on urine pH, BE, 35 to 54%, and EME, 32 to 49%. In one study, excretion data were obtained from subjects administered a bolus intravenous injection of cocaine followed by an intravenous infusion, supplying total doses of 253, 444, and 700 mg cocaine. Elimination half-lives averaged 0.8, 4.5, and 3.1 h for cocaine, BE, and EME, respectively. After intranasal application of 1.5 mg/kg, urine cocaine concentrations averaged 6.7 mg/L during the first hour, and BE concentrations peaked between 4 and 8 h at 35 mg/L. Oral ingestion of 25 mg cocaine by a single individual resulted in a peak urine BE concentration of 7.9 mg/L in the 6- to 12-h collection period, with a decline to 0.4 mg/L by 48 h. Oral consumption of coca tea of Peruvian origin containing approximately 4 mg of cocaine resulted in a peak urine BE concentration of 3.9 mg/L after 10 h in one individual. The cumulative urinary excretion of BE after approximately 48 h was 3.1 mg. Consumption of coca tea of Bolivian origin by the same individual, containing a similar amount of cocaine, resulted in a peak urine BE level of 4.9 mg/L at 3.5 h. The cumulative BE excreted in urine was 2.6 mg. The minor metabolites, including the *p*- and *m*-hydroxy metabolites, and also the pyrolysis product, AEME, have been detected in urine after cocaine administration.

Lysergic Acid Diethylamide

Lysergic acid diethylamide (LSD) is an indolealkylamine discovered by Albert Hoffman of Sandoz Laboratories in 1943. It may be synthesized from lysergic acid and diethylamine. Lysergic acid, a naturally occurring ergot alkaloid, is present in grain parasitized by the fungus *Claviceps purpurea*. A closely related alkaloid, lysergic acid amide, is present in morning glory seeds and the Hawaiian baby wood rose. In the 1950s, LSD was used as an aid in the treatment of alcoholism, opioid addiction, psychoneurosis, and sexual disorders, but currently it is classified under Schedule I of the federal Controlled Substances Act with no accepted medical use in the U.S. It is available illicitly as a powder, tablet, or gelatin capsule, or impregnated in sugar cubes, gelatin squares, blotter paper, or postage stamps.

Pharmacology

LSD is a potent centrally acting drug. The D-isomer is pharmacologically active while the L-isomer is apparently inactive. Neuropharmacological studies have shown that LSD exerts a selective inhibitory effect on the brain's raphe system by causing a cessation of the spontaneous firing of serotonin-containing neurons of the dorsal and median raphe nuclei. In this way, LSD acts as an indirect serotonin antagonist. However, inhibition of raphe firing is not sufficient to explain the psychotomimetic effects of LSD because the compound lisuride is a more potent inhibitor of the raphe system yet does not demonstrate hallucinogenic potential in humans. Therefore, other post-synaptic mechanisms such as action on glutamate or serotonin receptors may be involved. Also, there is evidence that LSD indirectly exerts effects on the cytoskeleton by reducing the amount of serotonin released by the raphe system. LSD produces sympathomimetic, parasympathomimetic, and neuromuscular effects, which include mydriasis, lacrimation, tachycardia, and tremor.

Absorption

LSD may be self-administered orally, nasally, or by parenteral ingestion; however, the oral route is the most common. Doses of 50 to 300 μg are ingested, with a minimum effective dose of 20 to 25 μg. Absorption is rapid and complete regardless of the route of administration. However, food in the stomach slows absorption when ingested. Effects are observed within 5 to 10 min, with psychosis evident after 15 to 20 min. Peak effects have been reported 30 to 90 min after dosing; effects decline after 4 to 6 h. The duration of effects may be 8 to 12 h.

Pharmacokinetic studies in humans are limited with much of the data dating from the 1960s. Following intravenous administration of 2 μg/kg, a peak plasma LSD concentration of 5 ng/ml was observed after 1 h. At 8 h, the plasma concentration had declined to 1 ng/ml. In much more recent studies a method using liquid chromatography with electrospray ionization and tandem mass spectrometric detection has been developed and validated for LSD and iso-LSD. Using this technique the lower limit for quantitative determination was 0.02 μg/L for LSD and iso-LSD. Peak plasma levels were slightly higher than earlier reports (case 1 plasma LSD = 0.31 μg/L, iso-LSD = 0.27 μg/L and in a second case LSD = 0.24 μg/L, iso-LSD = 0.6 μg/L in urine).

Distribution

Plasma protein binding of LSD is >80%. As the drug penetrates the CNS, it is concentrated in the visual brain areas and the limbic and reticular activating systems, correlating with perceived effects. LSD is also found in the liver, spleen, and lungs. The volume of distribution is reported to be low at 0.28 L/kg. Wagner et al. described a two-compartment open model for LSD with an elimination half-life of 3 h.

Metabolism and Excretion

LSD metabolism was investigated using MS-MS. Metabolites were determined using MS-MS. The main metabolite was 2-oxo-3-hydroxy-LSD (O-H-LSD) present in urine at concentrations of 2.5 and 6.6 μg/L, respectively, for case 1 and 2, but it was not detected at all in plasma. Nor-LSD was also found in urine at 0.15 and 0.01 μg/L levels. Nor-iso-LSD, lysergic acid ethylamide (LAE), trioxylated-LSD, lysergic acid ethyl-2-hydroxyethylamide (LEO), and 13- and 14-hydroxy-LSD and their glucuronide conjugates were detected in urine using specific MS-MS transitions.

The metabolism and elimination of LSD in humans has received limited study. Animal studies demonstrated extensive biotransformation via *N*-demethylation, *N*-deethylation, and hydroxylation to inactive metabolites. In humans, demethylation and aromatic hydroxylation occur to produce *N*-desmethyl-LSD and 13- and 14-hydroxy-LSD. Hydroxylated metabolites undergo glucuronidation to form water-soluble conjugates. Excretion into the bile accounts for approximately 80% of a dose. Concentrations of unchanged drug ranged from 1 to 55 ng/ml in the 24-h urine after ingestion of 200 to 400 μg LSD in humans. LSD or its metabolites were detectable for 34 to 120 h following a 300-μg oral dose in seven human subjects. The clearance of LSD in humans is unknown.

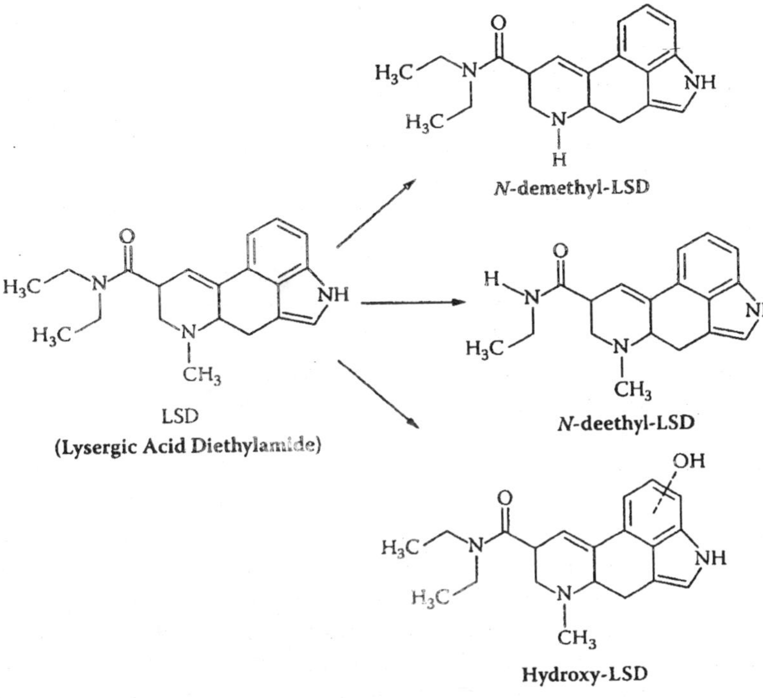

LSD
(Lysergic Acid Diethylamide)

N-demethyl-LSD

N-deethyl-LSD

Hydroxy-LSD

Fig. 17.6. Metabolic pathway of LSD.

Marijuana

The term "marijuana" refers to all parts of the plant *Cannabis sativa* L., whether growing or not: the seeds; resin extracted from any part of such plant; and every compound, salt, derivative, or mixture; but does not include the mature stalks, fiber produced from the stalks, or oil or cake prepared from the seeds. *Cannabis sativa* L. is an annual plant that grows in all parts of the world to a height of 16 to 18 ft. Commercially, it is cultivated for hemp production, with the bulk of the plant consisting of stalks with very little foliage, except at the apex. In contrast, the wild plant and those cultivated illegally possess numerous branches as the psychoactive ingredient is concentrated in the leaves and flowering tops. There may be significant differences in the gross appearance of marijuana plants due to climatic and soil conditions, the closeness of other plants during growth, and the origin of the seed. Marijuana is the crude drug derived from the plant *Cannabis sativa* L., a plant that is currently accepted as belonging to a family (Cannabaceae) that has only one genus (*Cannabis*) with only one species (*sativa*) that is highly variable. In 1980 the total number of natural compounds identified in *C. sativa* L. was 423. By 1995 the number had risen to 483, and recently 6 new compounds, 4 new cannabinoids and 2 new flavonoids, have been described. The major psychoactive constituent of marijuana is delta-9-tetrahydrocannabinol, commonly referred to as THC. Different parts of the plant contain varying concentrations of THC, with leaves containing <1% to 10% THC by weight, and hashish, a resin prepared from the flowering tops, containing approximately 15% THC. THC may be synthesized using citral and olivetol in boron trifluoride and methylene chloride. Although no reports have appeared within the published peer-reviewed literature, persistent reports from the enforcement community suggest that intensive cross-breeding has led to production of plants that have a THC content well over 20%. These "super" plants appear to be grown mainly along the Canadian–American border, primarily by Asian gangs.

Pharmacology

Marijuana is typically self-administered orally or by smoking in doses of 5 to 20 mg. It may produce a variety of pharmacological effects including sedation, euphoria, hallucinations, and temporal distortion. In addition, THC possesses activity at benzodiazepine, opioid, and cannabinoid receptors and also exerts effects on prostaglandin synthesis, DNA, RNA, and protein metabolism. Early workers thought that THC effects were nonspecific, but in the late 1980s a specific cannabinoid receptor was identified in the brains of rats. It is now apparent that there are two types of cannabinoid receptor—CB1 and CB2—and these receptors are the primary targets of endogenous cannabinoids (endocannabinoids). THC binds to both cannabinoid receptors. The CB 1 receptor is mostly found in the brain, while the CB2 receptor is found in immune tissues such as the spleen, thymus, and tonsils but not in the brain. Specific antagonists exist for each of the CB 1 and CB2 receptors.

Cannabinoid-coupled G protein–coupled receptors are involved in the control of many processes, including metabolic regulation, craving, pain, anxiety, bone growth, and immune function. The exogenous cannabinoids found in marijuana plants can also exert effects via G(i/o) proteins, negatively modulating cyclic AMP levels and activating the inward rectifying K(+) channels. Manipulation at either receptor site may have important clinical consequences and therapies based on cannabinoid–receptor interactions are under development. Cannabinoids mediate a decrease in blood pressure and can suppress cardiac contractility in hypertension. Conversely, if the CB1-mediated cardiodepressor and vasodilator effects of anandamide are enhanced (by blocking its hydrolysis), blood pressure tends to normalize. Many clinical developments taking advantage of these properties are likely to occur. By the time of publication of this book, rimonabant (Acompliat), a C1 blocking agent, will have been approved for weight loss by the FDA.

Absorption

Marijuana is commonly self-administered by the smoked route by rolling dried marijuana leaves in tobacco paper and smoking as a cigarette. Smoking results in rapid drug delivery from the lungs to the brain. However, loss of drug occurs during the smoking process due to pyrolysis and sidestream smoke. In an *in vitro* study in which loss due to sidestream smoke was minimized, Perez-Reyes et al. reported a 30% loss of THC due to pyrolysis. Sidestream THC losses of 40 to 50% have been reported. Once THC reaches the lungs, it is rapidly absorbed. Peak plasma THC concentrations of 100 to 200 ng/ml occur after 3 to 8 min and THC is present in blood after the first puff from a marijuana cigarette. Mean ± SD THC concentrations of 7.0 ± 8.1 ng/ml and 18.1 ± 12.0 ng/ml were observed after the first inhalation of low- or high-dose marijuana cigarettes (1.75%, 3.55%), respectively. Peak concentrations occurred at 9 min after the first puff. Lemberger et al. demonstrated that physiological and subjective measures of drug effects occurred simultaneously with the rise in blood THC concentrations.

After oral administration, THC is 90 to 95% absorbed. However, the oral route results in lower peak plasma concentrations at a later time. Wall et al. reported a mean peak plasma THC concentration of 6 ng/ml after ingestion of 20 mg. Wall et al. noted that peak plasma THC concentrations occurred 30 min after intravenous administration of 4 to 5 mg, with a mean concentration (n = 7) of 62 ng/ml. Reported values for the bioavailability of THC after smoking have ranged from 18 to 50%. This wide range reflects the large inter- and intrasubject variability that occurs in smoking dynamics. Altering the number, duration, and spacing of puffs, the length of time the inhalation is held and the inhalation volume or depth of puff may vary the amount of drug delivered. Measures to minimize the loss of side- and mainstream smoke as well as optimizing the temperature for drug volatilization will, in turn, increase the amount of drug available for delivery to the lungs. One facet of smoking that cannot be controlled by the smoker is drug deposition on non- or poorly absorbing surfaces within the body.

Deposition outside of the lungs is usually a function of drug particle or vapor size. Drug may be deposited in the nasopharyngeal region or the upper bronchial tree. This reduces the amount of drug reaching the lung alveoli where rapid absorption into the blood and subsequent transport to the brain occur. Ohlsson et al. compared the bioavailability of THC after intravenous, smoked, and oral administration. Eleven healthy subjects were administered 5 mg intravenously, 19 mg smoked, and 20 mg orally. Plasma concentrations rose rapidly after intravenous administration, reaching 161 to 316 ng/ml at 3 min and declining rapidly thereafter. Peak plasma concentrations also occurred at 3 min after smoking, with lower concentrations of THC ranging from 33 to 118 ng/ml. The plasma concentration time curve after smoking was similar to that obtained after intravenous administration but at lower concentrations. In contrast, low THC concentrations were found after oral administration, with much higher intersubject variability. The authors determined the bioavailability of THC to be 8 to 24% after smoking compared with 4 to 12% after oral ingestion.

Distribution

THC is 97 to 99% plasma protein bound with little present in red blood cells. Due to its lipophilicity, THC distributes rapidly into tissues. Highly perfused organs, such as the brain, accumulate THC rapidly after administration, whereas THC distributes more slowly into poorly perfused tissues such as fat. Harvey et al. reported finding maximum THC concentrations in the brains of mice 30 min after a single intravenous dose. The distribution of THC into various tissues and organs such as brain, liver, heart, kidney, salivary glands, breast milk, fat, and lung is reflected in the large volume of distribution (4 to 14 L/kg). Hunt and Jones proposed a four-compartment model to describe four tissue composites into which THC distributes after intravenous injection. They observed average half-lives of 1 min, 4 min, 1 h, and 19 h to describe these compartments. They concluded that a "*pseudoequilibrium*" is achieved between plasma and tissues 6 h after an intravenous dose. Thereafter, THC is slowly eliminated as THC diffuses from tissue to the blood. The terminal elimination half-life is approximately 1 day but has been reported to be 3 to 13 days in frequent users.

Metabolism and Excretion

Metabolism is the major route of elimination of THC from the body as little is excreted unchanged. In humans, over 20 metabolites have been identified in urine and feces. Metabolism in humans involves allylic oxidation, epoxidation, aliphatic oxidation, decarboxylation, and conjugation. The two

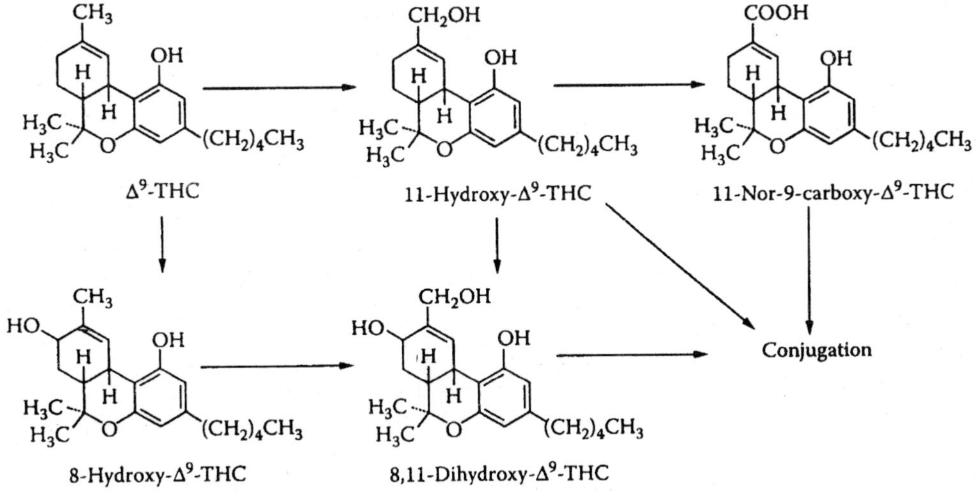

Δ^9-THC → 11-Hydroxy-Δ^9-THC → 11-Nor-9-carboxy-Δ^9-THC

Δ^9-THC → 8-Hydroxy-Δ^9-THC → 8,11-Dihydroxy-Δ^9-THC

11-Hydroxy-Δ^9-THC → 8,11-Dihydroxy-Δ^9-THC

11-Hydroxy-Δ^9-THC, 11-Nor-9-carboxy-Δ^9-THC, 8,11-Dihydroxy-Δ^9-THC → Conjugation

Fig. 17.7. Metabolic pathway of delta-9-THC.

monohydroxy metabolites 11-hydroxy (OH)-THC and 8-beta-hydroxy THC are active, with the former exhibiting similar activity and disposition to THC, while the latter is less potent. Plasma concentrations of 11-OH-THC are typically <10% of the THC concentration after marijuana smoking. Two additional hydroxy compounds have been identified, namely, 8-alpha-hydroxy-THC and 8,11-dihydroxy-THC, and are believed to be devoid of THC-like activity. Oxidation of 11-OH-THC produces the inactive metabolite, 11-nor-9-carboxy-THC, or THC-COOH. This metabolite may be conjugated with glucuronic acid and is excreted in substantial amounts in the urine.

The average plasma clearance is 600 to 980 ml/min with a blood clearance of 1.0 to 1.6 L/min, which is close to hepatic blood flow. This indicates that the rate of metabolism of THC is dependent on hepatic blood flow. Approximately 70% of a dose of THC is excreted in the urine (30%) and feces (40%) within 72 h. Because a significant amount of the metabolites are excreted in the feces, enterohepatic recirculation of THC metabolites may occur. This would also contribute to the slow elimination and hence long plasma half-life of THC. Unchanged THC is present in low amounts in the urine and 1 1-OH-THC accounts for only 2% of a dose.

The remainder of the urinary metabolites consists of conjugates of THC-COOH and unidentified acidic products. Following a single smoked 10-mg dose of THC, urinary THC-COOH concentrations peaked within 16 h of smoking, at levels of 6 to 129 ng/ml ($n = 10$). Huestis et al. reported a mean ($\pm$ SEM) urinary excretion half-life for THC-COOH of 31.5 $\pm$ 1 h and 28.6 $\pm$ 1.5 h for six healthy volunteers after administration of a single marijuana cigarette containing 1.75 or 3.55% THC, respectively. Passive exposure to marijuana smoke may also produce detectable urinary metabolite concentrations. Cone et al. exposed five volunteers to the smoke of 16 marijuana cigarettes (2.8% THC content) for 1 h each day for 6 consecutive days. After the first session, THC-COOH concentrations in urine ranged from 0 to 39 ng/ml. A maximum THC-COOH concentration of 87 ng/ml was detected in one subject on day 4 of the study.

THC may be ingested orally by consuming food products containing the seeds or oil of the hemp plant. Ingestion of 0.6 mg/day (equivalent to 125 ml hemp oil containing 5 μg/g of THC or 300 g hulled seeds at 2 μg/g) for 10 days resulted in urine THC-COOH concentrations of <6 ng/ml. The maximum urinary concentration of THC-COOH in another study after ingestion of hemp oil containing 0.39 to 0.47 mg THC/day for 5 days was 5.4 to 38.2 ng/ml ($n = 7$). After oral administration of a higher dose (7.5 and 14.8 mg THC/day) peak concentrations of THC-COOH ranged from 19.0 to 436 ng/ml. Controlled studies have shown that at the federally mandated cannabinoid cutoffs, it is possible but unlikely for a urine specimen to test positive after ingestion of manufacturer- recommended doses of low-THC hemp oils. On the other hand, patients taking Marinol, the synthetic form of THC approved by the FDA for the control of nausea and vomiting in cancer patients, will almost certainly test positive. Dronabinol or synthetic THC is present in Marinol capsules and ElSohly et al. found that within 24 h of administering a single 15-mg dose of dronabinol to four subjects, peak urine THC-COOH concentrations were between 189 and 362 ng/ml.

Opioids

Members of the group of natural, semisynthetic, or synthetic alkaloid compounds prepared from opium are referred to as "opioids." This group includes natural compounds usually denoted "opiates," such as morphine and codeine, and the synthetic and semisynthetic compounds such as oxycodone, buprenorphine, fentanyl, methadone, and tramadol. The pharmacological effects and pharmacokinetic parameters of these drugs share many common characteristics and are illustrated with the prototypic drug in this class, morphine.

Morphine is obtained from the latex of the opium poppy, *Papaver somniferum*. Morphine, codeine, and other opiates are extracted from a milky exudate that forms within 12 h when unripe seed capsules are incised. When dried, the material is called raw opium. The principal alkaloid in raw opium is morphine, constituting 8 to 19% of opium by dry weight. The actual percentage is highly dependent on growing conditions and location. Morphine is the analgesic of choice for the treatment of both chronic pain syndromes and acute myocardial infarction. Whether it will remain so for long is not clear. The results of recently published observational studies strongly suggest that in patients with acute coronary syndrome, the use of morphine, either alone or in combination with nitroglycerin, is associated with an increased mortality rate.

Morphine remains the prototypic mu-opioid analgesic. And, even though other opioids share similar structures, there is overwhelming proof that morphine is different from other similarly appearing agents. In the past, these differences had been explained by different pharmacokinetics, but now it appears that heroin and morphine act via different receptor mechanisms. As a result, the concept of multiple mu receptors has emerged. Multiple splice variants of the cloned mu-opioid receptor have been identified. Nonetheless, a relatively large volume of pharmacokinetic data exists describing morphine clinical applications, which are reviewed here. It is becoming increasingly obvious that knowledge of the molecular mechanisms involved in causing drug dependence and in providing pain relief is mandatory if there are to be clinical advances.

Morphine

Pharmacology

Morphine and other related opioids produce their pharmacological effects by binding to opiate receptors located throughout the body. Three types of opiate receptors μ (mu), κ (kappa), and δ (delta) — are recognized; they are approximately 70% homologous. Differences between receptors occur mainly at the N- and C-terminal ends. The mu receptor is thought to be the most important because it is where morphine (and like drugs) exerts its effect. When a mu receptor binds with an agonist, such as morphine, heroin, or oxycodone, a G protein attached to the third intracellular loop of the receptor is activated (opiate receptors have seven loops, also called transmembrane domains). The genes that determine the various receptor subtypes are located on different chromosomes. There are two mu, three kappa, and two delta subtypes. It is assumed that these receptors arise from post-translational modifications (i.e., they arise at a late stage in protein synthesis) because their genes have not been identified. A purported fourth opiate receptor, referred to as the sigma receptor, is now recognized as a completely unrelated entity.

Mu receptors are almost always located proximally, on the presynaptic side of the synapse. The periaqueductal gray is the region containing the most mu receptors, but they are also found in the superficial dorsal horn of the spinal cord, the external plexiform layer of the olfactory bulb, the nucleus accumbens (an area deeply implicated in the process of addiction), in some parts of the cerebral cortex, and in some of the nuclei of the amygdala. Mu receptors avidly bind enkephalins and beta-endorphin, but they have a low affinity for dynorphins (primarily a kappa receptor agonist).

The obvious clinical effects of morphine are papillary constriction due to its excitatory action on the parasympathetic nerves that supply the pupil. Respiratory depression also occurs because mu agonists exert a direct effect on brain stem respiratory centers, reducing their responsiveness to carbon dioxide. In addition, mu-stimulation depresses respiratory centers located in the pons. Small doses of morphine merely depress the respiratory rate, while large doses cause respiratory arrest, the accepted mechanism of death in cases of narcotic drug overdose. Nausea and vomiting are also associated with the use of mu receptor activation because opioids directly stimulate the chemoreceptor vomiting trigger zone in the medulla. Morphine provides effective and convenient pain relief, largely because there is no upper limit to the amount that can be given, provided enough time is allowed for tolerance to the respiratory effects to develop. Morphine, or compounds that bind the mu receptor, are also used to treat diarrhea and the cough associated with malignancy and tuberculosis. Heroin, which is converted to morphine within the body, was originally marketed by Bayer as a cough suppressant.

Activation of kappa receptors also produces analgesia, but it simultaneously induces nausea and dysphoria. Kappa receptors are located mainly on pain neurons located in the spinal cord and, to a lesser extent in the brain. They bind to an endogenously occurring ligand called dynorphin. The exact function of dynorphin is unknown, but evidence suggests that it is produced to counter the pleasurable effects of produced by cocaine and is, to some degree, neuroprotective. Some believe dynorphin may play an important role in determining an individual's risk for addiction. Blocking the actions of dynorphin helps to alleviate depression.

Delta receptor activation also produces analgesia, but it can also cause seizures as well. Delta receptors normally bind to a class of endogenous ligands known as enkephalins, but unlike mu receptors, information about delta receptors is limited. Enkephalins are peptides that are produced by the pituitary gland. Several different enkephalins have been identified. β-Enkephalin resembles opiates because when it binds to a delta receptor, it relieves pain.

Absorption

Morphine can be given orally, or by subcutaneous, intramuscular, or intravenous injection. Increasingly, as the purity of street heroin has risen, heroin is also being inhaled ("chasing the dragon"). Heroin is also administered epidurally, either as an individual dose or continuous infusion. Parenteral morphine is well absorbed, and in individuals with normal blood pressure, resultant plasma levels after subcutaneous, intramuscular, and intravenous injection are very similar. The oral bioavailability of morphine is quite low due to extensive first pass hepatic metabolism. A 10-mg bolus given to healthy volunteers undergoing elective surgery produced peak blood of 200 to 400 ng/ml 5 min after injection. After either intramuscular or subcutaneous injection, morphine plasma levels peak in 10 to 20 min. In healthy volunteers a dose of 10 mg/70 kg given intravenously produces a free morphine concentration of 80 ng/ml at 5 min, compared to a peak of 74 ng/ml at 15 min after the same dose was given as an intravenous bolus. Oral administration is a mainstay in the management of patients with cancer. In stable patients receiving sufficient oral morphine to produce acceptable analgesia, the mean trough serum morphine concentration is on the order of 18 ng/ml with roughly equal concentrations of the active metabolite M6G.

Distribution

The volume of distribution of morphine ranges from 2 to 5 L/kg in humans, although values as high as 7 L/kg have been reported. The wide variation could be explained by the health of the volunteers being studied. In patients with incompletely compensated heart failure and increased body water from any cause, higher values would be expected. Conversely, in patients with renal failure, where intravascular volume may be decreased, smaller values would be expected. Plasma protein binding of morphine in healthy humans ranges from 12 to 35% and appears to be independent of concentration over approximately a 1000-fold range, although a slight decrease (24 to 20% bound) was observed when the concentration was increased therapeutically by 60-fold. Morphine is bound mainly to albumin with approximately 5% bound to γ-globulin and 5% to α-1-acid glycoprotein. In healthy humans, the blood/plasma concentration ratio for morphine averages 1.02. This ratio was found to be consistent in the concentration range of 35 to 140 n*M*. The plasma half-life averaged 1.8 and 2.9 h in female and male surgical patients, respectively.

Morphine is relatively hydrophilic and therefore distributes slowly into tissues, where it may be detected in fat, even after death. Morphine crosses the blood–brain barrier, but not so freely as heroin and codeine, which possess an aromatic hydroxyl group at the C3 position. Morphine's passage across the blood–brain barrier is mediated by P-glycoprotein (P-gp) concentrated in brain capillary endothelium.

Drugs that interfere with P-gp, such as doxyrubrin, can alter brain morphine uptake and disposition. Lopermide, which is widely used to treat diarrheal disease, avidly binds the mu receptor but, because it does not bind to P-gp, it never enters the brain and never causes any of the psychological changes produced by morphine.

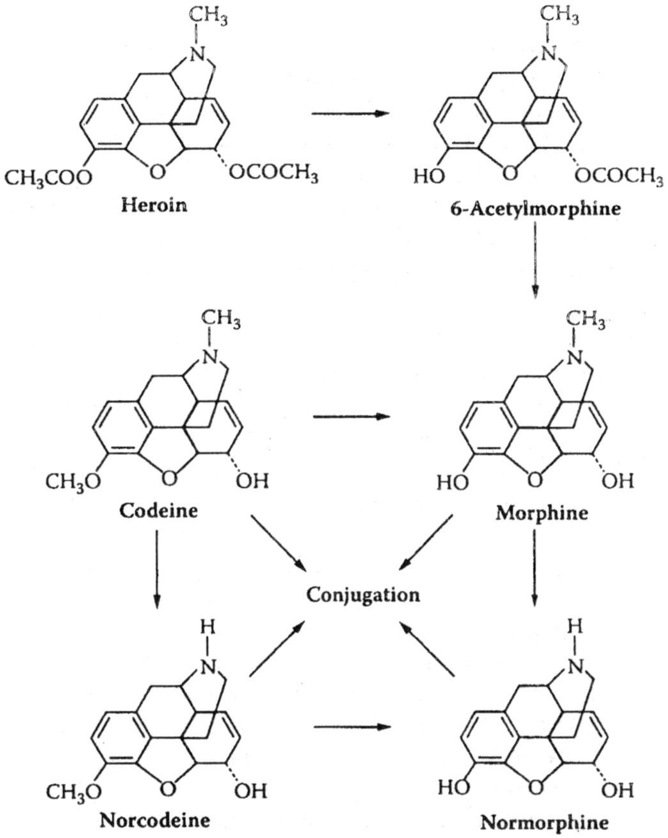

Metabolism and excretion

The major pathway for morphine metabolism is conjugation with glucuronic acid. The free phenolic hydroxyl group undergoes glucuronidation to produce morphine-3-glucuronide (M3G), a highly water-soluble metabolite. Metabolism occurs primarily in the liver with 90% of a dose excreted in the urine and 10% in the feces. There is extensive enterohepatic circulation of both conjugated and unconjugated morphine. Approximately 87% of a dose of morphine is excreted in the 72-h urine, 75% as M3G, 10% as free morphine, and the remainder as morphine-6-glucuronide, morphine-3-sulfate, normorphine, and conjugates. The clearance of morphine was found to vary between 1.2 and 1.9 L/min/70 kg in several studies of humans. M3G is the predominant metabolite in young children. The total body morphine clearance is 80% of an adult at 6 months of age. When the brains of experimental animals are directly injected with M3G, neuroexcitatory and anti-analgesic responses result, although this does not happen after system administration. Nonetheless, small amounts of M3G do cross the blood–brain barrier, and this may account for some reports of neuroexcitatory responses to morphine in humans. Attempts at correlating M3G plasma concentrations or M3G:morphine or M3G:M6G concentration ratios with the clinical activity of M3G have sometimes been successful, and sometimes not. To date, there are only two published studies describing the effects of injecting M3G directly into humans; both studies yielded equivocal results.

Fig. 17.8. Metabolic pathway of heroin and morphine.

M6G, on the other hand, is pharmacologically active and exerts important clinical opioid effects, especially when it is allowed to accumulate in the plasma of patients who have renal failure. However, after short-term morphine administration, the contribution of M6G to both analgesia and the occurrence of side effects is probably negligible. M6G may have peripheral analgesic effects. In a placebo-controlled, double blind, crossover study in ten healthy volunteers, M6G was given intravenously as a bolus followed by an infusion sufficient to maintain plasma concentrations of 500 ng/ml for 2 h. Analgesia was produced, but miotic effects were not, suggesting that the pain relief was a consequence of some peripheral effect exerted by M6G. A small amount of morphine, on the order of 5%, is *N*-demethylated by hepatic CYP3A4, and to a lesser extent CYP2C8, to form normorphine. This metabolite itself has pharmacological activity, but it is less potent than morphine and is present in lower concentrations.

Heroin

C.R. Wright first synthesized heroin, or 3,6-diacetylmorphine, from morphine in 1874. The Bayer Company of Germany advertised heroin as an antitussive in 1898. Under U.S. law (but not the laws of many other countries) heroin has no accepted medical use; it is classified as a Schedule I drug under the Controlled Substances Act of 1970.

Heroin is typically self-administered by intramuscular or intravenous injection and also by nasal insufflation ("*snorting*") or smoking. Peak heroin concentrations in blood are achieved within 1 to 5 min after intravenous and smoked administration and within 5 min after intranasal and intramuscular administration. In a study in which the method of smoked heroin delivery was optimized to reduce losses due to pyrolysis and sidestream smoke, Jenkins et al. reported similar pharmacokinetic profiles for the smoked and intravenous routes. Mean elimination half-lives for two subjects across three doses of heroin were 3.3 and 3.6 min, after smoked and intravenous administration, respectively. The mean residence time of heroin was less than 10 min after all doses by both routes. Cone et al. reported that the pharmacokinetic profile of intranasal heroin was equivalent to that for the intramuscular route. Mean elimination half-lives (hours plus or minus SD) were determined to be 0.09 ± 0.05, 0.07 ± 0.02, and 0.13 ± 0.07, following intranasal administration of 6 and 12 mg, and intramuscular administration of 6 mg of heroin, respectively. The relative potency of intranasal heroin was estimated to be approximately one half that of intramuscular administration.

Heroin may also be administered orally. In drug users this is an uncommon route since hydrolysis in the GI tract and loss due to first pass metabolism result in slow and inefficient delivery to the brain. Following low dose administration of 10 mg heroin hydrochloride, no heroin or 6-acetylmorphine was detected in blood. Peak morphine concentrations ranging from 2 to 15 ng/ml (mean = 8 ng/ml, $n = 6$) were achieved 7.5 min to 4 h after drug administration. In another study, 400 mg of heroin was orally administered, followed 359 min later by a second dose of 400 mg. In this study as well, heroin and 6-acetylmorphine were not detected in blood. Morphine and its conjugates were detected. Peak morphine concentrations were measured 1 to 2 h after the initial dose and were 0.73 and 1.34 mg/L in the two subjects. Girardin et al. administered heroin by three different routes to eight heroin addicts. The intramuscular route demonstrated linear pharmacokinetics for heroin and the metabolites 6-acetylmorphine (6-AM) and morphine. The oral route resulted in low blood concentrations of heroin and 6-AM but linear kinetics for morphine and its glucuronides.

It is known from *in vitro* studies that heroin is rapidly deacetylated to an active metabolite, 6-AM, which is then hydrolyzed to morphine. Spontaneous hydrolysis to 6-AM may occur under various conditions. Heroin is susceptible to base-catalyzed hydrolysis but will also hydrolyze in the presence of protic compounds such as ethanol, methanol, and aqueous media.

The addition of two acetyl-ester groups to the morphine molecule produces a more lipophilic compound. Experimental evidence suggests that heroin and morphine may exert their effects via different receptor mechanisms. Following intravenous infusion of 70 mg of heroin to human volunteers, 45% of the dose was recovered in urine after 40 h. More than 38% was recovered as conjugated morphine, approximately 4% as free morphine, 1% as 6-acetylmorphine, and 0.1% as heroin. Urinary elimination half-lives of 0.6, 4.4, and 7.9 h were reported for 6-AM, morphine, and conjugated morphine, respectively, after administration of 6 mg of heroin by the intramuscular route.

Methadone

Methadone is a synthetic opioid, clinically available in the U.S. since 1947. It exists in the dextro- and levo-rotatory forms with the levo-isoform possessing approximately 8 to 50 times more pharmacological activity. Methadone acts on the CNS and cardiovascular system producing respiratory and circulatory depression. Methadone also produces miosis and increases the tone of smooth muscle in the lower gastrointestinal tract while decreasing the amplitude of contractions. It is used clinically for the treatment of severe pain and in maintenance programs for morphine and heroin addicts.

Methadone is typically administered orally, with peak blood concentrations occurring after 4 h. Inturrisi and Verebely reported a peak plasma concentration of 75 ng/ml at 4 h after a single 15-mg oral dose. Concentrations declined slowly, with a half-life of 15 h, reaching 30 ng/ml by 24 h. A single 10-mg intravenous dose of methadone resulted in initial plasma concentrations of 500 ng/ml declining to 50 ng/ml after 1 to 2 h. Peak plasma concentrations (mean = 830 ng/ml) after 4 h were also observed with chronic oral administration of 100 to 200 mg/day. Concentrations of methadone reach a maximum in brain tissue approximately 1 to 2 h after an oral dose. Methadone is highly plasma protein bound (87%) with 70% bound to albumin. Methadone distributes rapidly to tissues, especially the lungs, liver, kidneys, and spleen. The volume of distribution is 4 to 5 L/kg.

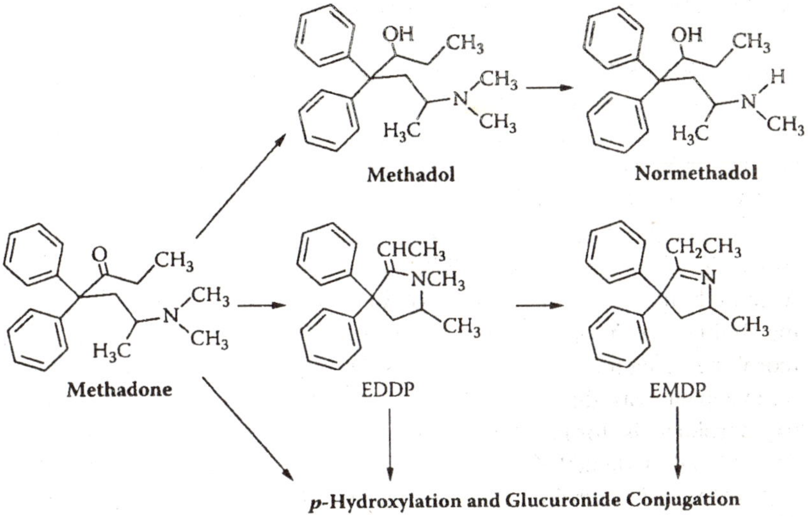

Fig. 17.9. Metabolic pathway of methadone.

Methadone is metabolized in the liver by *N*-demethylation to produce unstable metabolites, which undergo cyclization to form the metabolites 2-ethylidene- 1 ,5-dimethyl-3,3-diphenylpyrrolidine (EDDP) and 2-ethyl-5-methyl-3,3-diphenylpyrroline (EMDP). These metabolites and the parent drug undergo para-hydroxylation with subsequent conjugation with glucuronic acid. All three are excreted in the bile and are the major excretory products measured in the urine after methadone administration. Minor metabolites, methadol, and normethadol exhibit pharmacological activity similar to methadone but are produced in low concentrations. Metabolism to EDDP is achieved by multiple cytochrome P450 isoforms, namely, CYP2B6, 2C19, and 3A4. Michaelis–Menten data demonstrated that the highest V_{max} and lowest K_m occurred with CYP2B6. CYP2B6 and 2C19 showed stereoselective metabolism, with the former preferentially metabolizing *S*-methadone and the latter the R-enantiomer. Shiran et al. reported that methadone appears to inhibit CYP2D6 activity.

Large individual variations in the urine excretion of methadone are observed depending on urine volume and pH, the dose and rate of metabolism. Acidification of the urine may increase the urinary output of methadone from 5 to 22%. Typically, following a 5-mg oral dose, methadone and EDDP account for 5% of the dose in the 24-h urine. In those individuals on maintenance therapy, methadone may account for 5 to 50% of the dose in the 24-h urine and EDDP may account for 3 to 25% of the dose. (S)- and (R)-methadone and EDDP have been reported in saliva and methadone and (S)- and (R)-methadone in human breast milk.

Oxycodone

Oxycodone is a semisynthetic opioid derived from thebaine and used for oral pain relief. It is commonly formulated as an immediate-release medication with acetaminophen or aspirin. A controlled-release oxycodone formulation is used for the treatment of moderate to severe pain; it provides controlled drug delivery over 12 h. The oral bioavailability of this formulation is 60 to 87%. The results of clinical studies of patients with postoperative and cancer pain show that oxycodone has a potency 1.5 times that of morphine.

The absorption half-life of the immediate-release oral formulation is 0.4 h in healthy adults. In contrast the controlled-release form exhibits a biphasic absorption pattern with two apparent half- lives of 0.6 and 6.9 h. Peak plasma concentrations are achieved in approximately 1.6 h with the immediate release compared with 2 to 3 h with the controlled-release formulation. After a 10-mg oral dose of the immediate release formulation, peak plasma concentrations ranged from 13 to 46 ng/ml (mean = 30 ng/ml, n = 12). After the administration of 20 mg of the prolonged-release formulation the peak plasma concentration averaged 23 ng/ml in a group of 28 adults. The plasma half-life has been reported to be 4 to 6 h with a volume of distribution of 1.8 to 3.7 L/kg.

Oxycodone is metabolized in the liver by the cytochrome P450 isozymes and the elimination half-life is prolonged in individuals with liver disease, such as cirrhosis. Metabolism by *O*- and *N*-demethylation produces the metabolites oxymorphone and noroxycodone. The *O*-demethylated metabolite, oxymorphone, is a very powerful μ receptor agonist, providing ten times the relief of morphine in patients with cancer, and at one time it was believed that most of oxycodone's ability to relieve pain was due to oxymorphone formation. However, recent studies have shown that so little oxymorphone is formed that it cannot account for the relief afforded by the parent compound. Both the *O*- and *N*-demethylated forms are then conjugated with glucuronic acid. CYP2D6 metabolizes oxycodone and is encoded by a polymorphic gene with three mutations (*3, *4, and *5) with a combined 95% allelic frequency and approximately 10% prevalence. Less than 65% of a single dose is excreted in the urine over a period of 24 h with 13 to 19% comprising free oxycodone.

Hydrocodone

Hydrocodone is a semisynthetic opioid derived from codeine. It is utilized as an analgesic and antitussive available for oral administration, often in combination with acetaminophen or ibuprofen. As a rule, potent analgesics containing a methoxyl group at position 3 (e.g., hydrocodone, K_i = 19.8 n*M*) bind the mu receptor relatively weakly, but their *O*-demethylated metabolites (such as hydromorphone, K_i = 0.6 n*M*) bind more strangely. As with oxycodone, the possibility exists that some of their ability to relieve pain may actually derive from their active metabolites.

Hydrocodone has multiple actions, mainly involving the CNS and smooth muscle. Peak serum concentrations after single therapeutic doses are typically less than 30 ng/ml and occur within 1.5 h after drug administration. The plasma half-life has been reported to range from 3.4 to 8.8 h with a volume of distribution of 3.3 to 4.7 L/kg. In humans, hydrocodone is metabolized by *O*-demethylation (by the action of CYP2D6) and *N*-demethylation (by the action of CYP3A4) and also reduction of the 6-keto groups. This produces multiple metabolites including hydromorphone, norhydrocodone, hydrocodol, and hydromorphol. The last two metabolites exist as stereoisomers (6-alpha-hydrocodol is also known as dihydrocodeine). Hydromorphone and hydromorphol are then conjugated to form glucuronides. The unconjugated metabolites are believed to exhibit pharmacological activity and, therefore, may contribute to the actions of the drug. Hydrocodone is principally excreted by the kidneys. Approximately 26% of the drug from a single dose is eliminated in the 72-h urine, with less than 15% as unchanged drug.

Fentanyl

Fentanyl is a fast-acting potent synthetic opioid introduced in the U.S. in the early 1960s for use as an anesthetic supplement. It interacts with the opioid mu receptors located in the brain, spinal cord, and smooth muscle. Fentanyl is highly lipophilic and, therefore, crosses the blood–brain barrier rapidly.

Therapeutic use involves the CNS, producing pharmacological actions as pain relief and sedation. In addition to its use as an anesthetic agent, fentanyl is prescribed clinically to treat chronic pain. It is available in an oral transmucosal solid formulation and also as a transdermal delivery system (patches). In opioid nontolerant individuals effective analgesia occurs at blood concentrations of 1 to 2 ng/ml. Surgical anesthesia occurs at concentrations of 10 to 20 ng/ml.

The transmucosal formulation of fentanyl is designed to be dissolved slowly in the mouth, permitting absorption through the buccal mucosa, and a more prolonged absorption, after swallowing, in the GI tract. Bioavailability is dependent on the fraction of the dose absorbed by both routes. Typically 25% of the dose is rapidly absorbed through the buccal mucosa and approximately 33% of the remaining dose, which is swallowed, becomes systemically available. The time to reach peak blood concentrations after this form of drug delivery is generally 20 to 40 min after drug administration.

The transdermal system provides continuous systemic delivery of fentanyl for 72 h. The amount of drug released from the system per hour is proportional to the surface area. Following application of the patch to the skin, a depot of fentanyl concentrates in the upper skin layers. This is then available to the systemic circulation. There is an initial rise in blood fentanyl concentration after application followed by a leveling off that occurs 12 to 24 h later. Peak blood concentrations occur between 24 and 72 h after application. The skin does not appear to metabolize fentanyl when delivered transdermally.

Fentanyl is highly lipophilic. It is rapidly distributed to tissues such as the brain, heart, kidneys, and lungs, followed by slower movement into muscle and fat.

Fentanyl is approximately 80% bound to plasma proteins, principally α-1-acid glycoprotein. The volume of distribution reportedly ranges from 3 to 8 L/kg. The plasma half-life is 3 to 12 h. Fentanyl is metabolized in the liver and intestinal mucosa by cytochrome P450 3A4 isozyme by *N*-dealkylation to form the pharmacologically inactive metabolite norfentanyl. Hydroxylated inactive metabolites include hydroxyfentanyl and hydroxynorfentanyl. Fentanyl is primarily excreted in the urine with up to 85% of a single dose eliminated in 3 to 4 days. Norfentanyl is the principal compound detected in urine comprising 26 to 55% of a single dose.

Buprenorphine

Buprenorphine is derived from thebaine. It is a partial mu agonist with kappa antagonist activity. Buprenorphine has 25 to 50 times the potency of morphine. It is used to produce a longer-lasting analgesia than morphine. Effects of buprenorphine last longer because it is released more slowly from mu receptors than morphine. It is available as an injectable for intramuscular (IM) or intravenous administration in a 1-ml solution containing 0.3 mg buprenorphine (as buprenorphine HCl) for the relief of moderate to severe pain. It is also available to treat opioid dependence in the formulation of a tablet, alone or in combination with naloxone, in 2- or 8-mg doses to be administered sublingually (SL). The recommended sublingual daily dose is 12 to 16 mg/day.

Pharmacological effects occur within 15 min of IM administration, peaking at approximately 1 h and persisting for up to 6 h. After SL administration, peak pharmacological effects typically occur after 100 min. After an intravenous dose of 0.3 mg, plasma concentrations are typically less than 1 ng/ml. Sublingual maintenance therapy of 8 mg/day resulted in plasma buprenorphine concentrations of 1 to 8 ng/ml.

The bioavailability of the buprenorphine/naloxone tablet appears to be greater than the buprenorphine-alone formulation, with the former similar to the drug in liquid form. Buprenorphine is approximately 96% plasma protein bound, primarily to α- and β-globulin. The plasma half-life is 2 to 4 h with a volume of distribution of 2.5 L/kg. The drug undergoes *N*-dealkylation by CYP3A4 isozyme to norbuprenorphine, a pharmacologically active metabolite. This metabolite and parent are subject to glucuronidation. Buprenorphine is eliminated primarily in the feces as free drug with low concentrations occurring in the urine.

Tramadol

Tramadol has about one tenth the pain-relieving ability of morphine. There are two enantiomers, and both contribute to pain relief, but via different mechanisms. (+)-Tramadol and the metabolite (+)-*O*-desmethyl-tramadol, which is referred to as M1, are agonists of the mu opioid receptor. (+)-Tramadol inhibits serotonin reuptake and (–)-tramadol inhibits norepinephrine reuptake. This latter action enhances the inhibitory effects on pain transmission in the spinal cord. Because the actions of the two enantiomers are complementary, they are usually supplied as a racemic mixture. However, because it is a serotonin-reuptake blocker, interaction with other medications can lead to the occurrence of serotonin syndrome.

Tramadol is available as drops, capsules, and sustained-release formulations for oral use, suppositories for rectal use, and solution for intramuscular, intravenous, and subcutaneous injection. After oral administration, tramadol is rapidly and almost completely absorbed. Sustained-release tablets release the active ingredient over a period of 12 h, reach peak concentrations after 4.9 h, and have a bioavailability of 87 to 95% compared with capsules. One 100-mg dose given to healthy volunteers resulted in plasma levels of 375 ng/ml at 1.5 h. Tramadol is 20% bound to plasma protein and it is rapidly distributed in the body; it is mainly metabolized by *O*- and *N*-demethylation forming glucuronides and sulfates that are excreted by the kidney.

The mean elimination half-life is about 6 h. The *O*-demethylation of tramadol to M1, the main analgesic effective metabolite, is catalyzed by cytochrome P450 (CYP) 2D6, whereas *N*-demethylation to M2 is catalyzed by CYP2B6 and CYP3A4. The wide variability in the pharmacokinetic properties of tramadol can partly be ascribed to CYP polymorphism. *O*- and *N*-demethylation of tramadol as well as renal elimination are stereoselective.

Pharmacokinetic–pharmacodynamic characterization of tramadol is difficult because of differences between tramadol concentrations in plasma and at the site of action, and because of pharmacodynamic interactions between the two enantiomers of tramadol and its active metabolites.

Hydromorphone

Sold as Dilaudid in the U.S., hydromorphone is a semisynthetic, differing from morphine only by presence of a 6-keto group, and the hydrogenation of the double bond at the 7–8 position of the molecule. Like morphine, it acts primarily at the mu opioid receptors, and to a lesser degree at delta receptors.

As a hydrogenated ketone of morphine, it shares common pharmacologic properties with other opioid analgesics. These include the expected changes in the CNS, including increased cerebrospinal fluid pressure, increased biliary pressure, and increased parasympathetic activity. It can also produce transient hyperglycemia. It is generally viewed as a second tier analgesic and is not that widely prescribed.

Hydromorphone is well absorbed from the small intestine and is extensively metabolized in the liver, mainly to 3-glucuronide, which, like morphine, is devoid of analgesic effect but can cause significant neuroexcitation. It undergoes extensive first pass metabolism (62%), accounting for its relatively low bioavailability. A single 8-mg dose of hydromorphone yields blood concentrations of approximately 2 ng/ml, while a 12-mg time-release formulation gives plasma concentrations half as high.

Depending on the country where the drug is manufactured, a number of different time-release preparations are available. Palladone, a controlled-release preparation consisting of hydromorphone HCl pellets, was withdrawn from the U.S. market in 2005. When taken with alcohol the pellets rapidly released their contents leading to dangerously elevated peak plasma concentrations. Interaction with ethanol and "*dose dumping*" is not the only concern. Any CNS depressant may enhance the depressant effects of hydromorphone.

PHENCYCLIDINE

Phencyclidine, PCP, or 1-(1-phenylcyclohexyl) piperidine, is an arylcyclohexamine with structural similarities to ketamine. It is a lipophilic weak base with a pKa of 8.5. Phencyclidine was originally synthesized and marketed under the trade name Sernyl by Parke-Davis for use as an intravenously administered anesthetic agent in humans. Distribution began in 1963 but was discontinued in 1965 due to a high incidence (10 to 20%) of post-operative delirium and psychoses. However, its use continued as a veterinary tranquilizer for large animals until 1978, when all manufacture was prohibited and PCP was placed in Schedule II of the federal Controlled Substances Act (1970).

Illicit use of PCP as a hallucinogenic agent was first reported in San Francisco in 1967. It was first abused in oral form but then gained popularity in the smoked form as this mode of drug delivery allowed better control over dose. Because illicit synthesis is relatively easy and inexpensive, abuse became widespread in the 1970s and early 1980s. Today, use of PCP tends to be highly regionalized and located in certain areas of the U.S., notably the Washington D.C./Baltimore corridor, New York City, and Los Angeles.

Pharmacology

Phencyclidine binds with high affinity to sites located in the cortex and limbic structures of the brain. Binding results in blockade of *N*-methyl-D-aspartic acid (NMDA)-type glutamate receptors. The actions of glutamate and aspartate at the NMDA receptor allow movement of cations across the cell membrane. PCP exerts its action by binding to the glutamate receptor, thus preventing the flux of cations. PCP is also known to exert effects on catecholamines, serotonin, gamma-hydroxy butyric acid, and acetylcholine neurotransmitter release, but its role is incompletely defined. Due to its action on several systems, the physiological and behavioral effects of PCP are varied and depend on not only the dose, but also the route of administration and user's previous experience.

Absorption

Phencyclidine is typically self-administered by the oral, intravenous, or smoked routes. After oral administration to healthy human volunteers, the bioavailability was found to vary between 50 and 90%. In this study, peak plasma concentrations were achieved after 1.5 h and appeared to correlate with the time to reach maximum pharmacological effects. However, because there have been no comprehensive clinical controlled studies of phencyclidine, a correlation between PCP blood concentrations and pharmacological effects has not been definitively documented. Maximum serum PCP concentrations ranged between 2.7 and 2.9 ng/ml after 1 mg PCP administered orally.

PCP is commonly self-administered by the smoked route. Liquid PCP is soaked in parsley flakes and rolled as a cigarette; powdered PCP is sprinkled over a marijuana joint, or the end of a tobacco cigarette is dipped in liquid PCP and then smoked. Cook et al. studied the pharmacokinetic properties of PCP deposited on parsley cigarettes. Upon smoking, PCP is partially volatilized to 1-phenylcyclohexene (PC). These investigators found that 69 ± 5% of the PCP available in the cigarette was inhaled, 39% as PCP and 30% as PC. The pharmacological and toxicological properties of PC have not been established. Peak plasma concentrations of PCP were reached within 5 to 20 min. In 80% of the subjects, a second peak was observed in plasma PCP concentrations, occurring 1 to 3 h after the end of smoking. This may have been due to trapping of PCP in the mouth, where it could be released and absorbed by the GI tract or, alternatively, it could be due to absorption by the lung and bronchial tissue with slower release into the systemic circulation. Long-term users of PCP report feeling the effects of the drug within 2 to 5 min of smoking, with a peak effect after 15 to 30 min and residual effects for 4 to 6 h.

Distribution

Plasma protein binding of PCP in healthy individuals remains relatively constant between 60 and 70% over the concentration range of 0.007 to 5000 ng/ml. PCP binding to serum albumin accounts for only 24% of the binding, which suggests binding to another protein may occur to a significant extent. When studied *in vitro*, α_1-acid glycoprotein was also found to bind phencyclidine. The volume of distribution has been shown to be large, between 5.3 and 7.5 L/kg. providing evidence of extensive distribution to extravascular tissues.

Wall et al. administered 1.3 μg/kg of 3H-PCP intravenously to human volunteers and collected blood samples for 72 h. Data from this study suggested a two-compartment pharmacokinetic model with a plasma half-life for PCP of 7 to 16 h. Domino et al. further analyzed the data from Wall et al. and developed a more complex three-compartment PK model. The reported half-lives for each compartment were 5.5 min, 4.6 h, and 22 h. The specific tissues and organs represented by the multicompartment model were not identified. Half-lives of greater than 3 days have been reported in cases of PCP overdose.

Metabolism and Excretion

PCP is metabolized by the liver through oxidative hydroxylation. Unchanged PCP, two monohydroxylated and one dihydroxylated metabolite, have been identified in urine after oral and intravenous administration. The monohydroxlyated metabolites have been identified as 4-phenyl-4-(1-piperidinyl)-cyclohexanol (PPC) and 1-(1-phenylcyclohexyl)-4-hydroxypiperidine (PCHP). These metabolites are pharmacologically inactive in humans and PPC is present in both *cis*- and *trans*-isomeric forms. The *cis/trans* ratio was found to be 1:1.4 in human urine. The dihydroxylated metabolite was identified as 4-(4-hydroxypiperidino)-4-phenylcyclohexanol (HPPC). These metabolites are present in urine as glucuronide conjugates in addition to their unconjugated forms.

Approximately 30 to 50% of a labeled intravenous dose is excreted over a 72-h period in urine as unchanged drug (19.4%) and 80.6% as polar metabolites, mainly 4-phenyl-4-(1-piperidinyl) cyclohexanol. Only 2% of a dose is excreted in feces. After 10 days, an average of 77% of an intravenous dose is found in the feces and urine. Green et al. reported urine PCP concentrations between 40 and 3400 ng/ml in ambulatory users.

Urine pH is an important determinant of renal elimination of PCP. In a study in which urine pH was uncontrolled (6.0 to 7.5), the average total clearance of PCP was 22.8 ± 4.8 L/h after intravenous administration: In the same study, renal clearance was 1.98 ± 0.48 L/h. When the urine was made alkaline, the renal clearance of PCP was found to decrease to 0.3 ± 0.18 L/h. If the urine was acidified (pH 6.1) in the same subjects, renal clearance increased to 2.4 ± 0.78 L/h. Aronow et al. determined that if the urine pH was decreased to <5.0, renal clearance increased significantly to 8.04 ± 1.56 L/h. There is disagreement about the utility of urine acidification in the treatment of PCP overdose, even though excretion may be increased by as much as 100-fold. It should be noted that acidification may increase the risk of metabolic complications.

KETAMINE

Ketamine, a weakly basic compound structurally and pharmacologically similar to phencyclidine, is utilized in the U.S. to induce anesthesia. It is available in solution for intravenous or intramuscular injection. Since the drug is pharmacologically similar to PCP it has the potential of producing hallucinogenic effects and, therefore, in recent years has become a drug of abuse.

After intravenous administration of 175 mg/70 kg to five individuals, the average peak serum concentration was 1.0 mg/L achieved at 12 min. The concentration declined by 50% within 30 min. The plasma half-life is reported to be 3 to 4 h with a volume of distribution of 3 to 5 L/kg. Continuous infusion of 41 μg/kg/min after a 2-mg/kg bolus produced an average ($n = 31$) steady-state plasma concentration of 2.2 mg/L.

Two metabolites are formed that achieve serum concentrations similar to ketamine and may also exhibit the depressant effects of the parent compound. Norketamine is produced by *N-demethylation*. Norketamine is then dehydrogenated to form dehydronorketamine. Parent drug and metabolites are then subject to hydroxylation and conjugation. Approximately 2% of a single dose of ketamine is excreted in the 72-h urine as unchanged drug. In a recent study urine ketamine concentrations ranged from 6 to 7744 ng/ml (mean = 1083 ng/ml) in 33 subjects following illegal consumption.

INDEX